HANDBOOK OF DIET THERAPY

HANDBOOK OF DIET THERAPY

DOROTHEA TURNER

THE UNIVERSITY OF CHICAGO PRESS
CHICAGO & LONDON

Written and compiled for
the American Dietetic Association

International Standard Book Number: 0-226-81718-0
Library of Congress Catalog Card Number: 75-132788

The University of Chicago Press, Chicago 60637
The University of Chicago Press, Ltd., London

Published 1946
Fifth edition 1970
Second Impression 1971
Printed in the United States of America

CONTENTS

SECTION IV

EXPANDING OPPORTUNITIES IN THE PRACTICE OF DIET THERAPY

APPENDIXES

GLOSSARY OF DIETETIC TERMS, REVISED, 1965

INDEX

LIST OF TABLES

PREFACE

The purpose of the *Handbook of Diet Therapy* continues to be to aid in naming, defining, and describing therapeutic diets in terms of current dietetic principles. Up-to-date definitions of dietetic terminology have been included in the Revised Glossary of Dietetic Terms (1965) which appears in toto in this edition.

Since the aim of a normal dietary regimen is to maintain or to bring the patient to a state of nutritive sufficiency, it is to be expected that a therapeutic regimen should meet or exceed this goal. If a certain nutrient (sodium, for example) should be decreased for therapeutic purposes, other nutrients should remain at a level required for nutritive sufficiency. With this principle in mind, the therapeutic diet has again been regarded as a modification of the normal diet.

Therapeutic variants are largely quantitative in nature. For this reason, the normal diet and all therapeutic diets have been reassessed in quantitative terms, which will permit simple and relatively accurate modifications as well as a quick reappraisal of the over-all nutrient content. As in previous editions, a nutrient evaluation of each therapeutic diet appears as well as a sample menu pattern, and a description of the food groups and sample meals.

The changing content and bibliographies record the phenomenal growth of basic information on food composition and the use of food in therapy. New attention has been given to the 1968 revision of the *Recommended Dietary Allowances* and the greatly expanded compilations of data on many new food items. Current figures on fatty acid composition of foods, cholesterol, sodium and potassium analyses, and magnesium content of foods have been incorporated.

Since many important therapeutic diets require long-range changes in food habits, special attention has again been given to the patient's ability to make these changes. The chapter by Margaret Mead on "Interviewing the Patient" serves as an excellent introduction to this matter.

Greatly expanding facilities for health care in the nursing homes and home-care programs have brought about a vast need for improvements in the continuum of good patient care. Mildred Kaufman, in a chapter entitled "Expanding Opportunities in the Practice of Diet Therapy," discusses the need for an informative diet history, individualized diets, frequent assessment of food intake in the hospital, education of the patient, and improvements in communications between the physicians, the patients, and all community agencies and supporting workers in the community.

The intent of the *Handbook* has been to bring together new information heretofore scattered in various sources. In so doing, it is hoped that both professional workers and students will have a convenient reference and guide for use in dietetic practice.

SECTION I | NORMAL DIET

Chapter 1 *Nutritional Evaluation of a Basic Dietary Plan*

Since the aim of a dietary regimen is to maintain or bring the patient to a state of nutritive sufficiency, it is logical to assume that a therapeutic diet will be planned to meet or exceed the dietary allowances for a normal individual. On the other hand, there are instances in planning a therapeutic diet in which less than the normal requirement may be indicated, as in caloric or sodium restrictions. Other nutrients, in these instances, should remain at or above the levels of the normal diet. With this principle in mind, it follows that the therapeutic diet will be planned as a modification of the normal diet.

In the organization of a plan for practical use, the first step will be to outline and appraise a basic plan of food intake for the normal dietary regimen. Since most modifications for therapeutic purposes will be of a quantitative nature, in terms of calories, protein, or other nutrients, the basic plan of normal diet will be appraised in these terms to make possible quick and easily assessed adjustments.

To achieve this goal as concisely as possible, space will not be given to itemizing and calculating individual items in a diet. Instead, a basic pattern of diet will be outlined simply in terms of commonly used food groups. With this plan, foods may be combined into groups that are comparable enough in nutrient content to permit substitution within a group. This plan has the advantage of permitting variety in choice, minimizing dietary calculations, and insuring a good nutrient content.

Four food groups have been used in amounts required to meet the protein, mineral, and vitamin recommendations for the healthy individual. These four groups include the milk group, the vegetable and fruit group, the meat group, and the bread-cereal-potato-legume group. A fifth group—fats and sweets—has been considered separately, since this group adds comparatively little in protein, minerals, and vitamins but may instead be a major source of calories.

In the dietary patterns which follow, these groups have been outlined in the amounts necessary to meet the needs of the individual during childhood, adolescence, adult life, pregnancy and lactation, and after age fifty-five. In each case a nutrient evaluation has been made of the basic diet; each food group has been described; and a sample menu pattern and sample meals have been outlined as illustrations of the food plan.

In appraising the nutrient content of any dietary pattern, a question arises concerning the selection of figures on food composition for this purpose. In the past, nutritional accounting has been based on various tables of food composition. Widdowson and McCance (1)* have pointed out that there are two extreme schools of thought concerning food tables: "One tends to regard the figures in them as having the accuracy of atomic weight determinations; the other dismisses them as valueless on the ground that a foodstuff may be so modified by the soil, the season, or its rate of growth that no figure can be a reliable guide to its composition. The truth, of course, lies somewhere between these points of view."

To meet the need for representative values suitable for use in dietary calculations, the Food and Nutrition Board, National Research Council, and the Bureau of Human Nutrition and Home Economics, United States Department of Agriculture, in 1945 published *Tables of Food Composition in Terms of Eleven Nutrients* (2). Subsequent publications have now been superseded by *Composition of Foods—Raw, Processed, Prepared* (U.S. Department of Agriculture, Agriculture Handbook No. 8 [December, 1963]). Numerous foods not listed in the previous tables and different forms of food—especially frozen and cooked foods—as well as a number of foods of tropical or semitropical origin have brought the total items to nearly 2,500. In this publication, data are presented on energy,

* Numbers in parentheses refer to works cited in the References at the end of each chapter.

vitamins, and the minerals, calcium, phosphorus, and iron, per 100 gm. and per pound of product. New values for sodium and potassium have been incorporated together with data on selected fatty acids, cholesterol, and magnesium.

A condensed source of this information, relating to the 500 most commonly used foods in the United States, appears in the 1964 publication (3) entitled *Nutritive Value of Foods* (U.S. Department of Agriculture, Home and Garden Bulletin No. 72). In this publication items are described in common household measures and weights. For convenience these data are reproduced in Table 36.

TABLE 1

FOODS AVAILABLE FOR CONSUMPTION PER PERSON PER WEEK (8)

Vegetables and fruit		9.7 lb.
Dark-green and deep-yellow vegetables	0.6 lb.	
Citrus fruit	1.2 lb.	
Milk, cream, cheese		4.4 qt.
Eggs		0.6 doz.
Meat, poultry, fish		4.2 lb.
Separated fats and oils		0.9 lb.
Sugars		1.4 lb.
Flour, cereals, baked goods		2.8 lb.

Although figures taken from these tables serve a valuable function in making values on individual food items available, it would still be a laborious task to make detailed computations of menus over a prolonged number of days, unless use were made of a shortened method of dietary calculation. One such method has been developed jointly by The American Dietetic Association, the American Diabetes Association, and the U.S. Public Health Service (4). Foods have been combined into groups roughly equivalent in nutrient content. These groups have been called Exchanges and assigned the values shown in Table 20. Since the Exchanges have come into common use in making gross assessments of carbohydrate, protein, fat, and calories, these values have been used in the tables on normal diet which follow. The mineral and vitamin contents of the food groups have been grossly estimated from appraisal of the most commonly used foods in each group.

A *menu pattern* and *sample meals* have been outlined to illustrate

TABLE 2—EVALUATION OF A BASIC PLAN OF NORMAL DIET FOR AN ADULT (1,415–2,415 Calories; 70 Gm. Protein)

DAILY FOOD INTAKE	QUANTITY		CALORIES*	FOODSTUFFS			MINERALS		VITAMINS				
	Weight (Gm.)	Approximate Measure		Protein* (Gm.)	Fat* (Gm.)	Carbohydrate* (Gm.)	Ca (Mg.)	Fe (Mg.)	A (I.U.)	Ascorbic Acid (Mg.)	Thiamine (Mg.)	Riboflavin (Mg.)	Niacin (Mg.)
Milk, whole	488	1 pint	340	16	20	24	576	0.2	700	4	0.16	0.84	0.2
Egg	50	1 medium	75	7	5	...	27	1.1	590	...	0.05	0.15	Tr.
Meat, poultry, fish, cooked†	120	4 oz. E.P.§	300	28	20	...	16	3.4	35	...	0.40	0.25	5.9
Bread, whole-grain or enriched white‡	180	6 slices	420	12	...	90	123	4.6	Tr.	...	0.46	0.31	4.0
Cereal, whole-grain or enriched	20	½ cup, cooked	70	2	...	15	21	0.7	Tr.	...	0.07	0.05	0.7
Potato, cooked	100	1 small	70	2	...	15	5	0.5	Tr.	16	0.09	0.03	1.1
Vegetable (A)‖	150	2 servings	...	...	...	...	43	1.2	2,180	32	0.10	0.10	0.9
(B)#	50		20	1	...	4	12	0.5	1,660	5	0.03	0.03	0.4
Including deep green and yellow													
Fruit, citrus**	100	1 serving	40	...	...	10	18	0.1	140	40	0.05	0.01	0.1
Other fruit††	...	2 servings	80	...	...	20	14	0.8	945	9	0.04	0.06	0.8
Subtotal	...	...	1,415	68	45	178	855	13.1	6,250	106	1.45	1.83	14.1
Fats and oils§§	...	...	1,000	...	...	...	...	...	660	...	...	...	...
Sugar and sweets§§	...	...	...	...	...	...	...	...	...	...	...	...	...
Total‡‡	...	...	2,415‖‖	68	...	...	855	13.1‡‡	6,910	106	1.45	1.83	14.1

* Values for calories, carbohydrate, protein, and fat from the Food Exchange Lists Table 20, p. 000 have been used to evaluate foods and food groups.

† Weighting was adapted from *Meat Consumption Trends and Patterns* (U.S. Department of Agriculture, Agriculture Handbooks, No. 187 [Washington, D.C., July, 1960]). Weekly consumption estimated as 350 gm. beef, 280 gm. pork, 140 gm. poultry, and 70 gm. fish.

‡ 30 gm. (1 oz.) has been the weight assigned to one slice of bread in the exchange lists. It is recognized that variation is common. Adjustments should be made where usage varies.

§ Edible portion.

‖ Commonly used vegetables selected from the vegetable A group of the exchange lists were tomatoes, snap beans, spinach, asparagus, broccoli, cabbage, lettuce, and cucumber. It was estimated that these vegetables might be used 10 times weekly, averaging 150 gm. daily. Weighting was adapted from Agriculture Handbook No. 215, *Consumption, Trends, and Patterns for Vegetables* (U.S. Department of Agriculture, Economic and Statistical Analysis Division, Economic Research Service [July, 1961]).

It was assumed that the most commonly used vegetables from the vegetable B group of the exchange lists were peas, carrots, beets, and squash. It was estimated that these vegetables might be used 4 times weekly averaging 50 gm. daily. Weighting was adapted from Agriculture Handbook No. 215, *Consumption Trends and Patterns for Vegetables* (U.S. Department of Agriculture, Economic and Statistical Analysis Division, Economic Research Service [July, 1961]).

** Fresh orange, fresh grapefruit, canned orange juice, blended grapefruit and orange and frozen citrus juice were considered to be commonly used citrus fruits or juice. Weighting was adapted from *Consumption of Food in the United States*, Supplement for 1962 to Agriculture Handbook No. 62 (U.S. Department of Agriculture, Agricultural Marketing Service [October, 1963]).

†† Apple, banana, canned peaches, pineapple, pear, apricot, and plum were considered commonly used. Weighting was adapted from *Consumption of Food in the United States*, Supplement for 1962 to Agriculture Handbook No. 62 (U.S. Department of Agriculture, Agricultural Marketing Service [October, 1963]).

‡‡ Meets Recommended Dietary Allowances (Table 3) for an adult in good health except for iron level for women.

§§ Per capita consumption of fats and sweets has been estimated as 2 oz. separated fat or oil and 3 oz. sugar daily. *National Food Situation, NFS-108* (U.S. Department of Agriculture, Economic Research Service [May, 1964]).

‖‖ Caloric needs should be adjusted to individual requirements. For variations in need, see Table 3.

TABLE 2A

DESCRIPTION OF THE DAILY FOOD PLAN OF NORMAL DIET
(70 Gm. Protein, 1,415–2,415 Calories; Derived from Table 2)

Daily Food Plan	Description
MILK GROUP	
1 pint*	*One pint whole milk* contains 340 calories, 16 gm. protein, calcium, phosphorus, and the B complex in important amounts. One pint buttermilk made from whole milk or ½ pint evaporated milk are similar. *One pint skim milk* contains 180 calories, 18 gm. protein, and important amounts of calcium, phosphorus, and the B complex. If completely skimmed, no fat will be present, accounting for the 50 per cent decrease in calories. One pint of buttermilk made from skim milk or ½–⅔ cup (depending on brand) of non-fat milk solids is similar.
MEAT GROUP†	
5 meat equivalents	*One meat equivalent* is approximately equal to 1 oz. (edible portion—weighed after cooking) beef, veal, lamb, pork, poultry, fish, cheese, or 1 egg. The five equivalents may be distributed throughout the day as desired. Liver and other variety meats are exceptional sources of vitamin A, iron, and the B complex. Four ounces of cooked meat may contain about 28 gm. protein and 300 calories.
VEGETABLE AND FRUIT GROUP	
5 servings	*A dark-green or deep-yellow vegetable* is important each day for its vitamin A value. Asparagus, green beans, broccoli, carrots, green pepper, winter squash, pumpkin, and other greens make up this group. Carrots, winter squash, and pumpkin may contain about 35 calories per serving. The others will be negligible. *Other vegetables*, as beets, cabbage, cauliflower, celery, cucumber, eggplant, lettuce, mushrooms, onions, peas, tomatoes, or turnips contribute varied amounts of all nutrients. Beets, onions, peas, or turnips may contribute about 35 calories per ½ cup serving. Others will be negligible. *Citrus fruit or other fruit rich in vitamin C* is important each day. One orange or ½ cup juice, or ½ grapefruit or ½ cup juice, or 1 cup tomato juice or 1 cup strawberries or 1 cup red raspberries or ¼ cantaloupe or 1 large tangerine contains about 40 calories per serving and important amounts of vitamin C.

* 1 qt. of milk during last trimester of pregnancy; 1½ qts. of milk during lactation.

† If more meat is desired, 1 additional meat equivalent (edible portion—1 oz. cooked meat) may be substituted for 1 serving of the bread group without a significant change in calories. Other rearrangements or omissions should be assessed by reference to Tables 2 and 36.

TABLE 2A—*Continued*

Daily Food Plan	Description
VEGETABLE AND FRUIT GROUP—*Continued*	
5 servings—	*Other fruits,* such as 1 apple or 1 peach or 1 pear or 2 prunes or 4 halves apricots or 12 grapes or $\frac{1}{2}$ banana, contribute varied amounts of all nutrients and contain about 40 calories per serving. For other fruits see Table 26, page 000. If sugar or syrup is added, additional calories must be calculated.
BREAD-CEREAL-POTATO-LEGUME GROUP	
8 servings	*One serving provides approximately 70 calories,* important amounts of the B complex, and iron. One serving is equal to 1 slice enriched or whole-wheat bread, $\frac{1}{2}$ cup white potato, $\frac{1}{4}$ cup sweet potato, $\frac{1}{3}$ cup corn, $\frac{1}{2}$ cup cooked macaroni, noodles, spaghetti, rice, cornmeal, or $\frac{1}{2}$ cup cooked dried beans or peas, $\frac{1}{2}$ cup cooked cereal, or $\frac{3}{4}$ cup flake-type cereal or 2 graham crackers. For other equivalents see Table 27, page 000.
FATS AND SWEETS	*Without this group* the calories for the day approximate 1,245–1,415 (depending on whether skim milk is used). The 2 oz. separated fats and oils and 3 oz. sugar available per capita in the United States would add approximately 1,000 calories. Adjustments to fit individual needs may be made as follows: *If one level teaspoon fat or oil* is used on bread, in vegetables, or in cooking, about 45 calories may be added. One thin slice crisp bacon, 2 tablespoons light cream or 1 tablespoon heavy cream, 1 teaspoon mayonnaise or oil, 1 tablespoon cream cheese or French dressing, or 5 small olives or 6 small nuts, also contain 45 calories each. *One level teaspoon sugar, jelly, or honey* in cooking, on cereal, in fruit, or in coffee adds 20 calories. One-half cup ice cream, pudding, or gelatin dessert may add between 150 and 300 calories, and one serving cake or pie between 300 and 700 calories (see Table 36, p. 154, for additional caloric values).
IODIZED SALT	Iodized salt should be used in regions where iodine is lacking. Iodized salt is especially important in adolescence and pregnancy.

TABLE 2B

MENU PATTERN AND SAMPLE MEALS—NORMAL DIET FOR AN ADULT
(70 Gm. Protein; 1,415–2,415 Calories; derived from Tables 2 and 2A)

DAILY FOOD PLAN*	SAMPLE MENU PATTERN*	SAMPLE MEALS*
	A.M.	
MILK GROUP 1 pint† MEAT GROUP 5 meat equivalents‡ One equivalent equals 1 oz. meat (edible portion) weighed after cooking	½ cup citrus fruit or juice 1 egg 1 cup cooked enriched or whole-grain cereal or 1½ cups flake-type cereal with milk and sugar§ 1 slice enriched or whole-grain toast with spread§ Coffee or tea, if desired, with sugar§ and milk	Orange juice 1 egg 1 cup farina with milk and sugar§ 1 slice toast with spread§ Coffee or tea if desired
	Noon	
VEGETABLE AND FRUIT GROUP 5 servings or more BREAD-CEREAL-POTATO-LEGUME GROUP 8 servings‡ FATS AND SWEETS§ (Without this group the calories are approximately 1,415)	2 oz. meat, poultry, fish, cheese, or 2 eggs‡ ½ cup potato or substitute Dark-green or deep-yellow vegetable Other vegetable Fruit 2 slices enriched or whole-grain bread or alternate* with spread§ Milk	Broiled chicken breast Baked potato Broccoli Tomato and lettuce salad Baked apple 2 small hot rolls Milk
	P.M.	
	2 oz. meat‡ or substitute, as at noon Vegetable Fruit Milk Enriched or whole-grain bread 2 slices or alternate* with spread§ Dessert§	Vegetable soup Sandwich cheese and ham Sliced fresh peaches with ice cream§ Milk

* See Table 2A for alternates.

† The use of 1 pt. skim milk instead of 1 pt. whole milk will reduce the calories by 160. One quart of milk should be used daily during last trimester of pregnancy and 1½ qt. during lactation.

‡ If 1 additional meat equivalent (1 oz. E.P.) is desired, 1 serving of the bread group may be omitted with no important change in the calories. Other rearrangements or omissions should be reassessed by reference to Table 2.

§ Without sweets and fats, the diet contains about 1,415 calories. Per capita separated fats and sugar in United States average 1,000 calories. One teaspoon sugar, jelly, or honey adds 20 calories; 1 teaspoon fat or oil, 45 calories. A dessert like gelatin, ice cream, or pudding may add 150 to 300 calories. A dessert like cake or pie may add between 300 and 700 calories (see Table 36 in Appendix).

the "daily food plan" and some of the choices within each of the four food groups in the normal diet. Obviously, there is no "one" normal diet which must be consumed to insure a dietary sufficiency. Many foods may be combined in amounts which will meet individual needs. In selecting a basic plan, then, it would seem most suitable to combine commonly used foods in amounts which are the most generally acceptable.

Gross guides to the per capita consumption of food are available in the *National Food Situation* published quarterly by the Economic Research Service, U.S. Department of Agriculture, and in special reports from the Household Food Consumption Surveys, U.S. Department of Agriculture (5).

The kind and average quantity of foods available for consumption per person per week are summarized in Table 1, page 5. The nutrient evaluation by Stiebeling (6) indicated that these foods met or exceeded the Recommended Dietary Allowances (7). As such, then, they serve to suggest a framework for the basic plan.

In the basic plan of normal diet which follows (Table 2), the amounts of the milk group, the meat group, and the fruit and vegetable group closely approximate the "average diet" given in Table 1. Fats and sweets have been considered separately to permit modifications in calories, fat, and carbohydrate for various therapeutic purposes. A nutrient evaluation of the basic plan of normal diet appears in Table 2 and a menu pattern and sample meals in Tables 2A and 2B.

In setting up this framework for normal diet it is intended only that this pattern of eating be regarded as a flexible guide from which basic foods may be selected in proper amounts and with a wide variety of choice. It is not to be inferred that all individuals must use this exact allotment of foods. Modifications should be made for individuals as appropriate. A quick reassessment of nutrient content can then be made by a comparison with the basic plan in Table 2.

REFERENCES

1. Widdowson, E. M., and McCance, R. A. Food tables, Lancet, 1:230–32, 1943.
2. Bureau of Human Nutrition and Home Economics in cooperation with the National Research Council. Tables of food composition in terms of eleven nutrients. (U.S. Department of Agriculture, Miscellaneous Publications, No. 572.) 1945.

3. Consumer and Food Economics Research Division. Nutritive Value of Foods. (U.S. Department of Agriculture, Agricultural Research Service Home and Garden Bulletin No. 72.) 1964.
4. Caso, E. K. Calculation of diabetic diets, J. Am. Dietet. A., **26**: 575–83, 1950.
5. Household Food Consumption Survey, 1955. (U.S. Department of Agriculture, Agricultural Research Service Reports, Nos. 1–10.) 1957.
6. Stiebeling, H. K. Food and nutrient consumption trends and consumer problems: talk at American Institute of Nutrition, Chicago. (U.S. Department of Agriculture, Agricultural Research Service. Mimeo.) 1957.
7. Food and Nutrition Board, National Research Council. Recommended dietary allowances, revised, 1958. ("NAS-NRC Publications," No. 589.)

Chapter 2

Correlation of Basic Diet with Recommended Dietary Allowances

The next step will be to compare the plan of diet with nutrient needs. Two guides to nutrient sufficiency are desirable: one for the needs in good health and one for the requirements in disease states. At the present time, only an accepted guide to the former has been established.

In 1943, the Food and Nutrition Board of the National Research Council prepared the first established guide to the needs of healthy individuals covering recommended allowances from infancy to old age (3). These allowances have been revised approximately every five years as advances in knowledge have provided data for making better estimates. They have become the accepted guide for the United States.

RECOMMENDED DIETARY ALLOWANCES (Revised 1968)*

It is important to keep in mind the purposes of the Recommended Dietary Allowances. If their purpose is misinterpreted, one is led to the erroneous conclusion that the recommendations are too high. They are set at levels which will maintain good nutrition in practically all healthy persons in the United States and are intended to serve as goals in planning food supplies and as guides for the interpretation of food consumption records of groups of people. It must be stressed that since the recommendations are intended to meet the full needs of practically everybody, they will be considerably higher than some persons will need.

The Recommended Dietary Allowances should not be interpreted as nutritional requirements for individuals. However, they may be used as recom-

* Reprinted by permission from the *Journal of the American Dietetic Association*, vol. 54 (February 1969). © 1969 by The American Dietetic Association.

TABLE 3

Recommended Daily Dietary Allowances[a], Revised 1968

AGE[b]					FAT-SOLUBLE VITAMINS			WATER-SOLUBLE VITAMINS							MINERALS				
From—Up to	WEIGHT	HEIGHT	KCALORIES	PROTEIN	Vitamin A activity	Vitamin D	Vitamin E activity	Ascorbic acid	Folacin[c]	Niacin	Riboflavin	Thiamine	Vitamin B_6	Vitamin B_{12}	Calcium	Phosphorus	Iodine	Iron	Magnesium
								Infants											
years	*kg.(lb.)*	*cm.(in.)*		*gm.*	*I.U.*	*I.U.*	*I.U.*	*mg.*	*mg.*	*mg. equiv.*[d]	*mg.*	*mg.*	*mg.*	*mcg.*	*gm.*	*gm.*	*mcg.*	*mg.*	*mg*
Birth—1/6	4(9)	55(22)	kg. × 120[e]	kg. × 2.2	1,500	400	5	35	0.05	5	0.4	0.2	0.2	1.0	0.4	0.2	25	6	40
1/6 —1/2	7(15)	63(25)	kg. × 110[e]	kg. × 2.0	1,500	400	5	35	0.05	7	0.5	0.4	0.3	1.5	0.5	0.4	40	10	60
1/2 —1	9(20)	72(28)	kg. × 100[e]	kg. × 1.8	1,500	400	5	35	0.1	8	0.6	0.5	0.4	2.0	0.6	0.5	45	15	70
								Children											
1 —2	12(26)	81(32)	1,100	25	2,000	400	10	40	0.1	8	0.6	0.6	0.5	2.0	0.7	0.7	55	15	100
2 —3	14(31)	91(36)	1,250	25	2,000	400	10	40	0.2	8	0.7	0.6	0.6	2.5	0.8	0.8	60	15	150
3 —4	16(35)	100(39)	1,400	30	2,500	400	10	40	0.2	9	0.8	0.7	0.7	3	0.8	0.8	70	10	200
4 —6	19(42)	110(43)	1,600	30	2,500	400	10	40	0.2	11	0.9	0.8	0.9	4	0.8	0.8	80	10	200
6 —8	23(51)	121(48)	2,000	35	3,500	400	15	40	0.2	13	1.1	1.0	1.0	4	0.9	0.9	100	10	250
8 —10	28(62)	131(52)	2,200	40	3,500	400	15	40	0.3	15	1.2	1.1	1.2	5	1.0	1.0	110	10	250
								Males											
10 —12	35(77)	140(55)	2,500	45	4,500	400	20	40	0.4	17	1.3	1.3	1.4	5	1.2	1.2	125	10	300
12 —14	43(95)	151(59)	2,700	50	5,000	400	20	45	0.4	18	1.4	1.4	1.6	5	1.4	1.4	135	18	350
14 —18	59(130)	170(67)	3,000	60	5,000	400	25	55	0.4	20	1.5	1.5	1.8	5	1.4	1.4	150	18	400
18 —22	67(147)	175(69)	2,800	60	5,000	400	30	60	0.4	18	1.6	1.4	2.0	5	0.8	0.8	140	10	400
22 —35	70(154)	175(69)	2,800	65	5,000	—	30	60	0.4	18	1.7	1.4	2.0	5	0.8	0.8	140	10	350
35 —55	70(154)	173(68)	2,600	65	5,000	—	30	60	0.4	17	1.7	1.3	2.0	5	0.8	0.8	125	10	350
55 —75+	70(154)	171(67)	2,400	65	5,000	—	30	60	0.4	14	1.7	1.2	2.0	6	0.8	0.8	110	10	350
								Females											
10 —12	35(77)	142(56)	2,250	50	4,500	400	20	40	0.4	15	1.3	1.1	1.4	5	1.2	1.2	110	18	300
12 —14	44(97)	154(61)	2,300	50	5,000	400	20	45	0.4	15	1.4	1.2	1.6	5	1.3	1.3	115	18	350
14 —16	52(114)	157(62)	2,400	55	5,000	400	25	50	0.4	16	1.4	1.2	1.8	5	1.3	1.3	120	18	350
16 —18	54(119)	160(63)	2,300	55	5,000	400	25	50	0.4	15	1.5	1.2	2.0	5	1.3	1.3	115	18	350
18 —22	58(128)	163(64)	2,000	55	5,000	400	25	55	0.4	13	1.5	1.0	2.0	5	0.8	0.8	100	18	350
22 —35	58(128)	163(64)	2,000	55	5,000	—	25	55	0.4	13	1.5	1.0	2.0	5	0.8	0.8	100	18	350
35 —55	58(128)	160(63)	1,850	55	5,000	—	25	55	0.4	13	1.5	1.0	2.0	5	0.8	0.8	90	18	300
55 —75+	58(128)	157(62)	1,700	55	5,000	—	25	55	0.4	13	1.5	1.0	2.0	6	0.8	0.8	80	10	300
Pregnancy			+ 200	65	6,000	400	30	60	0.8	15	1.8	+0.1	2.5	8	+0.4	+0.4	125	18	450
Lactation			+1,000	75	8,000	400	30	60	0.5	20	2.0	+0.5	2.5	6	+0.5	+0.5	150	18	450

[a] The allowance levels are intended to cover individual variations among most normal persons as they live in the United States under usual environmental stresses. The recommended allowances can be attained with a variety of common foods providing other nutrients for which human requirements have been less well defined. See text for more detailed discussion of allowances and of nutrients not tabulated.

[b] Entries on lines for age range 22-35 years represent the reference man and woman at age 22. All other entries represent allowances for the midpoint of the specified age range.

[c] The folacin allowances refer to dietary sources as determined by *Lactobacillus casei* assay. Pure forms of folacin may be effective in doses less than 1/4 of the RDA.

[d] Niacin equivalents include dietary sources of the vitamin itself plus 1 mg. equivalent for each 60 mg. of dietary tryptophan.

[e] Assumes protein equivalent to human milk. For proteins not 100 per cent utilized, factors should be increased proportionately.

mendations for individuals with the clear understanding that the amounts recommended may be in excess of the individual requirement. The important point is that it must not be assumed that an individual will suffer from malnutrition if he does not obtain the Recommended Dietary Allowances, and diets must not be called deficient for an individual when he does not obtain the recommended allowances.

A second point that should be noted is that the Recommended Dietary Allowances are intended for use in the United States, under current conditions of living. They, therefore, take into account the climatic conditions, the economic status, the distribution of the population, and various other factors which make them particularly suitable for the United States.

CALORIC ALLOWANCES

For purposes of estimating a recommended allowance for calories, a "reference" man and woman are described as weighing 154 and 128 lb., respectively. Age 22 years was selected, since there is evidence that weight gain after this age is likely to be fat. In the present revision, the daily allowances have been reduced to 2,800 and 2,000 kcalories, respectively. This assumes that physical activity is light, that is, neither sedentary nor heavy physical labor. It is our feeling that a better level of health would be reached if the population were more physically active, and there is growing evidence that a sedentary life is one of the causes contributing to degenerative arterial disease and obesity, with their many complications. We would prefer to see physical activity increased, rather than caloric intake further reduced (Table 4).

TABLE 4

EXAMPLES OF ENERGY EXPENDITURE FOR REFERENCE MAN AND WOMAN

Activity	Time (Hrs.)	Man		Woman	
		Rate (Kcal/Min)	Total	Rate (Kcal/Min)	Total
Sleeping and reclining*	8	1.1	530	1.0	480
Sitting†	7	1.5	630	1.1	460
Standing‡	5	2.5	750	1.5	450
Walking§	2	3.0	360	2.5	300
Other‖	2	4.5	540	3.0	360
			2,810		2,050

* Essentially basal metabolic rate.

† Includes normal activity carried on while sitting, e.g., reading, driving automobile, eating, playing cards, and desk or bench work.

‡ Includes normal indoor activities while standing and walking intermittently in limited area, e.g., personal toilet, moving from one room to another, etc.

§ Includes purposeful walking, largely outdoors, e.g., home to commuting station to work site, and other comparable activities.

‖ Includes intermittent activities in occasional sports, exercises, limited stair climbing or occupational activities involving light physical work. This category may include week-end swimming, golf, tennis, or picnics using 5–20 kcalories per minute for a limited time.

Adjustments for age take into account that linear growth is virtually complete by age twenty-one for the male and by age seventeen for the female, although in the United States, the average person continues to gain in body weight until about sixty years of age. An increase in muscle mass may continue during the third decade, particularly in individuals who are undergoing rigorous physical training. Statistical data indicate that the most favorable health expectations are associated with conditions under which weight as normally achieved by age twenty-two is maintained throughout life.

Energy requirements decline progressively after the years of early adulthood because of a decrease in resting metabolic rate, as well as lessened physical activity. While the approximate rate of decline of resting metabolism is known to be 2 per cent per decade in adults, it is difficult to estimate the decrease in reduction in physical activity associated with advancing age. In the present revision, these adjustments for age are less than those in the 1964 allowances and take into account the fact that many individuals who are already sedentary do not further decrease their activity as they grow old. During pregnancy, an additional caloric allowance not exceeding 200 kcalories per day is considered sufficient.

The caloric allowances for infants during the first year have been set at levels which reflect the general pattern of food intake of thriving infants. Caloric allowances are made on a body-weight basis, i.e., 120 kcalories per kilogram at birth reduced to 100 kcalories per kilogram by the end of the first year of life.

Allowances for individual children should be derived by observation of activity and quality of growth as determined not only by weight but by the extent of deposits of subcutaneous fat.

CARBOHYDRATE AND FAT

More attention is given in the new revision to carbohydrate and fats—particularly fats, because of the increased interest in the relationship between lipid and carbohydrate intake and atherosclerosis. Although it is possible to adapt to diets very low in carbohydrates, individuals accustomed to normal diets need at least 100 gm. carbohydrate per day to avoid ketosis, excessive protein break down, and other undesirable metabolic responses. It must be remembered that the storage capacity for carbohydrate in the body as glycogen is normally less than 1,800 kcalories. Therefore, when carbohydrate is not provided in sufficient quantity in the diet, it must be derived in large part from either dietary or body protein.

In 1966, fats accounted for approximately 41 per cent of the calories available for consumption in the retail market in the United States. Data indicate that the proportion of total fat in the diet from animal sources is decreasing while that from vegetable sources is increasing. Many studies indicate that the percentage of fat calories in the United States diet is too high and that the trend toward a lower fat intake containing more linoleic acid is desirable. Although we have some data indicating that the requirement for essential fatty acids is relatively low, we are unable to make any recommendation, either as to the total fat in the diet or the proportion of linoleic acid which should be recommended.

PROTEIN ALLOWANCES

Theoretically, it should be possible to calculate a recommended protein intake on the basis of amino acid composition data. However, the lack of quantitative information about the essential amino acid requirement in relation to total nitrogen, the variability of different types of food in the diet, and the question of the availability of amino acids in foods limit this method of calculation (Table 5). The protein allowances are based on the assumption that the efficiency of utilization of proteins in the United States diet is 70 per cent that of the ideal protein. Using this method of calculation, the total requirement for ideal protein for the 70-kg. reference man per day is 35 gm. Allowing a 30 per cent variability factor gives a figure of 45.5 gm. per day. Applying the utilization factor of 70 per cent for food protein, the protein allowance becomes 65 gm. per day for the "reference" man, or approximately 0.9 gm. protein per kilogram body weight per day.

The recommended protein for infants was derived by a different method. A great majority of the infants in the United States receive formula diets as a

TABLE 5

CALCULATION OF THE RECOMMENDED PROTEIN ALLOWANCE FOR THE REFERENCE MAN

Basal kcaloric requirement for 70 kg. reference man	=	1,750
Requirement for ideal protein per day = 20 mg. per basal kcalorie = 1,750 × 20 = 35,000 mg.	=	35.0 gm.
Allowance (30 per cent) for individual variability in a large population = $\frac{30}{100}$ × 35.0	=	10.5 gm.
Total		45.5 gm.
Assuming 70 per cent utilization of food protein, total daily allowance for reference man = $\frac{100}{70}$ × 45.5 gm.	=	65.0 gm.
Allowance per kilogram of body weight = $\frac{65.0}{70}$	=	0.9 gm.

partial or total substitute for mother's milk. It is assumed that a baby, breast-fed by a healthy, well-nourished mother, with normal lactation, consumes an adequate amount of protein, and the efficiency of utilization of mother's milk is assumed to be 100 per cent. Based on the composition of human milk, the protein allowance for infants is 1.8 gm. per 100 kcalories. If proteins of lower quality than those of human milk are fed to infants, the intake should be proportionately higher and the allowance per kilogram body weight should be increased by correcting for lower protein utilization. This explains the apparent discrepancy in the table between the allowance of 25 gm. protein for the one-to-two-year age group as compared with only 16 gm. protein in the six-months-to-one-year age group. If infants under one year are being fed regular mixed diets, it would be advisable to apply the quality correction factor of 100:70 to the lower figures based on human milk protein. It must be emphasized that if the dietary protein is less than 8 per cent of the calories as provided by human milk, it is not possible to feed the infant enough food to meet protein needs.

VITAMIN ALLOWANCES

An allowance has been given for vitamin E for the first time. Recent evidence indicates that vitamin E deficiency may result in symptoms in infants. The vitamin E requirement does not appear to be related directly to body weight or to caloric intake, but rather to the factor body weight in kilograms to the 0.75 power which has been designated as physiologic or metabolic body size. The recommended allowances are expressed in international units as determined by the factor 1.25 times the body weight in kilograms to the 0.75 power. For the "reference" man, the recommended allowance is 30 I.U. per day.

The allowance for ascorbic acid has been reduced from 70 mg. to 60 mg. per day for the adult man and to 55 mg. per day for the adult woman. This was done only after a thorough reconsideration of the literature and a study of recent isotopic work. Studies of body pools by means of ^{14}C isotopes permit measurement of the actual utilization of ascorbic acid by healthy men, indicating a mean utilization of 21.5 mg. per day with a standard deviation of 8.1 mg. The allowance is set at 60 mg., or four standard deviations from the mean, in order to allow for individual variations and for the perishability of ascorbic acid.

The allowance of 35 mg. ascorbic acid for infants is about the same amount supplied daily from 850 ml. of mother's milk (in the United States). The tyrosinemia and tyrosyluria observed in young infants fed high-protein diets are diminished by supplements of ascorbic acid. Therefore, infants receiving formulas containing two to three times the protein content of human milk may need up to 50 mg. of ascorbic acid daily during the first few weeks of life.

Folacin is another nutrient for which a recommendation is being made for the first time. There is increasing evidence that folacin deficiency may be more important in the United States than was thought a few years ago. There still remains considerable uncertainty about the available folacin in foods and the amount destroyed by cooking, which may be quite variable, and we have but limited knowledge as to the efficiency of absorption of the various forms of folacin in food. Therefore, the recommended allowance has been set at 0.4 mg. from dietary sources, based on the *L. casei* method of assay. This is higher than that needed if folacin is administered as a pure synthetic compound. An intake of 0.1 mg. of synthetic folacin per day meets the requirement for the normal adult.

The allowance for niacin has been slightly decreased and is expressed as previously, i.e., in terms of niacin equivalents. The niacin equivalent is defined as 1 mg. niacin or 60 mg. dietary tryptophan. The minimum requirement for niacin equivalents to prevent pellagra has been placed at 4.4 per 1,000 kcalories per day, or at a minimum of 9 equivalents when the caloric intake is less than 2,000 kcalories. The recommended allowance is 6.6 per 1,000 kcalories and not less than 13 equivalents, when the caloric intake is less than 2,000 kcalories. During pregnancy, there is an increased conversion of tryptophan to niacin, although this does not necessarily indicate that niacin needs are increased. The allowance is increased by 2 equivalents per day, based on the recommended increase in caloric intake.

The recommended allowances for riboflavin have been recalculated on the basis of metabolic body size as represented by body weight in kilograms taken to the 0.75 power. In practice, there are no remarkable differences in the recommended allowances whether they are calculated on the basis of metabolic body size, caloric intake, or protein allowance.

As a result of a thorough restudy of the literature, it is concluded that 0.33 mg. per 1,000 kcalories represents a minimal thiamine requirement and a figure of 0.4 mg. per 1,000 kcalories has been selected to take care of individual variation. The same requirement is obtained from estimates of the urinary excretion of thiamine metabolites. It is, therefore, estimated that 0.5 mg. per 1,000 kcalories will maintain thiamine nutriture under normal conditions in the United States, and this forms the base of the current recommendations. Because it is possible that older persons use thiamine less efficiently, a recommendation of 1.0 mg. per day is made for older adults, even though they may be consuming less than 2,000 kcalories daily. The literature suggests an increased need for thiamine during pregnancy, although the magnitude of this increase is uncertain. An additional amount of 0.2 mg. per day is recommended during pregnancy, in accordance with the increased caloric recommendation. For the infant, the thiamine content of human milk is variable and is influenced by the mother's thiamine intake. Mature human milk provides 0.015 mg. thiamine per 100 ml., as compared with 0.04 mg. per 100 ml. in cow's milk.

A recommended allowance for vitamin B_6 has also been established for the first time. "Vitamin B_6" is a collective term for a group of naturally occurring pyridines that are metabolically and functionally interrelated and are present in varying amounts in different food products. Since the vitamin B_6 content of foods is not usually included in tables of food composition, estimates of the intake of vitamin B_6 from food sources are uncertain. Recent repletion studies in young adults indicate that on diets supplying 100 gm. protein per day, the amount of B_6 required is about 1.25 mg. per day. Higher amounts of protein appear to require more vitamin B_6. In order to supply a reasonable margin of safety and allow for daily intakes of 100 gm. or more of protein, the recommended allowance for adults has been set at 2.0 mg. per day.

Vitamin B_{12} also is tabulated for the first time. An allowance of 5 mcg. obtained from the food supply is based on observations that at this level, absorption is 30 per cent or less. A dietary intake at this level will insure replacement of normal losses. A diet containing 15 mcg. per day will gradually replenish body stores if they have been depleted. Average American diets appear to meet these needs.

MINERALS

With reference to calcium and phosphorus, a calcium-phosphorus ratio of one to one is recommended, except for early infancy when a two-to-one ratio seems desirable. The recommended allowances are unchanged in the present revision and continue higher than the suggested practical allowances adopted by the FAO/WHO Expert Group in 1962 (2). The recommended allowances are based on the losses in urine, feces, and sweat and the calcium available for absorption from food, which is assumed to average around 40 per cent. On this basis, the recommended allowances are 800 mg. calcium and 800 mg. phosphorus.

In considering the phosphorus allowance for the infant, the ratio of calcium to phosphorus in human milk is two to one while that in cow's milk is approximately 1.2 to one, and it is recognized that the high phosphorus intake, such as provided by cow's milk, may contribute to the occurrence of hypocalcemic tetany during the first few weeks of life. Current evidence supports the recommendation that in early infancy, the calcium: phosphorus ratio in the diet should be 1.5:1. For older infants, the phosphorus is raised to about 80 per cent of the calcium allowance, or to a ratio to calcium similar to cow's milk. This is a practical consideration, since infants of this age generally receive cow's milk as their dietary staple.

Iodine is tabulated for the first time. The recommended dietary allowance is about 5 mcg. per 100 kcalories or about 100 to 150 mcg. per day for adults. Endemic goiter does not occur where adult iodine intakes are above 75 mcg. per day.

With reference to iron, the evidence of the widespread occurrence of iron deficiency anemia in the United States has led to a great deal of recent research work and re-evaluation of the recommendation for iron. The greatest problem is in connection with the availability of iron from various foods and the individual variability due to various factors in connection with the absorption of iron. Iron exchange studies indicate losses in normal men of about 1.0 mg. per day. In the female, there is an additional loss accompanying menstruation which averages about 0.5 mg. per day. Pregnancy also increases requirements to about 3.5 mg. per day, and in the latter part of pregnancy, this may rise to 4 mg. per day. During lactation, the loss of iron is approximately 0.5 to 1.0 mg. per day. During adolescence, the requirement for girls, to meet the needs of rapid growth and ensuing menstruation, is 0.5 to 0.6 mg. per day. Estimates of iron that must be retained by children and adolescent boys during growth range from 0.2 to 1.0 mg. per day. The absorption of iron is a complex process, influenced by the behavior of the intestinal mucosa, the amount of available iron in the food ingested, the chemical form, the presence of dietary substances which interact with iron to influence its availability, and gastrointestinal secretions which modify absorption. The recommended allowance is based on 10 per cent absorption of food iron. For men, the allowance of 10 mg. per day is readily attained, but the 18-mg. recommendation for females with kcalorie intakes of around 2,000 is difficult to meet. If attained, it will permit sufficient accumulation of iron stores to avoid the need for iron therapy in pregnancy. It is recognized that further fortification of the diet with iron, such as increasing the iron level in enriched bread and flour and other enriched or fortified cereal products, may be required to provide the recommended allowance for women on ordinary diets.

Magnesium is included in the new revision for the first time, with the recommended allowance based on balance studies. It has been set at 350 mg. per day for adult men and 300 mg. for adult women. These levels will maintain positive balance.

The importance and essentiality of trace elements is recognized, but there is insufficient data to establish allowances for such items as chromium, cobalt, manganese, zinc, and selenium.

Sodium, potassium, and chloride are also discussed in connection with body fluids, but no recommended allowances have been formulated for these elements.

Finally, attention is also called to the importance of water, although the multiple factors that determine water losses preclude setting a general value for a minimum water requirement. Under ordinary circumstances, a reasonable allowance is 1 ml. per kcalorie for adults and 1.5 ml. per kcalorie for infants.

Special attention to water needs also must be given to infants on high-protein formulas and to all persons in hot environments.

BODY SIZE

In adapting caloric allowances for differences in size, weight may be used as a basis provided the subjects are not overweight or underweight. Table 6 can serve as a guide for this adjustment. Heights and weights as recorded are without shoes or clothing.

TABLE 6*

DESIRABLE WEIGHTS FOR HEIGHT

HEIGHT† (INCHES)	WEIGHT† IN POUNDS	
	Men	Women
60	....	109 ± 9
62	....	115 ± 9
64	133 ± 11	122 ± 10
66	142 ± 12	129 ± 10
68	151 ± 14	136 ± 10
70	159 ± 14	144 ± 11
72	167 ± 15	152 ± 12
74	175 ± 15	....

* Modified from Table 80, Hathaway and Ford, 1960, *Height and Weight of Adults in the U.S.* (Home Economics Research Report, No. 10, ARS, USDA.)

† Heights and weights are "without shoes and other clothing." To convert inches to centimeters, multiply by 2.54. To convert pounds to kilograms, multiply by 0.454.

REFERENCES

1. FOOD AND NUTRITION BOARD, NATIONAL RESEARCH COUNCIL. Recommended dietary allowances, 7th revised edition, 1968. ("NAS-NRC Publications," No. 1694.)
2. FOOD AND AGRICULTURE ORGANIZATION AND WORLD HEALTH ORGANIZATION. Calcium requirements. ("WHO Technical Report Series," No. 230, "FAO Nutrition Meetings Report Series," No. 30, 1962.)

Chapter 3 | Modification of Basic Diet at Various Phases of Life

DIET DURING PREGNANCY AND LACTATION

There is an increased need above the normal maintenance allowances for protein, minerals, vitamins, and calories during pregnancy and lactation. (See Table 3.)
mended Dietary Allowances, 6th Revised Edition, 1964 [1].)

During pregnancy increased energy needs arise due to the building of new tissue in placenta and fetus, the increased work load associated with the movement of the mother, and the increase in basal metabolic rate in the second and third trimesters. It is suggested in the Recommended Dietary Allowances that 200 calories per day be added to meet this need. The suitability of this allowance should be evaluated at frequent intervals by a physician, nurse, or nutritionist.

During lactation, the increase in energy requirements is proportional to the quantity of milk produced. Since this varies widely for each individual, adjustment may be made by approximating 120 calories for each 100 ml. of milk produced. Assuming an average milk yield of 850 ml. per day for between one and four months, it is proposed that an allowance of 1,000 calories per day be afforded during the period of lactation.

In the post-partum period the mother may increase her activities by the care of the infant and return to household duties. If such an increase occurs, additional calories should be provided whether breast feeding takes place or not.

Increases in protein need come about as a result of the growth of the fetus and accessory tissues. Although evidence for a high protein diet is limited, the Food and Nutrition Board recommends an addi-

TABLE 7

Nutrient Content of Diet for Use During Pregnancy and Lactation‡‡

(Protein 82 Gm.; Calories 1,645–2,645)

Daily Food Intake	Quantity		Calories**	Foodstuffs			Minerals		Vitamins				
	Weight (Gm.)	Approximate Measure#		Protein (Gm.)‖‖	Fat (Gm.)‖‖	Carbohydrate (Gm.)‖‖	Ca (Mg.)	Fe (Mg.)	A (I.U.)	Ascorbic Acid (Mg.)	Thiamine (Mg.)	Riboflavin (Mg.)	Niacin (Mg.)
Milk, whole‡‡	976	1 quart	680	32	40	48	1,152	0.4	1,400	8	0.32	1.68	0.4
Egg	50	1 medium	75	7	5	....	27	1.1	590	....	0.05	0.15	Tr.
Meat, poultry, or fish, cooked*	120	4 oz. edible portion	300	28	20	....	16	3.4	35	....	0.40	0.25	5.9
Bread, whole-grain or enriched white†	150	5 slices	350	10	....	75	103	3.7	Tr.	....	0.37	0.25	3.2
Cereal, whole-grain or enriched white	20	½ cup	70	2	....	15	21	0.7	Tr.	....	0.07	0.05	0.7
Potato, cooked	100	1 small	70	2	....	15	5	0.5	Tr.	16	0.09	0.03	1.1
Vegetable (A)‡	150	2 servings	....	....	....	....	43	1.2	2,180	32	0.10	0.10	0.9
(B)§	50		20	1	....	4	12	0.5	1,660	5	0.03	0.03	0.4
Including green and yellow													
Fruit, citrus	100	1 serving	40	....	....	10	18	0.1	140	40	0.05	0.01	0.1
Fruit, other‖	....	1 serving	40	....	....	10	7	0.4	473	5	0.02	0.03	0.4
Subtotal	....	....	1,645	82	65	177	1,404	12.0	6,478	106	1.50	2.58	13.1
Vitamin D concentrate‡‡	....	....	....	....	....	....	....	....	....	....	....	....	....
Separated fats and sweets††	....	....	1,000	....	....	....	....	....	660	....	....	....	....
Total§§	....	....	2,645	82	....	....	1,404	12.0§§	7,138	106	1.50	2.58	13.1

* Estimate based on weekly consumption of 350 gm. beef, 280 gm. pork, 70 gm. fish, and 140 gm. poultry. *Meat Consumption Trends and Patterns* (U.S. Department of Agriculture, Agricultural Marketing Service, Agricultural Economics Division, Agriculture Handbook, No. 187 [Washington, D.C., July ,1960]).

† Each slice of bread has been considered to weigh 30 gm. (1 oz.) as in the values assigned to the exchange lists. It is recognized, however, that sliced bread may range between 20 and 30 gm. in weight. Adjustments should be made where usage varies.

‡ In making this estimate, it was considered that the commonly used vegetables A, tomatoes, snap beans, spinach, asparagus, broccoli, cabbage, lettuce, and cucumber, might be used 10 times weekly. Weighting was adapted from Agriculture Handbook, No. 215, *Consumption Trends and Patterns for Vegetables* (U.S. Department of Agriculture, Economic and Statistical Analysis Division, Economic Research Service [July, 1961]).

§ It was assumed that the most commonly used vegetables from the vegetable B group of the exchange lists were peas, carrots, beets, and squash. It was estimated that these vegetables might be used 4 times weekly averaging 50 gm. daily. Weighting was adapted from Agriculture Handbook, No. 215, *Consumption Trends and Patterns for Vegetables* (U.S. Department of Agriculture, Economic and Statistical Analysis Division, Economic Research Service [July, 1961]).

‖ Apples, bananas, canned peaches, pineapples, pears, apricots, and plums were considered commonly used. Weighting was adapted from *Consumption of Food in the United States*, Supplement for 1962 to Agriculture Handbook, No. 62 (U.S. Department of Agriculture, Agricultural Marketing Service [October, 1963]).

Weights and measures assigned to the Exchanges are indicated in Tables 21–29.

** Calories are rounded off to the nearest 5.

†† Per capita consumption of fats and sweets has been estimated as 2 oz. separated fat or oil and 3 oz. sugar daily. *National Food Situation, NFS-108* (U.S. Department of Agriculture, Economic Research Service [May, 1964]).

‡‡ 400–800 I.U. vitamin D may be obtained from fortified milk or a concentrate. During lactation 1½ quarts of milk should be used to provide extra protein and other nutrient levels proposed in the Recommended Dietary Allowances (Table 3). The use of skim milk would reduce the calories in 1 quart by approximately 340.

§§ The total minerals, vitamins, and protein will approximate the recommended dietary allowances (Table 3), with the exception of iron. Liver and other iron-rich foods may be used to augment this level. Caloric needs should be adjusted to the individual.

‖‖ Values for calories, carbohydrate, protein, and fat from the Food Exchange Lists, Table 20, p. 000, have been used to evaluate foods and food groups.

TABLE 7A*

MENU PATTERN AND SAMPLE MEALS DURING PREGNANCY AND LACTATION†
(82 Gm. Protein and 1,645–2,645 Calories; Derived from Table 7)

DAILY FOOD PLAN‡	SAMPLE MENU PATTERN‡	SAMPLE MEALS‡
	A.M.	
MILK GROUP 1 qt. whole milk# MEAT GROUP 5 ounces or equivalent‖ Cooked beef, pork, veal, lamb, poultry or fish	1 citrus fruit or ½ cup juice ½ cup cooked cereal or ¾ cup flake-type with milk and sugar§ 1 slice enriched or whole-grain toast with spread§ Milk—1 glass	½ grapefruit ¾ cup flakes with milk and sugar§ 1 slice toast with spread§ Milk—1 glass
	Noon	
VEGETABLE AND FRUIT GROUP 4 servings or more A dark-green or deep-yellow vegetable daily for vitamin A value A citrus fruit or other fruit rich in vitamin C daily	2 oz. meat, poultry, fish, cheese or 2 eggs‖ Vegetable 2 slices enriched or whole-grain bread or substitute Milk—1 glass	Sandwich: 2 slices meat 2 slices bread Sliced tomatoes and lettuce Milk—1 glass
	P.M.	
BREAD-CEREAL-POTATO-LEGUME GROUP 7 servings FATS AND SWEETS (Without this group the diet contains 1,645 calories) 10 teaspoons fat or oil contain 450 calories 10 teaspoons sugar, jelly, or honey contain 200 calories	3 oz. meat,‖ poultry, fish or substitute ½ cup potato or substitute Dark-green or deep yellow vegetable Other vegetable Fruit 2 slices enriched or whole-grain bread with spread§ or substitute Milk—1 glass	Meat loaf Baked potato Asparagus tips Cabbage slaw Fresh strawberries 2 hot rolls with spread§ Milk—1 glass
	Between	
Vitamin D#	Milk—1 glass	Milk—1 glass

* The Recommended Dietary Allowances (Table 3) during pregnancy may be met by this pattern, with the exception of iron. Liver and other iron rich foods may be used to augment this level.

† During lactation 1½ quarts of milk per day would provide the extra protein and other nutrients required to meet the Recommended Dietary Allowances.

‡ For alternates within each food group see Tables 21–29.

§ 1 teaspoon sugar adds 20 calories; 1 teaspoon fat or oil adds 45 calories. Desserts like ice cream, pudding, and gelatin may add 150–300 calories. For additional caloric values see Table 36. Adjustments in this group should be made to suit caloric needs of the individual patient.

‖ If additional meat is desired, one serving of the bread group (as 1 slice bread) may be omitted for each 1 oz. meat added, without changing the caloric value or reducing nutrient content. Other rearrangements or omissions should be assessed by reference to the values in Table 7.

\# The use of skim milk would reduce calories in 1 quart of milk by 360.
If 400 I.U. of vitamin D is not contained in 1 quart of milk a concentrate should be prescribed.

tional allowance of 20 gm. protein per day above the normal requirement. It is noted, however, that normal gestation seems to occur with less than this added amount.

The protein requirement for lactation may be estimated from the fact that a liter of breast milk contains approximately 12 gm. protein. If the efficiency of conversion of dietary protein to milk protein approaches 50 per cent, an additional requirement of 25 gm. might be projected. Since milk production may actually exceed a liter per day, the Recommended Dietary Allowances indicate an additional 40 gm. protein during lactation. It is recognized that lower protein intakes are common in other parts of the world and that acceptable growth occurs during the first six months of life. Whether continuous low levels of protein intake are detrimental to the mother is not clear.

These recommendations for increased protein and other nutrients may be met, with the exception of iron, by adding to the basic dietary plan for the normal diet 1 pint of milk during pregnancy and 1 quart of milk during lactation. Without the fats and sweets, the basic dietary pattern indicated in Table 7 will approximate 1,645 calories and 82 grams of protein. A further reduction of 340 calories may be attained with the use of skim milk. If the milk is not fortified with 400 International Units vitamin D per quart, an additional supplement should be prescribed. An example of a menu pattern together with sample meals is indicated in Table 7A. Any modifications in the kind and amount of foods or food groups in a resultant diet may be reassessed by reference to Table 7.

DIETS DURING INFANCY, CHILDHOOD, AND ADOLESCENCE

Relatively more calories, protein, minerals, and vitamins are recommended per unit of weight during the growth period of an individual. A wide range of normality exists in the development pattern. Data on heights and weights of children and youth in the United States have been compiled by Hathaway (2). The compilation includes general tables giving height-weight data from research studies on children and youth from thirty-four states and the District of Columbia; height-weight standards used in appraisal of growth and nutritional status; special tables relating height-weight-age data to some factors affecting growth patterns; and an annotated list of references, which furnishes pertinent details of methodology and supplementary information concerning the studies from which data have been quoted. Mean figures indicating height and weight appear in Table 3.

Allowances for energy needs of infants during the first year range from 130 calories per kg. at birth to 100 calories per kg. by the end of the year. There are wide individual variations in physical activity in both infants and children. Inactive children may become obese with less than these allowances; very active children may require more. For this reason much caution should be used in selecting a value for any one individual.

Major differences in growth rates between boys and girls after age nine also contribute to wide individual differences. Appropriate allowances for individual children must be derived from observation of growth, appetite, activity, and body fatness. Figures 1 and 2, pages 16 and 17, may be used as a general guide to caloric adjustments for body size.

Protein need during growth must be relatively higher than that of the adult to provide for the formation of new tissues. The evidence from studies of young children indicates that their protein metabolism is similar to that of the adult except for the larger amount required for growth.

The protein allowances proposed for children after infancy provide approximately 10 per cent of the caloric intake as protein. The dietary protein ordinarily comes from a variety of sources including 25 to 50 per cent of the total from animal sources or other high quality protein. This can be expected to provide approximately twice the minimal need for the average child and allow a reasonable margin for growth. The bases for the Recommended Dietary Allowances for minerals and vitamins, fats and carbohydrates are discussed in the text of Publication 1146, *A Report of the Food and Nutrition Board*, 6th revised edition, 1964 (National Academy of Sciences, National Research Council).

Although the relative amounts of each food consumed will vary during the child's developmental period, the selection of food is derived ordinarily from the commonly consumed foods and food groups indicated in the basic dietary patterns. For example, the Recommended Daily Allowances for protein indicate a variation in

TABLE 8

NUTRIENT CONTENT OF DIET FOR CHILD BETWEEN FOUR AND SIX YEARS OF AGE

(64 Gm. Protein; 1,355–1,700 Calories)

DAILY FOOD INTAKE	QUANTITY		CALORIES**	FOODSTUFFS			MINERALS		VITAMINS				
	Weight (Gm.)	Approximate Measure#		Protein (Gm.)‖‖	Fat (Gm.)‖‖	Carbohydrate (Gm.)‖‖	Ca (Mg.)	Fe (Mg.)	A (I.U.)	Ascorbic Acid (Mg.)	Thiamine (Mg.)	Riboflavin (Mg.)	Niacin (Mg.)
Milk, whole	976	1 quart	680	32	40	48	1,152	0.4	1,400	8	0.32	1.68	0.4
Egg	50	1 medium	75	7	5	...	27	1.1	590	...	0.05	0.15	Tr.
Meat, poultry, or fish, cooked*	60	2 oz. edible portion	150	14	10	...	8	1.7	18	...	0.20	0.13	3.0
Bread, whole-grain or enriched white†	90	3 slices	210	6	...	45	62	2.3	Tr.	...	0.23	0.16	2.0
Cereal, whole-grain or enriched	20	½ cup	70	2	...	15	21	0.7	Tr.	...	0.07	0.05	0.7
Potato, cooked	100	1 small	70	2	...	15	5	0.5	Tr.	16	0.09	0.03	1.1
Vegetable (A)‡	150	2 servings	...	...	...	...	43	1.2	2,180	32	0.10	0.10	0.9
(B)§	50		20	1	...	4	12	0.5	1,660	5	0.03	0.03	0.4
Including green and yellow													
Fruit, citrus	100	1 serving	40	...	...	10	18	0.1	140	40	0.05	0.01	0.1
Fruit, other‖	...	1 serving	40	...	...	10	7	0.4	473	5	0.02	0.03	0.4
Vitamin D concentrate§§	...	...	...	...	...	...	...	...	...	...	...	...	...
Separated fats and sweets††	...	...	...	...	...	...	...	...	...	...	...	...	...
Total‡‡	...	...	1,355	64	55	147	1,355	8.9‡‡	6,461	106	1.16	2.37	9.0

* Estimate based on weekly consumption of 175 gm. beef, 140 gm. pork, 35 gm. fish, and 70 gm. poultry. *Meat Consimption Trends and Patterns* (U.S. Department of Agriculture, Agricultural Marketing Service, Agricultural Economics Division, Agriculture Handbook, No. 187 [Washington, D.C., July 1960]).

† Each slice of bread has been considered to weigh 30 gm. (1 oz.) as in the values assigned to the exchange lists. Sliced bread, however, may range between 20 and 30 gm. in weight. Adjustments should be made where usage varies.

‡ In making this estimate, it was considered that the commonly used vegetables A, tomatoes, snap beans, spinach, asparagus, broccoli, cabbage, lettuce, and cucumber, might be used 10 times weekly. Weighting was adapted from Agriculture Handbook, No. 215, *Consumption Trends and Patterns for Vegetables* (U.S. Department of Agriculture, Economic and Statistical Analysis Division, Economic Research Service [July, 1961]).

§ It was assumed that the most commonly used vegetables from the vegetable B group of the exchange lists were peas, carrots, beets, and squash. It was estimated that these vegetables might be used 4 times weekly averaging 50 gm. daily. Weighting was adapted from Agriculture Handbook, No. 215, *Consumption Trends and Patterns for Vegetables* (U.S. Department of Agriculture, Economic and Statistical Analysis Division, Economic Research Service [July, 1961]).

‖ Apples, bananas, canned peaches, pineapples, pears, apricots, and plums were considered commonly used. Weighting was adapted from *Consumption of Food in the United States*, Supplement for 1962 to Agriculture Handbook No. 62, U.S. Department of Agriculture (Agricultural Marketing Service [October, 1963]).

\# Weights and measures assigned to the Exchanges are indicated in Tables 21–29.

** Calories are rounded off to the nearest 5.

†† 1 teaspoon sugar adds 20 calories; 1 teaspoon fat or oil adds 45 calories. Such desserts as ice cream, pudding, and gelatin may add 150–300 calories. For additional caloric values see Table 36.

‡‡ Meets Recommended Dietary Allowances (Table 3) for child in good health except for iron.

§§ 400–800 I.U. vitamin D may be obtained from fortified milk or a concentrate.

‖‖ Values for calories, carbohydrate, protein, and fat from the Food Exchange Lists, Table 20, have been used to evaluate foods and food groups.

TABLE 8A

Menu Pattern and Sample Meals for Child Between Four and Six Years of Age

(64 Gm. Protein; 1,355–1,700 Calories; Derived from Table 8)

Daily Food Plan*	Sample Menu Pattern*	Sample Meals*
Milk Group	A.M.	
1 qt. milk Meat Group	1 citrus fruit or ½ cup juice ½ cup cereal with sugar‡ 1 slice toast with spread‡ 1 glass milk	Orange juice Enriched farina with sugar‡ Toast with spread‡ 1 glass milk
3 equivalents† (One equivalent is equal to 1 oz. cooked beef, veal, pork, lamb, liver, poultry, fish, cheese or one egg)	Noon	
Vegetable and Fruit Group 4 servings A dark-green or deep-yellow vegetable is important for vitamin A	2 oz. meat, poultry, fish, cheese or 2 eggs ½ cup potato or substitute Dark-green or deep-yellow vegetable Dessert‡ 1 slice enriched or whole-grain bread with spread‡ Milk—1 glass	Broiled ground beef Baked potato Carrot rings Ice cream Bread with spread‡ Milk—1 glass
A citrus fruit or other fruit rich in vitamin C is important daily	P.M.	
Bread-Cereal-Potato-Legume Group 5 servings Fats and Sweets (Without this group the diet contains 1,355 calories)	1 egg or 1 oz. cheese, meat, poultry, or fish Vegetables, raw or cooked Fruit 1 slice enriched or whole-grain bread with spread‡ Milk—1 glass	Liver in tomato sauce Shredded lettuce Baked apple Bread with spread‡ Milk—1 glass
5 teaspoons fat or oil add 225 calories	Between	
4 teaspoons sugar, jelly or honey add 80 calories	Milk—1 glass	Milk—1 glass

* For alternates within each food group see Tables 21–29.

† If additional meat is desired, one serving of bread group (as 1 slice bread) may be omitted for each 1 oz. meat added, without changing the caloric value or reducing nutrient content. Other rearrangements or omissions should be assessed by reference to the values in Table 8.

‡ 1 teaspoon sugar adds 20 calories; 1 teaspoon fat or oil adds 45 calories. Such desserts as ice cream, pudding, and gelatin may add 150–300 calories. For additional caloric values see Table 36.

TABLE 9

NUTRIENT CONTENT OF DIET FOR AN ADOLESCENT BETWEEN TWELVE AND FIFTEEN YEARS OF AGE

(Protein 82 Gm.; Calories 1,645–2,645)

DAILY FOOD INTAKE	QUANTITY		CALORIES**	FOODSTUFFS			MINERALS		VITAMINS				
	Weight (Gm.)	Approximate Measure#		Protein (Gm.)‖‖	Fat (Gm.)‖‖	Carbohydrate (Gm.)‖‖	Ca (Mg.)	Fe (Mg.)	A (I.U.)	Ascorbic Acid (Mg.)	Thiamine (Mg.)	Riboflavin (Mg.)	Niacin (Mg.)
Milk, whole	976	1 quart	680	32	40	48	1,152	0.4	1,400	8	0.32	1.68	0.4
Egg	50	1 medium	75	7	5	...	27	1.1	590	...	0.05	0.15	Tr.
Meat, poultry, or fish, cooked*	120	4 oz. edible portion	300	28	20	...	16	3.4	35	...	0.40	0.25	5.9
Bread, whole-grain or enriched white†	150	5 slices	350	10	...	75	103	3.7	Tr.	...	0.37	0.25	3.2
Cereal, whole-grain or enriched white	20	½ cup	70	2	...	15	21	0.7	Tr.	...	0.07	0.05	0.7
Potato, cooked	100	1 small	70	2	...	15	5	0.5	Tr.	16	0.09	0.03	1.1
Vegetable (A)‡	150	2 servings	...	...	...	...	43	1.2	2,180	32	0.10	0.10	0.9
(B)§ Including green and yellow	50		20	1	...	4	12	0.5	1,660	5	0.03	0.03	0.4
Fruit, citrus	100	1 serving	40	...	...	10	18	0.1	140	40	0.05	0.01	0.1
Fruit, other‖	...	1 serving	40	...	...	10	7	0.4	473	5	0.02	0.03	0.4
Subtotal	...	...	1,645	82	65	177	1,404	12.0	6,478	106	1.50	2.58	13.1
Vitamin D concentrate‡‡	...	...	...	...	...	...	...	...	...	...	...	...	...
Separated fats and sweets††	...	...	1,000	...	...	...	...	...	660	...	...	...	...
Total§§	...	...	2,645	...	...	...	1,404	12.0§§	7,138	106	1.50	2.58	13.1

* Estimate based on weekly consumption of 350 gm. beef, 280 gm. pork, 70 gm. fish, and 140 gm. poultry. *Meat Consumption Trends and Patterns* (U.S. Department of Agriculture, Agricultural Marketing Service, Agricultural Economics Division, Agriculture Handbook, No. 187 [Washington, D.C., July, 1960]).

† Each slice of bread has been considered to weigh 30 gm. (1 oz.) as in the values assigned to the exchange lists. It is recognized, however, that sliced bread may range between 20 and 30 gm. in weight. Adjustments should be made where usage varies.

‡ In making this estimate, it was considered that the commonly used vegetables A, tomatoes, snap beans, spinach, asparagus, broccoli, cabbage, lettuce, and cucumber, might be used 10 times weekly. Weighting was adapted from Agriculture Handbook, No. 215, *Consumption Trends and Patterns for Vegetables*, (U.S. Department of Agriculture, Economic and Statistical Analysis Division, Economic Research Service [July, 1961]).

§ It was assumed that the most commonly used vegetables from the vegetable B group of the exchange lists were peas, carrots, beets, and squash. It was estimated that these vegetables might be used 4 times weekly averaging 50 gm. daily. Weighting was adapted from Agriculture Handbook, No. 215, *Consumption Trends and Patterns for Vegetables* (U.S. Department of Agriculture, Economic and Statistical Analysis Division, Economic Research [July, 1961]).

‖ Apples, bananas, canned peaches, pineapples, pears, apricots, and plums were considered commonly used. Weighting was adapted from *Consumption of Food in the United States*, Supplement for 1962 to Agriculture Handbook, No. 62 (U.S. Department of Agriculture, Agricultural Marketing Service [October, 1963]).

Weights and measures assigned to the Exchanges are indicated in Tables 21–29.

** Calories are rounded off to the nearest 5.

†† Per capita consumption of fats and sweets have been estimated as 2 oz. separated fat or oil and 3 oz. sugar daily. *National Food Situation, NFS-108* (U.S. Department of Agriculture, Economic Research Service [May, 1964]).

‡‡ 400–800 I.U. vitamin D may be obtained from fortified milk or a concentrate.

§§ Meets Recommended Dietary Allowances (Table 3) for adolescents in good health except for iron level for girls.

‖‖ Values for calories, carbohydrate, protein, and fat from the Food Exchange Lists, Table 20, have been used to evaluate foods and food groups.

TABLE 9A*

Menu Pattern and Sample Meals for an Adolescent between Twelve and Fifteen Years of Age
(82 Gm. Protein and 1,645–2,645 Calories; Derived from Table 9)

Daily Food Plan‡	Sample Menu Pattern‡	Sample Meals‡
Milk Group	**A.M.**	
1 qt. whole milk# **Meat Group** 5 ounces or equivalent§ Cooked beef, pork, veal, lamb, poultry or fish	1 citrus fruit or ½ cup juice ½ cup cooked cereal or ¾ cup flake-type with milk and sugar† 1 slice enriched or whole-grain toast with spread† Milk—1 glass	½ grapefruit ¾ cup flakes with milk and sugar† 1 slice toast with spread† Milk—1 glass
	Noon	
Vegetable and Fruit Group 4 servings or more A dark-green or deep-yellow vegetable daily for vitamin A value A citrus fruit or other fruit rich in vitamin C daily	2 oz. meat, poultry, fish, cheese or 2 eggs§ Vegetable 2 slices enriched or whole-grain bread or substitute Milk—1 glass	Sandwich: 2 slices meat 2 slices bread Sliced tomatoes Milk—1 glass
	P.M.	
Bread-Cereal-Potato-Legume Group§ 7 servings **Fats and Sweets†** (Without this group the diet contains 1,645 calories) 10 teaspoons fat or oil contain 450 calories 10 teaspoons sugar, jelly, or honey contain 200 calories	3 oz. meat, poultry, fish or substitute§ ½ cup potato or substitute Dark-green or deep-yellow vegetable Other vegetable Fruit 2 slices enriched or whole-grain bread with spread† or substitute Milk—1 glass	Meat loaf Baked potato Asparagus tips Cabbage slaw Fresh strawberries 2 hot rolls with spread† Milk—1 glass
	Between	
Vitamin D**	Milk—1 glass	Milk—1 glass

* The Recommended Dietary Allowances (Table 3) during adolescence may be met by this pattern, with the exception of iron. Liver and other iron rich foods may be used to augment this level.

† 1 teaspoon sugar adds 20 calories; 1 teaspoon fat or oil adds 45 calories. Desserts like ice cream, pudding, and gelatin may add 150–300 calories. For additional caloric values see Table 36. Adjustments in this group should be made to suit caloric needs of the individual patient.

‡ For alternates within each food group see Tables 21–29.

§ If additional meat is desired, one serving of the bread group (as 1 slice bread) may be omitted for each 1 oz. meat added, without changing the caloric value or reducing nutrient content. Other rearrangements or omissions should be assessed by reference to the values in Table 9.

The use of skim milk would reduce calories by 360.

** 400 I.U. vitamin D should be used as a concentrate if not contained in milk.

protein need between 40 and 100 gm., depending upon the age and size of the child. In younger children the 32 gm. protein provided in 1 quart of milk will insure a surplus of animal protein. With 1 egg and 1 oz. meat in addition, it would be possible to provide two-thirds of the protein as animal protein in a diet including 65 gm. protein daily.

A combination of foods given a child between four and six years of age might approximate that given in Table 8. A daily food pattern and sample meals have been illustrated in Table 8A. The nutrient evaluation of the plan in Table 8 meets or exceeds the Recommended Dietary Allowances, 1968 (Table 3).

It is not intended or expected that all children will conform to any one exact pattern of eating. However, if any omissions or gross changes in the basic pattern of eating are made, it is desirable to reassess the resultant nutrient content of the diet by reference to appropriate tables.

A menu pattern and sample meals for an adolescent between twelve and fifteen years of age are outlined in Table 9A. If omissions or gross changes are made in this basic plan, a reassessment of the resultant diet should be made by reference to Table 9.

DIETS AFTER FIFTY-FIVE YEARS OF AGE

Energy requirements decline progressively after the years of early adulthood in part because of a decrease in basal metabolic rate and in part because of a reduction in physical activity. It has been proposed in the Recommended Dietary Allowances (Table 3) that caloric allowances be reduced by 5 per cent per decade between ages 35 and 55 and by 8 per cent per decade from ages 55 to 75. A further decrease of 10 per cent is recommended for age 75 and beyond. However, it is most difficult to estimate precisely the degree of reduction in physical activity in any one individual. For this reason, the Allowances should serve only as a reference, with deviations being determined by the individual's total health status.

With advancing age, the total food consumption will fall markedly in line with the decrease in caloric needs. The total body protein (or "active metabolic mass") also falls with age. The extent to which this is a natural accompaniment of aging, of a change in food habits, or of decreased activity is not certain. The efficiency of protein utilization may decrease, with age. In view of the lack of clear evidence the protein allowance in the Recommended Dietary Allowances has been made 1 gm. per kg. per day for adults of all ages. Other nutrient needs for minerals and vitamins also remain at the level of the young adult.

A reduction in caloric needs will point primarily to a need for reduction in such food groups as the bread and cereal, and fats and sweets if the greatest advantage is to be taken of foods high in good quality protein and other nutrients. For this purpose the basic plan of diet indicated for the young adult in Table 2 will be appropriate with the curtailment of fats and sweets. The basic plan provides approximately 1,415 calories and 70 gm. protein. Modifications in this plan should be made to accommodate the size and health status of the older individual. Any gross omission or change in the resultant plan should be reassessed by reference to Table 2.

A description of the basic dietary pattern containing 1,415 calories may be obtained from Table 2. Sample menu pattern and sample meals are outlined in Table 10. Appropriate modification should be made in fats and sweets to achieve the goal for any one individual.

The following publications for popular use are available from The American Dietetic Association, 620 North Michigan Avenue, Chicago, Illinois, 60611:

Give Yourself a Break contains questions and answers on food for teen-agers with hints for weight control. A single copy is available for 3 cents; or fifty copies for $1.25.

Eating is Fun—For Older People Too is a 28-page booklet directed to the administrator or manager of a residential home for older people or a nursing home. It contains ideas for planning menus, sample lunches and suppers, comments on modified diets, and tips on saving money. The cost is 50 cents per copy; or $17.50 for fifty copies.

Forget Birthdays and Enjoy Good Eating is a folder for the older person who wants sound advice on food selection for healthful living. A single copy is 3 cents; fifty copies, $1.25.

Food Facts Talk Back is a booklet designed to combat food misinformation. Questions and answers cover common misconceptions. Single copies are available at 50 cents each; 50 copies may be obtained for $17.50.

TABLE 10

Menu Pattern and Sample Meals for Individual Fifty-five Years or Over

(70 Gm. Protein; 1,415–1,615 Calories; Derived from Table 2)‡

Daily Food Plan	Sample Menu Pattern	Sample Meals
	A.M.	
Milk Group† 1 pint milk Meat Group† 5 equivalents (One equivalent equals 1 oz. edible portion of cooked beef, veal, lamb, poultry, fish, cheese or 1 egg)	1 citrus fruit or ½ cup juice ½ cup cooked cereal or ¾ cup flake-type cereal with milk and sugar* 1 slice enriched or whole-grain toast with spread* Coffee or tea if desired*	½ cup orange juice ¾ cup flake-type cereal with milk and sugar* Toast with spread* Coffee or tea if desired*
	Noon	
Vegetable and Fruit Group† 5 servings or more A dark-green or deep-yellow vegetable is important for vitamin A value A citrus fruit or other fruit rich in vitamin C is important daily	Meat, poultry, fish or cheese (3 oz. edible portion) ½ cup potato or substitute† Dark-green or deep-yellow vegetable Fruit 1 slice enriched or whole-grain bread with spread* Milk	Browned meat pattie Baked potato Broccoli Tossed lettuce and tomato salad* Applesauce Bread with spread* Milk
	P.M.	
Bread-Cereal-Potato-Legume Group† 8 servings Fats and Sweets (Without this group the diet contains 1,415 calories) 3 teaspoons fat or oil add 135 calories 3 teaspoons sugar, jelly, or honey add 60 calories	2 oz. edible portion of meat, poultry, fish, cheese or 2 eggs ½ cup potato, or rice, or substitute† Vegetables Fruit 2 slices enriched or whole-grain bread or substitute† Milk	Vegetable soup with crackers† Tuna casserole† Mixed salad greens* Peach custard* 1 slice bread with spread* Milk
	Between	Bedtime
	Milk 2 Graham crackers†	Milk 2 Graham crackers†

* 1 teaspoon sugar adds 20 calories; 1 teaspoon fat or oil adds 45 calories. Desserts like ice cream, pudding, or gelatin may add 150–300 calories. Cake or pie may add 300–700 calories. For additional caloric values see Table 36.

† See Tables 21–29 for other alternates within each food group. Five soda crackers (2 inches square) or 2 Graham crackers may be used as an alternate for 1 slice bread.

‡ The nutrient content of the above plan corresponds to the Recommended Dietary Allowances for the older individual.

The Best of Health to You includes normal nutrition for the adult. Meals, menus, and modifications for weight control are designed for the adult. Single copy is 5 cents; fifty copies, $1.75.

REFERENCES

1. Food and Nutrition Board, National Research Council. Recommended dietary allowances. 7th revised edition, 1968. ("NAS-NRC Publications," No. 1694.)
2. Hathaway, M. L. Heights and weights of children and youth in the United States. ("U.S. Department of Agriculture Home Economics Research Reports," No. 2.) 1957.

SECTION II | MODIFICATIONS OF THE NORMAL DIET

As stated previously, the aim of the normal dietary regimen is to maintain, or bring the patient to, a state of nutritive sufficiency. If, in illness, deterioration has occurred in the digestive or metabolic processes or in the utilization of nutrients, nutritional needs may increase. On the other hand, there are instances in which a decrease is indicated, as in sodium or calories. In such instances, all other nutrients should remain at or above the needs for nutritive sufficiency. From this it is logical to assume that a therapeutic diet may be regarded as a modification of the normal diet. With this principle in mind, two basic guides will be called for, from which appropriate adaptations may be made: first, a guide to the recommended nutrient allowances for healthy individuals and, second, a plan of eating which will meet these needs. Appropriate adaptations may then be made from this to suit the special purposes of therapeutic diets.

Recently a revision of a guide to the nutrient needs of healthy individuals has been prepared by the Food and Nutrition Board of the National Research Council, covering the needs of individuals from infancy to old age. This guide, called *Recommended Dietary Allowances*, 7th Revised Edition, 1968, has been reproduced and discussed on pages 12–18b in the text.

The next step will be to develop a flexible plan of eating which will approximate this level of nutrient content. To achieve this goal as concisely as possible, a basic daily pattern of diet has been outlined simply, in terms of commonly used and available food groups. For this purpose, foods have been divided into the four food groups which supply the major portion of the day's needs for protein, minerals, and vitamins. These four groups include the milk group, the meat group, the bread-cereal-potato-legume group, and the vegetable and fruit group. A fifth group, fats and sweets, has been noted separately because this group contributes a major source of calories but comparatively small amounts of protein, mineral, and vitamins. In this manner it will be possible to think in terms of a small number of food groups with approximately similar nutrient characteristics rather than many individual food items. This plan has the advantage of requiring a minimum of effort on the part of the dietitian, nurse, or physician in suggesting appropriate variety on a modified diet or in re-totaling the nutrient content of a diet if certain omissions or additions are made to the basic plan for therapeutic purposes.

The selection and definition of the therapeutic diets which follow have been made in terms of dietetic principles rather than in terms of diseases or names of physicians in order that more accurate, flexible, and nutritionally appropriate dietary programs may be prescribed for the therapeutic goals established by the physician. The definitions of diets are taken from the *Revised Glossary of Dietetic Terms* prepared by committees of the Diet Therapy Section of The American Dietetic Association. In bringing this material up to date, some changes in definitions have been made as a result of special study and review by member-contributors.

In each therapeutic diet which follows, a definition has been stated; a basic plan of daily food intake has been evaluated for nutrient content; deviations from the Recommended Dietary Allowances for normal diet have been noted; a description of the daily food plan has been presented in terms of food groups; a menu pattern and sample meals have been derived from this, and, where appropriate, foods to restrict have been noted. It is not intended, however, that these patterns should be used without appropriate adaptations for individual needs. It is hoped only that the description of each diet has been made sufficiently concise and flexible that it will be possible easily to formulate diets suitable for individual needs and with full awareness of the nutrient content.

Chapter 4 | *Modifications in Consistency*

LIQUID DIETS

Liquid diets are of two kinds—the full liquid and the clear liquid. The full liquid diet consists of a variety of foods that are liquid or that liquefy at body temperature. Milk, plain frozen desserts, pasteurized eggs, fruit juice, vegetable juice, cereal gruels, and broth may be used. Finely homogenized meat or liver may be added to the broth or tomato juice to advantage. If this is not done, dried brewer's yeast will serve to improve the iron, protein, and B complex of this diet. Such a diet becomes a modification of a normal diet as far as physical consistency is concerned. The criterion is that it pour.

The foods enumerated in Table 11 will supply 80 gm. protein, 1,780 calories, and minerals and vitamins which approximate or exceed the Recommended Allowances for normal diet with the exception of iron and thiamine. If more or less of any nutrient is desired for a particular purpose, changes may easily be made by reference to the values given in Table 11 for each of the food groups. A reassessment of the resultant diet may then be made by re-totaling the nutrient content.

Description of the daily plan of food intake has been made in Table 11A, followed by a sample menu pattern and sample meals in Table 11B. Innumerable combinations may be made of these foods. The outlines should be considered examples only.

The clear liquid diet has been defined in the Glossary of Dietetic Terms as one that supplies clear fluids but is of little nutritional benefit. Only fat-free broth, tea, and coffee with sugar but without milk

TABLE 11

NUTRIENT CONTENT OF FULL LIQUID DIET
(80 Gm. Protein; 1,780 Calories)

DAILY FOOD INTAKE	QUANTITY		CALORIES	FOODSTUFFS			MINERALS		VITAMINS				
	Weight (Gm.)	Approximate Measure		Protein (Gm.)	Fat (Gm.)	Carbohydrate (Gm.)	Ca (Mg.)	Fe (Mg.)	A (I.U.)	Ascorbic Acid (Mg.)	Thiamine (Mg.)	Riboflavin (Mg.)	Niacin (Mg.)
Milk‖	1,464	1½ qt.	1,020	48	60	72	1,728	0.6	2,100	12	0.48	2.52	0.6
Egg	100	2 medium	150	14	10	…	54	2.3	1,180	…	0.10	0.30	Tr.
Cereal, refined enriched	40	(dry weight) 4 level tablespoons	140	4	…	30	42	1.4	Tr.	…	0.14	0.10	1.4
Fruit juice, citrus	100	½ cup	40	…	…	10	18	0.1	140	40	0.05	0.01	0.1
Tomato juice	200	1 cup	40	2	Tr.	8	14	1.8	1,600	32	0.10	0.06	1.6
Cocoa, dry	10	4 level teaspoons	30	2	2	5	13	1.0	Tr.	…	0.01	0.05	0.2
Sugar	15	1 level tablespoon	60	…	…	15	…	…	…	…	…	…	…
Plain gelatin	3	1 level teaspoon	12	3	Tr.	…	…	…	…	…	…	…	…
Bouillon cube	4	1 cube	5	1	Tr.	Tr.	…	…	…	…	…	…	…
Fats or oils	25	5 level teaspoons	225	…	25	…	…	…	220*	…	…	…	…
Subtotal†	…	…	1,722	74	97	140	1,869	7.2	5,240	84	0.88	3.04	3.9
Finely strained liver‡	60	2 oz.	60	8	2	1	4	3.4	14,400	6	0.03	1.20	4.6
Total§	…	…	1,782	82	99	141	1,873	10.6§	19,640	90	0.91	4.24	8.5

* If 5 gm. butter or fortified margarine is included.

† Does not meet levels of iron, vitamin A, or thiamine in Recommended Dietary Allowances (Table 3) for adult in good health.

‡ Strained liver or other strained meat for baby foods serves conveniently for combination with broth.

§ Approaches Recommended Dietary Allowances (Table 3) for adults in good health except for iron and thiamine.

‖ If a high protein drink is desired, 1–1½ cups non-fat, dry milk solids (100 gm.) may be added to each 1 qt. of fluid milk, thereby adding approximately 34 mg. protein and 330 calories to each quart.

TABLE 11A

Description of the Daily Food Plan for the Full Liquid Diet*

(80 Gm. Protein; 1,780 Calories; Derived from Table 11)

Daily Food Plan	Description
MILK GROUP	
1½ qt. fluid whole milk†	*One and ½ qt. fluid whole milk* contain approximately 50 gm. protein and 1,000 calories. Three-fourths quart of evaporated milk or 1½ cups whole milk solids may be used as a substitute.‡
MEAT AND EGG GROUP	
2 oz. finely homogenized meat or 2 eggs or variations	*Two eggs* contain 14 gm. protein and 150 calories. Two ounces finely homogenized meat will contain approximately 14 gm. protein and 60 calories. Liver is of exceptional value in iron, vitamin A, and the B complex. However, other finely homogenized meats may be combined with bouillon or broth and served in soup. Meat and eggs may be interchanged.
VEGETABLE AND FRUIT GROUP	
	The puree or juice from spinach, asparagus, carrots, tomatoes, string beans, or celery may be used. Mild-flavored vegetables are commonly served in soups. Other vegetable purees or juices may be used if tolerated by the patient. Calories from this source are negligible. *Citrus or tomato juice* daily provides an important source of vitamin C. A half-cup of citrus juice or 1 cup tomato juice provides approximately 40 calories.
CEREAL-POTATO GROUP	
1 or more servings	*One cup strained, cooked cereal* or 1 cup strained potato contains approximately 140 calories as well as a source of iron and the B complex. Combinations may be made with milk in gruels or soups.
FATS AND SWEETS	
	Three teaspoons sugar contribute approximately 60 calories and serve as flavoring for cocoa or gruel. Five teaspoons fat or oil provide approximately 225 calories and serve as flavoring for gruels or soup.
MEAT SUPPLEMENT	
	Two ounces finely homogenized calf liver supplies 8 gm. protein, 60 calories, and an important source of iron and the B complex. It may be added to bouillon or tomato juice. If this is not used, additional meat and eggs will supply iron, protein, and the B complex.

* If any omissions or changes are made in this food plan, it should be reassessed for nutrient content.

† If 1–1⅓ cups (depending on the brand) non-fat milk solids are added to the 1½ quarts fluid milk, approximately 34 gm. protein and 330 calories will be added to the value of this group.

‡ This fluid whole milk containing non-fat milk solids may be used in beverages, strained cereal gruels, strained soups, ice cream, and desserts such as soft custard and rennet desserts, where high protein drinks or desserts are needed.

or cream are allowed. Occasionally small amounts of ginger ale, clear fruit, or vegetable juice, and gelatin may be added. This diet would be used for very brief periods of time when it is necessary to minimize the amount of fecal material in the colon.

Tube feedings may be prepared from a mixture of foods modified in consistency to the point at which the mixture may be passed through a tube. Such feedings may vary from a finely homogenized mixture of foods selected from the "regular or house diet" to food combinations carefully designed to serve particular therapeutic purposes. Barron *et al.* (15 and 16) demonstrated the successful use of

TABLE 11B

MENU PATTERN AND SAMPLE MEALS FOR A FULL LIQUID DIET*
(80 Gm. Protein;‡ 1,780 Calories;‡ Derived from Table 11 and 11A)

SAMPLE MENU PATTERN†	SAMPLE MEALS†
A.M.	
½ cup citrus juice	Citrus juice
Cereal gruel (made from 2 tablespoons dry cereal) and milk containing non-fat milk solids with sugar, butter, or margarine	Cream of wheat gruel Sugar and butter or margarine
Coffee or tea if desired	Coffee with milk and sugar
Noon	
Broth with finely homogenized liver or other meat‡	Broth with finely homogenized liver‡
Ice cream, rennet dessert, gelatin dessert, or soft custard	Soft custard
Milk containing non-fat milk solids	Milk
P.M.	
Strained milk soup or cereal gruel‡	Strained potato soup‡
Ice cream, or dessert as at noon	Ice cream
Milk containing non-fat milk solids	Cocoa

Between

Midmorning, midafternoon, and bedtime: tomato juice or soup with finely homogenized liver, or additional eggs in desserts. Milk beverage, ice cream, and soft desserts serve as between-meal nourishments. One glass of whole milk to which ⅓ cup instant non-fat dry milk, sugar, and flavoring is added may serve as a "high protein drink."

* If any omissions or changes are made in this food plan, it should be reassessed for nutrient content, by reference to Table 11.

† Foods to restrict: Obviously, anything that has not been finely homogenized or will not pour has been omitted. Although meat, poultry, fish, vegetables, and fruits have been greatly reduced in amount, it would be possible to use more, provided that the food is finely homogenized and diluted to the extent of pouring. Pepper, cloves, mustard, and nutmeg are the spices commonly avoided.

‡ See Table 11A for alternates and for total amounts of foods to be used daily in order to include 80 gm. protein and 1,780 calories.

a small mechanical pump to pass well-blenderized, liquefied natural foods through small plastic tubing at a slow, constant rate. A highly nutritious combination of foods which may be used for this purpose may be derived from the foods outlined in the Full Liquid Diet, Table 11. Commercial products derived from natural foods and supplemented with various nutrients are also available.

SOFT AND LOW-FIBER DIETS

The soft and low-fiber diets follow the normal diet pattern, with modifications in consistency, that is, including liquid foods and those solid foods which contain a restricted amount of indigestible carbohydrate and no tough connective tissue. If the only modification required is that a diet be made mechanically soft, this may be accomplished by cooking, mashing, pureeing, or homogenizing the foods used in a normal diet. If consideration must also be given to indigestible carbohydrate, connective tissue, or flavor, the following modifications may be made.

Indigestible carbohydrates.—These carbohydrates are substances that make up the cell-wall structure of plants, consisting of varying amounts of cellulose, hemicellulose, lignin, pectic substances, gums, and mucin. A number of foods have been analyzed for their cellulose, hemicellulose, and lignin content by Williams and Olmsted (1), by Olmsted and Williams (2), and by Hummel, Shepherd, and Macy (3). Figures for total fiber have been included in the compilation by Chatfield and Adams (4) and in *Composition of Foods—Raw, Processed, Prepared* (U.S. Department of Agriculture, Agriculture Handbook No. 8 [1963]). Information on hemicelluloses, celluloses, and lignins, as well as pectins, gums, and related substances, have been compiled by Hardinge, Swarner, and Crooks (18).

A reduction of the indigestible carbohydrate content of the diet may be effected by the use of refined breads and cereals, immature vegetables, and fruits from which the skins and seeds have been eliminated. During cooking, both the pectic substances and the cellulose are disintegrated (5). For this reason, cooked vegetables and fruits are sometimes used instead of the raw. In extreme instances, still greater reduction in indigestible carbohydrates may be effected by the use of pureed vegetables and fruits or the juice only of the vegetable or fruit.

TABLE 12

NUTRIENT CONTENT OF SOFT AND LOW-FIBER DIET
(90 Gm. Protein; 2,075 Calories)

DAILY FOOD INTAKE	QUANTITY		CALORIES‖	FOODSTUFFS			MINERALS		VITAMINS				
	Weight (Gm.)	Approximate Measure		Protein# (Gm.)	Fat# (Gm.)	Carbohydrat# (Gm.)	Ca (Mg.)	Fe (Mg.)	A (I.U.)	Ascorbic Acid (Mg.)	Thiamine (Mg.)	Riboflavin (Mg.)	Niacin (Mg.)
Milk, whole	976	1 quart	680	32	40	48	1,152	0.4	1,400	8	0.32	1.68	0.4
Egg	50	1 medium	75	7	5	...	27	1.1	590	...	0.05	0.15	Tr.
Meat, poultry, fish, cooked†	150	5 oz. E.P.	375	35	25	...	20	4.3	44	...	0.50	0.31	7.4
Bread, white, enriched	150	5 slices	350	10	...	75	103	3.7	Tr.	...	0.37	0.25	3.2
Cereal, refined, enriched	20	½ cup	70	2	...	15	21	0.7	Tr.	...	0.07	0.05	0.7
Potato, cooked	100	1 small	70	2	...	15	5	0.5	Tr.	16	0.09	0.03	1.1
Vegetable cooked:													
A‡	100	one serving	...	...	...	...	31	1.1	1,310	19	0.09	0.10	0.6
B§	100	one serving	35	2	...	7	24	1.0	3,320	10	0.06	0.06	0.8
Fruit juice, citrus	100	½ cup	40	...	...	10	18	0.1	140	40	0.05	0.01	0.1
Fruit, other, cooked**	...	2 servings	80	...	...	20	14	0.8	945	9	0.04	0.06	0.8
Subtotal	...	...	1,775	90	70	190	1,415	13.7	7,749	102	1.64	2.70	15.1
Separated fats and oil	20	4 level teaspoons	180	...	20	...	...	...	220	...	...	...	...
Sugar	30	6 level teaspoons	120	...	...	30	...	...	...	...	...	...	...
Total*	...	...	2,075	90	90	220	1,415	13.7	7,969	102	1.64	2.70	15.1

* The mineral, vitamin, and protein content of this basic plan will meet or exceed the Recommended Dietary Allowances (Table 3) for a man in normal good health (70 kg.) or a woman (58 kg.) with the exception of iron. If necessary iron-rich foods could be used more frequently to bring about an increase to meet individual caloric needs. Adjustments should be made as appropriate.

† Weighting was adapted from *Meat Consumption Trends and Patterns* (U.S. Department of Agriculture, Agricultural Marketing Service, Agricultural Economics Division, Agriculture Handbook No. 187 [Washington, D.C., July, 1960]).

‡ An average of snap beans, spinach, asparagus, and tomato juice.

§ An average of cooked carrots, beets, peas, and squash.

‖ Calories rounded off to nearest 5.

\# Values for carbohydrate, protein, and fat from exchange lists.

** Apple sauce, pear, peach, apricot, plum.

TABLE 12A

DESCRIPTION OF THE DAILY FOOD PLAN FOR THE SOFT AND LOW-FIBER DIET*

(90 Gm. Protein; 2,075 Calories; Derived from Table 12)

Daily Food Plan†	Description
MILK GROUP	
1 qt. fluid whole milk	*One quart of fluid whole milk* contains 680 calories and 32 gm. protein. One pint evaporated milk or 1 cup whole milk solids may be substituted for 1 qt. fluid whole milk.
MEAT AND EGG GROUP	
6 meat equivalents	*One meat equivalent* is approximately equal to 1 oz. cooked (edible portion) beef, veal, pork, lamb, poultry, fish, cheese, or 1 egg. Each equivalent contributes approximately 7 gm. protein and 75 calories. Liver and other glandular meats are exceptional sources of iron, vitamin A, and the B complex.
VEGETABLE AND FRUIT GROUP	
4 servings	*A dark-green or yellow vegetable* daily is important for vitamin A value. Asparagus, carrots, green beans, yellow squash, pumpkin, spinach, and other greens are in this group. Additional vegetables commonly used include beets, peas, summer squash, and tomato juice or tomato puree. Other vegetables may be used as tolerated by the patient. Yellow squash, pumpkin, carrots, beets, and peas contain approximately 35 calories per serving. The others are negligible in calories.
	One-half cup citrus juice or 1 cup tomato juice daily will contribute an important part of the vitamin C needed daily. Approximately 40 calories per serving come from this source.
	Other fruits without skins or small seeds may be used. One serving of sweetened fruit may contain between 75 and 100 calories.
CEREAL-BREAD-POTATO GROUP	
7 servings	*One serving provides* approximately 70 calories and is equal to 1 slice enriched bread, ½ cup potato, ½ cup cooked macaroni, noodles, spaghetti, rice, cornmeal or ½ cup cooked cereal or ¾ cup refined flake-type cereal. For other equivalents in calories see Table 27. Other substitutes may be added as tolerated by the individual.
FATS AND SWEETS	
	Without this group the diet contains approximately 1,800–2,100 calories. Six teaspoons sugar, jelly, or honey add about 120 calories. Four teaspoons fat or oil add about 180 calories. For additional calories in desserts see Table 36.

* If any omissions or changes are made in this food plan, it should be reassesssed for total nutrient content by reference to Table 12.

† *Foods to restrict:* This diet has become increasingly liberalized and individualized to the extent that restrictions which would apply to all patients would be difficult to name (14). However, foods highly flavored with pepper, cloves, mustard, and possibly nutmeg are commonly omitted. Foods which are "overfried" or overcooked to the extent of becoming potential mechanical irritants are also commonly omitted. Foods such as bran, corn, dried beans, nuts, raisins, and fruits with small seeds and skins are also commonly avoided in view of the relatively high fiber content.

The trend, however, has been a more liberal one, due in large part to the observation (6) that vegetable purees are notoriously unpopular and that many patients refuse to eat them. The use of immature vegetables such as frozen or canned young vegetables resulted in a more palatable diet and happier patients, who benefited from eating vegetables that had been refused in their pureed state.

There has also been a trend to the use of a wider variety of fruits

TABLE 12B

MENU PATTERN AND SAMPLE MEALS FOR SOFT AND LOW-FIBER DIET
(90 Gm. Protein; 2,075 Calories; Derived from Tables 12 and 12A)

SAMPLE MENU PATTERN*	SAMPLE MEALS*
A.M.	
½ cup citrus juice or 1 cup tomato juice	Tomato juice
1 egg	1 egg
½ cup cooked refined cereal or ¾ cup flake-type with milk and sugar†	Cream of wheat with milk and sugar†
1 slice enriched toast with spread†	Toast with spread†
Coffee or tea if desired	Coffee
Noon	
3 oz. tender meat, poultry, fish, or cheese	Roast beef
½ cup potato or alternate	Mashed potato
Cooked vegetables such as asparagus, carrots, spinach, yellow squash, pumpkin, or other greens; other vegetables may be used as tolerated	Asparagus tips
Fruit (no skin or seeds)	Sliced peaches
1 slice enriched bread with spread†	Enriched bread with spread†
1 glass milk	1 glass milk
Dessert†	Plain cake†
P.M.	
Cream soup	Cream soup
2 oz. (edible portion) cooked meat, poultry, fish, cheese, or 2 eggs	Tuna with rice casserole
1 cup rice, spaghetti, noodles, potato, or alternate*	1 slice enriched bread or alternate*
Cooked vegetables (as at noon)	Peas
1 glass milk	1 glass milk
1 slice enriched bread with spread† or alternate*	
Dessert†	Ice cream†
Between	
Milk beverage	Milk shake

* See Table 12A for alternates and total amounts to use daily.

† Six teaspoons sugar (120 calories) and 4 teaspoons fat (180 calories) may be used during the day, or, if a substitution is desired for the 300 calories calculated in sugar and fat, ½ cup ice cream, plain pudding, custard, or gelatin dessert may add 150–300 calories. One serving plain cake may add 200–300 calories (see Table 36 for additional caloric values).

and vegetables, including some raw fruits. Removal of skins and seeds is usually specified, however. Peeled apples, pears, peaches, apricots, and bananas are frequently recommended.

Connective tissue.—Whether meat is tender or less tender is due chiefly to the relative quantity of connective tissue present. Connective tissue in meat consists of white or collagenous fibers and yellow elastic fibers called elastin. The total amount of connective tissue depends not only on the extent to which the muscle has been exercised but somewhat on the age. In general, older animals have denser, tougher connective tissue than do younger ones, although the toughness may be lessened in an older animal that has been confined and fattened.

This quantitative difference in the amount of connective tissue present forms the basis for an appropriate cookery process. Tenderness of meat may be increased by cooking with moist heat to convert the collagen in the connective tissue to gelatin and also by the use of low-temperature cookery to reduce or lessen the toughening or hardening of soluble proteins. The total effect of these two reactions depends on the composition of the meat, its acidity, the temperature, and the rate at which it is cooked (7).

Flavor.—Muscle tissue contains such non-protein nitrogenous products as creatine, creatinine, purines, and other products which are thought to stimulate the flow of gastric juices. The most important non-nitrogenous extractive from a quantitative viewpoint is lactic acid (8). In the usual mixed diet, the effect of this factor is minimized, and this consideration becomes of less importance; however, if it is desirable to limit the extractives, poultry as well as meat, meat broths, consommé, and gravy will have to be restricted. In this case adequate compensation for protein and other nutrients provided by meat may be made by the proportional increase in other protein-containing foods.

In recent years the trend in the use of a wide variety of meats has been a liberal one. Beef, veal, pork, lamb, liver, poultry, and fish are all commonly used. Exceptions are generally in terms of the special needs of an individual patient.

Strongly flavored vegetables, such as onions, leeks, radishes, dried beans, and vegetables of the cabbage family—Brussels sprouts, cauliflower, broccoli, and turnips—have commonly been omitted.

Here again it has been found (6) that many patients can and do eat some of the strongly flavored or "gas-forming vegetables" without particular discomfort if the vegetables are properly prepared. To prevent the decomposition of sinigrin and any other substances yielding disagreeable products that may be present, such vegetables should be heated quickly, to destroy enzymes that catalyze decomposition; the kettle kept uncovered, to prevent the water from becoming acid; the cooking period made as short as possible; and the vegetable drained and served immediately when it is done. Vegetables contain both volatile and non-volatile acids, and these acids are released largely in the first few minutes of cooking. A closed kettle retains not only the volatile sulfur compounds which mar odor and flavor but also volatile vegetable acids, which favor decomposition of the sulfur compounds present (9). With proper cooking, it may be desirable, therefore, to eliminate only those vegetables that the individual patient cannot tolerate rather than to eliminate all strongly flavored vegetables.

It is now less common to restrict all spices. Schneider, DeLuca, and Gray (10) have studied the effect of spice ingestion upon the mucosa of fifty patients with active duodenal or gastric ulcer craters. In periods of up to 180 days, it was found that cinnamon, allspice, mace, thyme, sage, paprika, and caraway seed administered with food did not exert a harmful effect upon the stomach as judged by the rate of ulcer healing and clinical symptomatology, the gastroscopic appearance of the stomach before and after the ingestion of spices, and the effect on gastric secretion of pepsin. Black pepper, chili pepper, cloves, mustard seed, and possibly nutmeg were considered gastric irritants.

Beverages.—Coffee contains caffeine, fat, coffalic acid, and chlorogenic acid, which, on oxidation, yields caffeic acid. The chlorogenic acid differs from tannins in that it does not precipitate proteins and is therefore not astringent. The percentage of caffeine varies from $\frac{2}{3}$–$2\frac{1}{2}$ per cent, with an average of $1\frac{1}{4}$ per cent (11). The main change during roasting consists in the production of aromatic, brown, and oily substances. This oil consists of 50 per cent furfurol alcohol, small quantities of valerianic acid, phenol, pyridine, and a nitrogenous aromatic substance. A cup of strong coffee contains about 0.1–0.15 gm. of caffeine. A cup of coffee has also been found to contain about 1 mg. of niacin, as well as small amounts of thiamine and riboflavin.

Tea contains caffeine (1.4–3.5 per cent), tannins (1–30 per cent), and traces of theobromine, theophylline, xanthine, and volatile oils. A cup of strong tea prepared from 1 teaspoon of dried leaves contains about 0.1 gm. of caffeine. A quick infusion extracts practically all the caffeine but only part of the tannins. The customary brief infusion is therefore recommended. Tea also contains traces of riboflavin and niacin.

Cocoa contains $1\frac{1}{2}$–$4\frac{1}{2}$ per cent theobromine, a trace of caffeine, 31 per cent carbohydrate, 9 per cent protein, and approximately 10 per cent fat.

Nutrient content.—In the past it was common practice to put more emphasis on "foods to avoid" and less on "foods to eat," with the result that this group of diets has been singled out by Duncan (12) and Pollack *et al.* (13) as one of the hazards of hospitalization, resulting in nutritional deficiency and delayed convalescence. Any such deficiency is unnecessary and can be avoided if care is given to the proper selection and amount of food used.

Milk, eggs, meat, poultry or fish, vegetables, and fruit may be used in amounts sufficient to meet or exceed the Recommended Dietary Allowances. This is particularly important for those individuals who have been ill for some time and who may have had undue dietary restrictions, resulting in an inadequate intake of nutrients. In addition, changes due to the disease itself may impose further nutritional demands to hasten healing of tissue or to compensate for poor absorption. Such extra requirements would justify an increase in all the food groups, above the level recommended for the normal diet. For example, when this diet is used for reduction of gastric acidity, the number of meals and distribution may be given in 6 or more small feedings per day. Since protein containing foods are effective in buffering the acidity of the stomach, it would be advantageous to fortify fluid milk with sufficient non-fat milk solids at least to double the natural protein content of milk, thus making the total approximately 65 gm. protein per quart. In this instance, it is well to add sufficient eggs, citrus juice, and other foods to exceed the Recommended Dietary Allowances (Table 3) for the normal individual. Special adaptations to suit the needs of any one individual may be made with a full awareness of the total nutrient content by referring to Table 12.

The nutrient content of the soft and low-fiber diet is indicated in Table 12, which shows approximately 90 gm. protein and 2,075 calories. With the exception of iron, minerals and vitamins exceed the levels indicated in the Recommended Dietary Allowances (Table 3) for the normal individual. A description of the daily food plan and a sample menu pattern and sample meals appear in Tables 12A and 12B. It is intended that appropriate adaptations of this plan be made in food selection or in calories and other nutrients to suit individual needs. However, if changes or omissions are made in any of the food groups, a reassessment of the nutrient content should be made by reference to Table 12.

The validity of correlations between food and gastrointestinal symptomatology has been critically reviewed in a report of the Joint Committee on Diet as Related to Gastrointestinal Function of The American Dietetic Association and the American Medical Association (17). Consideration is given to the chemical and physical composition of a food before its ingestion, the effect of that food in altering the gastrointestinal contents, the effect of the food or its products on the digestive tube itself, and the clinical significance of such an effect. The evidence available, the gaps in our knowledge, and the need for further research are pointed out.

REFERENCES

1. Williams, R. D., and Olmsted, W. H. The effect of cellulose, hemicellulose, and lignin on the weight of the stool: a contribution to the study of laxation in man, Nutrition, **11**:433–49, 1936.
2. Olmsted, W. H., and Williams, R. D. Carbohydrates of certain vegetables and fruits, Proc. Soc. Exper. Biol. & Med., **40**:586, 1939.
3. Hummel, F. C., Shepherd, M. L., and Macy, I. G. Effect of changes in food intakes upon the lignin, cellulose, and hemicellulose content of diets, J. Am. Dietet. A., **16**:199–207, 1940.
4. Chatfield, C., and Adams, G. Proximate composition of American food materials. (U.S. Department of Agriculture Circular No. 549.) 1940.
5. Simpson, J. I., and Halliday, E. G. Chemical and histological studies of the disintegration of cell-membrane materials in vegetables during cooking, Food Research, **6**:189–206, 1941.
6. Krause, M. V. Some modern concepts concerning hospital diets, J. Am. Dietet. A., **20**:610–12, 1944.

7. COMMITTEE ON PREPARATION FACTORS, NATIONAL COOPERATIVE MEAT INVESTIGATIONS. Meat and meat cookery. Chicago: National Live Stock and Meat Board, 1942, p. 76.
8. *Ibid.*, p. 32.
9. HALLIDAY, E. G., and NOBLE, I. T. Food chemistry and cookery. Chicago: University of Chicago Press, 1943, p. 35.
10. SCHNEIDER, M. A., DELUCA, V., JR., and GRAY, S. J. The effect of spice ingestion upon the stomach, Am. J. Gastroenterol., **26**:722–32, 1956.
11. SOLLMANN, T. A. A manual of pharmacology. Philadelphia and London: W. B. Saunders Co., 1942, pp. 265–67.
12. DUNCAN, G. C. Some nutritional hazards of the hospitalized patient, J. Am. Dietet. A., **25**:330–38, 1949.
13. POLLACK, H., and HALPERN, S. L., with the collaboration of the COMMITTEE ON THERAPEUTIC NUTRITION, FOOD AND NUTRITION BOARD, NATIONAL RESEARCH COUNCIL. Therapeutic nutrition. (Publication No. 234.) 1952.
14. Is there a rationale for the bland diet? J. Am. Dietet. A., **33**:608–9, 1957.
15. BARRON, J., and FALLIS, L. S. Tube feeding with natural foods in elderly patients, J. Am. Geriatrics Soc., **4**:400–401, 1956.
16. BARRON, J., PRENDERGAST, J. J., and JOCZ, M. W. Food pump: new approach to tube feeding, J.A.M.A., **161**:621–22, 1956.
17. REPORT OF THE JOINT COMMITTEE ON DIET AS RELATED TO GASTROINTESTINAL FUNCTION OF THE AMERICAN DIETETIC ASSOCIATION AND THE AMERICAN MEDICAL ASSOCIATION. Diet as related to gastrointestinal function, J. Am. Dietet., A. **38**:425–32, 1961.
18. HARDINGE, M. G., SWARNER, J. B., and CROOKS, H. Carbohydrate in foods, J. Am. Dietet. A., **46**:197–204, 1965.

Chapter 5 | Modifications in Calories

CALORIE-RESTRICTED DIETS

The low-calorie diet is a modification of the normal diet pattern in that the prescribed allowance has a caloric value below the total maintenance energy requirement for the day, thus providing for a depletion of body fat. Protein, minerals, and vitamins remain at or above those given in *Recommended Dietary Allowances*, 7th Revised Edition, 1968 (Table 3).

Caloric allowance.—Since weight may be lost on any level of calories below the number required to maintain the actual weight of an individual, it becomes a matter of arriving at an allowance below maintenance that is tolerable to the patient and that permits a rate of weight loss satisfactory to both the physician and the patient. In making an accurate estimate of caloric needs for maintenance of the actual body weight, a reliable record of activity during a 24-hour period and of the food intake would be helpful. In lieu of this, a gross estimate of caloric need may be made by using 12–15 calories per pound as an approximation of the needs of a sedentary adult. Thus a woman weighing 150 pounds might need between 1,800 and 2,250 calories to maintain her actual weight. A more reliable estimate of caloric expenditure may be made by reference to the values compiled by Passmore and Durnin from direct observations of energy expenditure under various conditions of work, recreation, and rest (see Table 44).

In estimating the rate of weight loss which might be expected, a deficit of 500 calories per day under maintenance needs may be used as a gross guide. Such a deficit may be expected to bring about a loss in body weight in the range of 1 pound per week. The exact loss on the scale, however, will be influenced by factors affecting water balance, heat loss, metabolism, activity, and the presence of disease. Most women lose weight satisfactorily on diets between 1,000 and 1,500 calories and most men on diets between 1,500 and 2,000.

Nutrient content.—The patterns of diet and the modifications outlined in Tables 13, 13A, 13B, and 13C for a calorie-restricted diet for an adult, an adolescent, or for use during pregnancy and lactation are all based upon amounts of the essential food groups which approximate levels of protein, minerals, and vitamins indicated in the Recommended Dietary Allowances, 7th Revised Edition, 1968 (Table 3). These plans have the advantage of being the most likely to provide for the maintenance of good nutritional health, and as such, they provide the basis for a long-term dietary program of weight control.

If, in each instance, foods for the dietary program are derived from well-liked, familiar foods which suit various ethnic and cultural habits, the likelihood of the patient's maintaining a permanent program of weight control and a feeling of well being is greatly increased. This individualization should be possible in large degree with the wide variety of alternates suggested within each essential food group; if, however, any changes are made in the amounts of the essential food groups, the nutrient content of the total diet should be reassessed by reference to Tables 2, 7, 8, or 9.

The dietitian's efforts in assisting patients call for a well-coordinated program that begins with insight gained from an adequate dietary history, and provides the modification needed for weight control and the long-term guidance which will lead to new food preferences, new methods of food preparation, and a new way of life which includes satisfying and enjoyable meals. The widening areas of responsibility of the dietitian are described by Kaufman and Mead (see Chaps. 12 and 13).

Preparation.—It will be necessary to take advantage of ways of cooking and flavoring foods that do not depend on the use of fats and sweets, unless these have been planned as part of the regimen. The suggestions (p. 55) are only a few of many possibilities for obtaining flavorful food.

TABLE 13

DESCRIPTION OF FOOD PLAN FOR CALORIE-RESTRICTED DIETS FOR AN ADULT
(70 Gm. Protein; 1,415 Calories; Derived from Normal Diet, Table 2)

Daily Food Plan	Description
MILK GROUP	
1 pt. milk	*One pint milk* contains 340 calories. One pint skim milk contains 180 calories, 18 gm. protein, and important amounts of calcium, phosphorus, and the B complex. One pint of buttermilk made from skim milk or $\frac{1}{2}$–$\frac{2}{3}$ cup non-fat dry milk (depending on brand) may be substituted for this.
MEAT GROUP	
5 meat equivalents	*One meat equivalent* is approximately equal to 1 oz. (edible portion, weighed after cooking) beef, veal, lamb, pork, poultry, fish, cheese, or 1 egg. The five equivalents may be distributed throughout the day as desired. Liver and other variety meats are exceptional sources of vitamin A, iron, and the B complex. One ounce of cooked meat or 1 egg may contain approximately 7 gm. protein and 75 calories.
VEGETABLE AND FRUIT GROUP	
5 servings	*A dark-green or deep-yellow vegetable* is important each day for its vitamin A value. Asparagus, green beans, broccoli, carrots, green peppers, winter squash, pumpkin, and other greens make up this group. Carrots, winter squash, and pumpkin contain about 35 calories per $\frac{1}{2}$ cup serving. The others will be negligible.
	Other vegetables, such as beets, cabbage, cauliflower, celery, cucumber, eggplant, lettuce, tomatoes, mushrooms, onions, peas, or turnips, contribute varied amounts of all nutrients. Beets, onions, peas, or turnips may contribute about 35 calories per $\frac{1}{2}$ cup serving. Others will be negligible.
	Citrus fruit or other fruit rich in vitamin C is important each day. One orange or $\frac{1}{2}$ cup juice or $\frac{1}{2}$ grapefruit or $\frac{1}{2}$ cup juice or 1 cup tomato juice or 1 cup strawberries or 1 cup red raspberries or $\frac{1}{4}$ cantaloupe or 1 large tangerine contains about 40 calories per serving and important amounts of vitamin C.
	Other fruits, such as 1 apple or 1 peach or 1 pear or 2 prunes or 4 apricot halves or 12 grapes or $\frac{1}{2}$ banana, contribute varied amounts of nutrients and contain about 40 calories per serving. For equivalent amounts of other fruits see Table 26. If sugar or syrup is included, additional calories must be calculated.

TABLE 13—*Continued*

Daily Food Plan	Description
BREAD-CEREAL-POTATO-LEGUME GROUP	
8 servings	*One serving provides approximately 70 calories,* important amounts of the B complex, and iron. One serving is equal to 1 slice enriched or whole-grain bread, ½ cup white potato, ¼ cup sweet potato, ⅓ cup corn, ½ cup cooked macaroni, noodles, spaghetti, rice, cornmeal, ½ cup cooked dried beans or peas, ½ cup cooked cereal, ¾ cup flake-type cereal, 2 Graham crackers, or 5, 2-inch-square soda crackers. For other equivalents see Table 27.
FATS AND SWEETS	
	Without this group the calories for the day approximate 1,415. If 1 level teaspoon fat or oil is used on bread, in vegetables, or in cooking, about 45 calories will be added. One thin slice crisp bacon, 2 tablespoons light cream or 1 tablespoon heavy cream, 1 teaspoon mayonnaise or oil, 1 tablespoon cream cheese or French dressing, 5 small olives, or 6 small nuts contain about 45 calories each.
	One level teaspoon sugar, jelly, or honey in cooking, on cereal, on fruit, or in coffee adds 20 calories. One-half cup ice cream, pudding, or gelatin dessert may add between 150 and 300 calories; and 1 serving cake or pie between 300 and 700 calories (see Table 36 for additional caloric values).

MODIFICATIONS OF THE CALORIE-RESTRICTED DIET

1,200-*calorie diet for an adult.*—If 3 servings of the bread-potato cereal-legume group are omitted from the Daily Food Plan indicated above, the diet will become approximately 1,200 calories. Iron and the B complex will be correspondingly lowered. Reference may be made to Table 3, Recommended Dietary Allowances to determine whether this reduction is appropriate.

If 1 pint skim milk is used instead of whole milk, the diet will approximate 1,245 calories.

1,415 *calories, using additional meat.*—If more meat is desired, 1 additional meat equivalent (1 oz. edible portion, cooked meat) may be substituted for 1 serving of the bread group without a significant change in calories. Other rearrangements or omissions should be assessed by reference to Table 2.

1,800-*calorie diet.*—In this case 350 calories may be added from any of the food groups desired by the patient: 350 calories may be added from the use of 4 oz. meat group, or from 4 servings of the bread group, or from additional fats and sweets. Additional caloric values may be noted from Table 36.

TABLE 13A

Menu Pattern and Sample Meals for a Calorie-restricted Diet for an Adult

(70 Gm. Protein; 1,245–1,415 Calories; Derived from Table 2)

Daily Food Plan†	Sample Menu Pattern	Sample Meals
	A.M.	
MILK GROUP 1 pt. whole milk* MEAT GROUP 5 equivalents‡ (One equivalent equals 1 oz. edible portion of cooked beef, veal, lamb, pork, poultry, fish, cheese, or 1 egg)	1 citrus fruit or $\frac{1}{2}$ cup juice 1 egg 2 slices toast Coffee or tea if desired	Sliced orange Poached egg 2 slices toast Milk Coffee or tea if desired
	Noon	
VEGETABLE AND FRUIT GROUP 5 servings A dark-green or deep-yellow vegetable daily for vitamin A value A citrus fruit or other fruit rich in vitamin C daily	2 oz. (2 equivalents) lean meat, poultry, or fish $\frac{1}{2}$ cup potato or substitute Dark-green or deep-yellow vegetable Other vegetable 2 slices enriched or whole-grain bread or alternate 1 glass milk 1 fruit	Broiled ground lean meat Baked potato Spinach Tomato and lettuce salad with special dressing§ 2 hot rolls 1 glass milk $\frac{1}{4}$ cantaloupe
	P.M.	
BREAD-CEREAL-POTATO-LEGUME GROUP 8 servings FATS AND SWEETS (Without this group the diet contains 1,415 calories)‖	2 oz. (2 equivalents) lean meat, poultry, fish, cheese or 2 eggs Vegetable 1 glass milk 3 slices enriched or whole-grain bread or alternate	Sandwich: 1 slice cheese 1 slice meat 2 slices bread Tossed salad with special dressing§ 1 glass milk 2 Graham crackers

* If skim milk is used, 160 calories may be deducted.

† See Tables 21–29 for alternates or equivalents within each food group.

‡ If additional meat is desired, 1 meat equivalent (1 oz. lean meat) may be added, and 1 serving from bread group omitted. Other rearrangements or omissions should be reassessed by reference to Tables 2 and 3.

§ See text, p. 55, for discussion of food preparation.

‖ If 1 level teaspoon sugar, jelly, or honey is used, approximately 20 calories will be added. If 1 level teaspoon fat or oil is included, approximately 45 calories will be added. A dessert, such as ice cream, pudding, or gelatin dessert, may add 150–300 calories; pie or cake may add 300–700 calories (see Table 36 for additional caloric values).

TABLE 13B

Menu Pattern and Sample Meals for a Calorie-restricted Diet During Adolescence

(80 Gm. Protein; 1,650 Calories; Derived from Table 9)

Daily Food Plan*	Sample Menu Pattern	Sample Meals
	A.M.	
Milk Group 1 qt. whole milk‖ Meat Group 5 equivalents† (One equivalent equals 1 oz. edible portion cooked beef, veal, lamb, pork, poultry, fish, cheese, or 1 egg)	1 citrus fruit or $\frac{1}{2}$ cup juice 1 egg $\frac{1}{2}$ cup cooked, enriched, or whole-grain cereal or $\frac{3}{4}$ cup flake-type cereal or alternate One slice enriched or whole-grain toast 1 glass milk	$\frac{1}{2}$ grapefruit Poached egg on toast $\frac{3}{4}$ cup flake-type cereal 1 glass milk
	Noon	
Vegetable and Fruit Group 5 servings A dark-green or deep-yellow vegetable daily for vitamin A value A citrus fruit or other fruit rich in vitamin C daily	2 oz. (2 equivalents) lean meat, poultry, fish, cheese or 2 eggs Vegetable 1 fruit 2 slices enriched or whole-grain bread or alternate 1 glass milk	Sandwich: 2 slices lean meat 2 slices bread Heart of lettuce with special dressing‡ Fresh pear 1 glass milk
	P.M.	
Bread-Cereal-Potato-Legume Group 7 servings Fats and Sweets§ (Without this group the diet contains 1,650 calories)	2 oz. (2 equivalents) lean meat, poultry, fish, or cheese $\frac{1}{2}$ cup potato or substitute Dark-green or deep yellow vegetable 1 slice bread or substitute 1 fruit 1 glass milk	Lean roast beef Potato Frozen green beans with sweet-sour sauce‡ 1 small hot roll Baked apple 1 glass milk
	Between	
	1 glass milk with 2 Graham crackers	1 glass milk with 2 Graham crackers

* See Table 13 for variety in selection within each food group.

† If additional meat is desired, 1 oz. lean meat may be added and 1 serving of the bread group omitted without alteration in calories. Other rearrangements or omissions should be reassessed by reference to Tables 2, 3, and 36.

‡ See text, p. 55, for discussion of food preparation.

§ If 1 level teaspoon sugar, jelly, or honey is used, 20 calories will be added. If 1 level teaspoon fat or oil is used, 45 calories will be added (see Table 36 for additional caloric values).

‖ If skim milk is used, calories in diet may be reduced to approximately 1,300.

TABLE 13C

MENU PATTERN AND SAMPLE MEALS FOR A CALORIE-RESTRICTED DIET DURING PREGNANCY AND LACTATION
(80 Gm. Protein; 1,300–1,650 Calories; Derived from Table 7)

DAILY FOOD PLAN*	SAMPLE MENU PATTERN	SAMPLE MEALS
	A.M.	
MILK GROUP 1 qt. whole milk‖ MEAT GROUP 5 equivalents† (One equivalent equals 1 oz. edible portion cooked beef, veal, lamb, pork, poultry, fish, cheese, or 1 egg)	1 citrus fruit or ½ cup juice 1 egg ½ cup cooked, enriched, or whole-grain cereal or ¾ cup flake-type cereal or alternate One slice enriched or whole-grain toast 1 glass milk Coffee or tea if desired	½ grapefruit Poached egg on toast ¾ cup flake-type cereal 1 glass milk Coffee or tea if desired
	Noon	
VEGETABLE AND FRUIT GROUP 5 servings A dark-green or deep-yellow vegetable daily for vitamin A value A citrus fruit or other fruit rich in vitamin C daily	2 oz. (2 equivalents) lean meat, poultry, fish, cheese or 2 eggs Vegetable 2 slices enriched or whole-grain bread or alternate 1 glass milk	Sandwich: 2 slices lean meat 2 slices bread Heart of lettuce with special dressing‡ 1 glass milk
	P.M.	
BREAD-CEREAL-POTATO-LEGUME GROUP 7 servings FATS AND SWEETS (Without this group the diet contains approximately 1,650 calories)§	2 oz. (2 equivalents) lean meat, poultry, fish, or cheese ½ cup potato or substitute Dark-green or deep-yellow vegetable Other vegetable 1 slice bread or substitute 1 fruit 1 glass milk	Lean roast beef Potato Frozen green beans with sweet-sour sauce‡ Raw carrot sticks A small hot roll Baked apple 1 glass milk
	Between	
	1 glass milk with 2 Graham crackers	1 glass milk with 2 Graham crackers

* See Table 13 for variety in selection within each food group.

† If additional meat is desired, 1 oz. lean meat may be added and 1 serving of the bread group omitted without alteration in calories. Other rearrangements or omission should be reassessed by reference to Tables 2, 3, and 36.

‡ See text, p. 55, for discussion of food preparation.

§ If 1 level teaspoon sugar, jelly, or honey is used, 20 calories will be added. If 1 level teaspoon fat or oil is used, 45 calories will be added (see Table 36 for additional caloric values).

‖ If skim milk is used, calories in diet may be reduced to approximately 1,300.

Aluminum foil serves to protect meat, poultry, or fish from fat and oil during baking or roasting or in frying in the same pan used for the family. Salt, pepper, spices, and herbs, onion, garlic, or green pepper may be used as desired. Meat or fish simmered or baked in a tomato sauce (canned tomatoes, green pepper, mushrooms, onions, garlic, salt, spices, or herbs) also is a convenient method of cooking without added fat or oil.

Vegetables may be cooked together for flavor or boiled in bouillon. Mint, spices, or herbs provide variety in flavor; or small amounts of dried cheese, such as Parmesan, Romano, or American, may be added to the vegetable at the table. A hot, French-type dressing may also be used to add interest to cooked vegetables. This may be made from tomato juice or tomato puree flavored with lemon or vinegar, grated onion, celery, garlic, salt, horse-radish, spices, and herbs to suit the taste. Artificial sweetener may be added if desired. This dressing serves as a good French-type dressing on salads also. The calories are negligible. Mineral oil is not a satisfactory product for use in salad dressing. Curtis (1) has calculated that each ounce of mineral oil will dissolve 140,000 I.U. of carotene at body temperature and 120,000 I.U. at room temperature. Since it has been shown also that the ingestion of liquid petrolatum or mineral oil is capable of interfering with absorption of vitamin D, calcium, phosphorus, and vitamin K, it has been concluded by the Council on Foods and Nutrition of the American Medical Association (2) that there can be no justification for the incorporation of mineral oil in foods.

Desserts may be prepared by combining the milk and eggs from the food allowance into eggnog, flavoring with extract, and sweetening with an artificial sweetener. This may be baked as custard or frozen as eggnog ice cream. The addition of the fruit allowance to this dessert will add further variety. Rennet tablets added to flavored milk will also provide attractive milk desserts. Fruit whips may be made from the fruit allowance, unsweetened gelatin, or egg white.

If a patient must eat in a restaurant or cafeteria, it is generally more satisfactory to select plain foods such as roasted or broiled meat rather than stews or fricassees, to select salads without dressing and plain fresh fruits rather than other desserts.

Maintenance diet.—After reaching the desirable weight, it will become necessary to establish a level of calories on which weight is maintained. Obviously, it will not be possible to go back to the old habits of eating and inactivity without regaining weight. A gross guide to the level of calories needed may be deduced from the rate of weight loss and the caloric intake during the final period of reducing. For example, if the patient has been losing at the rate of ½ pound per week in the final weeks of reducing, it is probable that an additional 200–300 calories per day will be sufficient to maintain his weight.

The following sources of supplementary material for popular use are available from The American Dietetic Association, 620 North Michigan Avenue, Chicago, Illinois 60611.

The Best of Health to You contains meal patterns for adults with suggestions for modifications which will reduce calories. Fifty copies cost $1.25.

Step Lively and Control Weight includes foods for an adult for one day and sample meals illustrating 1,800 calories, 1,500 calories, and 1,200 calories. Fifty copies cost $1.25.

Give Yourself a Break, provides questions and answers on food for the teen-ager. Hints on weight control are outlined. Fifty copies cost $1.25.

Available from the U.S. Department of Agriculture, Superintendent of Documents, Government Printing Office, Washington, D.C. 20402, is *Food and Your Weight*, Home and Garden Bulletin No. 74, revised, 1964. This pamphlet contains suggestions for reducers as well as for those who want to gain weight. Caloric needs, meals and menus, and calories are included.

HIGH-CALORIE DIET

The high-calorie diet is a prescribed food allowance which has a caloric value above the total energy requirement per day, thus providing for storage of fat. Proteins, minerals, and vitamins are at or above the levels in the normal diet.

Appraisal of the home dietary intake.—A deficit in the caloric content of the patient's customary food intake is frequently accompanied by a deficiency in proteins, minerals, or vitamins. This means that the dietitian is faced with the problem of obtaining reliable information regarding the over-all nutritive content of the usual food intake.

Caloric allowance.—The levels of caloric intake to be recommended may vary, depending upon the individual's energy requirement for maintenance and the rate of weight gain desired. A guide to caloric allowances for the normal individual at moderate activity has been recommended by the Food and Nutrition Board of the National Research Council (Table 3). More specific estimates under various conditions of work, recreation, and exercise have been compiled by Passmore and Durnin (3). (See Table 44.)

A gross guide to the number of calories that must be added above the level of calories required for maintenance of body weight is the allowance of 500 additional calories per day. This increase may permit a gain of approximately 1 pound of body tissue per week. However, the exact gain may vary, depending upon the degree of activity and upon factors affecting metabolism, heat loss, the water balance, and the presence of disease.

Dietary recommendations.—Since food habits are most easily and permanently changed when consideration is given to the ethnic and cultural pattern of eating, the simplest place to start is with a food diary in which the patient has recorded his self-chosen food intake. The sufficiency of this diet for various nutrients may be assessed by reference to the outlines of normal diet in Tables 2, 7, 8, and 9.

The next step that will be of the greatest nutritional advantage to the patient will involve the addition of any foods from the essential four groups which may be in deficit and which are sufficiently acceptable to the patient to permit the use of additional amounts. Several practical suggestions for supplementing the diet by 500 calories are listed here.

Milk Group
500 calories

A milk beverage containing about 500 calories may be prepared by adding $\frac{1}{2}$–$\frac{3}{4}$ cup (depending on the brand) non-fat dry milk solids (180 calories) to 1 pint of whole milk (340 calories). The addition of flavoring, such as 1 tablespoon sugar (60 calories) and 2 teaspoons cocoa (35 calories), will add another 100 calories.

If the milk is preferred plain, the non-fat dry milk solids may be incorporated into such foods as cottage cheese, mashed potato, macaroni, and cereals.

Or

MEAT-EGG-BREAD GROUP
500 calories

A sandwich containing approximately 500 calories may be prepared by using two slices of meat or cheese (150 calories); 1 tablespoon mayonnaise or fat spread for bread (135 calories); and 2 slices bread (140 calories). One egg in beverage, dessert, or plain will add about 75 calories.

Or

CEREAL-AND-MILK GROUP
500 calories

Cereal and milk with a banana or other fruit may provide about 500 calories if used as follows:

One cup cooked cereal or $1\frac{1}{2}$ cups flake-type cereal (140 calories) may be served with 1 cup whole milk (170 calories) to which $\frac{1}{4}$–$\frac{1}{3}$ cup (depending on the brand) non-fat dry milk solids (90 calories) has been added. One tablespoon sugar (60 calories) and a sliced banana (80 calories) will bring the total to approximately 500 calories. For some individuals this serves as an enjoyable bedtime snack.

Or

FATS AND SWEETS

For calories obtained from additional desserts and sweets or from fat and oils see Table 36.

Distribution of meals throughout the day.—In some instances, an increase in the number of feedings may be indicated. In others, a decrease in the number of feedings per day will result in a better appetite and an increase in total food consumption. Lundgren and Hammarsten (4) report that the amount of edible tray waste decreased significantly when the quantity of between-meal nourishment was reduced. Keeton (5) has also reported highly significant increases in caloric intake when the number of meals was reduced to one or two per day.

Plan of diet.—For a sample menu and plan of meals see the appropriate plan of normal diet. Supplements as suggested above may then be added; or other possibilities may be developed by reference to Table 36.

If a high-caloric modification of a therapeutic or a liquid or soft diet is desired, the respective evaluations, menu patterns, and meal plans should be noted, and adaptations made to suit individual needs.

REFERENCES

1. Curtis, A. C. The mineral oil vitamin A problem, Virginia M. Monthly, **69**:235–36, 1942.
2. Council on Foods and Nutrition, American Medical Association. Mineral oil (liquid petrolatum) in foods, J.A.M.A., **123**:967–69, 1943.
3. Passmore, R., and Durnin, J. V. G. A. Human energy expenditure, Physiol. Rev., **35**:801–40, 1955.
4. Lundgren, E. M., and Hammarsten, J. F. Effect of between-meal nourishments on tray food waste, J. Am. Dietet. A., **25**:873–74, 1949.
5. Keeton, R. W. Influence of distribution of meals on appetite in the sick, J. Am. Dietet. A., **26**:336–44, 1950.

Chapter 6 | *Modifications in Fat Intake*

A food allowance may be modified in terms of a prescribed level of fat, in terms of the percentage of fat calories, or in terms of the amount of, or ratio between, fatty acids. Other nutrients should remain at a level suitable for nutritive sufficiency.

"AVERAGE" FAT CONSUMPTION IN THE UNITED STATES

The kind and extent of the changes that would be necessary in making modifications in the level of fat, the proportion of calories from fat, or the amounts of and ratio between fatty acids may be judged in some degree from the contribution of various food groups in the average diet in the United States (Table 14).

An average of 155 gm. fat per person per day was available for consumption in the United States, according to data collected in the 1955 food consumption survey (1), thus accounting for approximately 44 per cent of the total calories. It should be noted, however, that no deductions were made in the survey for food discarded.

Stiebeling (2) has estimated the nutritive content of the average diet to be as follows: calories, 3,200; fat, 155 gm.; protein, 103 gm.; calcium, 1.2 gm.; iron, 18 mg.; vitamin A value, 8,540 I.U.; thiamine, 1.6 mg.; riboflavin, 2.3 mg.; niacin, 10 mg.; ascorbic acid, 106 mg. This "average," however, should be regarded only as a statistical average. Obviously, wide differences will occur in individual food habits.

BASIC DIET: 20–35 GM. FAT

The reduction of fat to approximately 20 gm. may be accomplished by omission of separated fats and oils; by the use of lean meat; by substitution of poultry and fish low in fat for part of the customary meat and cheese; by use of skim milk; and by reduction of nuts and baked goods.

The basic plan in Table 15 indicates the kinds and amounts of the food groups that will provide approximately 20 gm. fat, 80 gm. protein, and 1,200 calories. By following values indicated in Table

TABLE 14*

TOTAL FAT AND SELECTED FATTY ACIDS IN DIETS, BY FOOD GROUP, HOUSEHOLDS IN THE UNITED STATES
(Average per Person per Day from Food Used at Home in Week, April–June, 1955)

Food Group†	Total Fat (Gm.)	Saturated Fatty Acids (Gm.)	Oleic Acid (Gm.)	Linoleic Acid (Gm.)
Beef, veal, lamb	22.1	11.0	8.8	0.4
Pork (excluding bacon, salt pork)	15.1	6.0	7.6	1.5
Poultry, fish	4.4	1.2	1.6	0.8
Bacon, salt pork	13.4	5.4	6.7	1.3
Lard	9.2	3.7	4.6	0.9
Other shortening	9.0	2.2	5.8	0.7
Oils, salad dressing	9.3	1.9	2.8	4.6
Margarine	10.4	2.6	6.4	0.8
Butter	10.6	7.0	2.9	0.4
Milk, cream, ice cream, cheese	28.0	18.5	7.6	1.0
Eggs	5.6	2.0	2.5	0.4
Other foods (purchased baked goods, nuts, fruits, vegetables, etc.)	18.0	3.6	9.0	3.6
Total	155.1	65.1	66.3	16.4

* From *Food Consumption and Dietary Levels of Households in the United States: Some Highlights from the Household Food Consumption Survey, Spring, 1955* (U.S. Department of Agriculture, Agricultural Research Service, ARS 62-6 [Washington: Government Printing Office, 1957], 0-433306).

† Estimates of quantities of foods "brought into the kitchen" appear on p. 5 in text.

15, the total fat may be reduced from 155 gm. in the average diet to 20 gm.; the saturated fatty acids from 65 to 5 gm.; and the polyunsaturated acids (chiefly linoleic acid) from 16.4 to 2.0. To increase the calories without significant alterations in the fat or fatty acid levels, further additions would have to be made in sugar and sweets, fruits, vegetables, and grains.

Totals or ratios of saturated, oleic, and polyunsaturated fatty acids may be varied by using different kinds and amounts of fats and oils. Modifications may be made by reference to typical fatty acid analyses of some fats and oils of animal and plant origin in Table 16.

TABLE 15

Fat, Fatty Acids, and Cholesterol in a Basic Diet Containing 1,215–1,350 Calories and 20–35 Gm. Fat

Daily Food Intake‖‖	Quantity		Calories	Foodstuffs						Minerals		Vitamins					Cholesterol (Mg.)
						Fatty Acids											
							Unsaturated										
	Wt. (Gm.)	Approximate Measure		Protein (Gm.)	Fat (Gm.)	Saturated (Gm.)	Oleic (Gm.)	Linoleic (Gm.)	Carbohydrate (Gm.)	Ca (Mg.)	Fe (Mg.)	A I.U.	Ascorbic Acid (Mg.)	Thiamine (Mg.)	Riboflavin (Mg.)	Niacin (Mg.)	
Skim milk	492	1 pint	180	18	Tr.	......	......	......	26	596	0.2	20	4	0.20	0.88	0.4	15
Egg*	25	½ egg	40	3	3	1.0	1.5	Tr.	Tr.	14	0.6	295	......	0.03	0.08	Tr.	140
Cooked lean meat, poultry, fish or cottage cheese†	180	6 oz. E. P.	295	42	9	3.2	3.1	1.2	......	88	3.4	140	......	0.21	0.34	11.3	105
Bread, white enriched or cereal##	180	6 or 7 slices	490	16	6	1.2	3.2	0.8	90	125	4.4	Tr.	......	0.45	0.31	4.2	......
Potato, white	100	1 small	70	2	......	......	......	......	15	5	0.5	Tr.	16	0.09	0.03	1.1	......
Vegetable (A)‡	150	2 servings	......	......	......	......	......	......	......	43	1.2	2,180	32	0.10	0.10	0.9	......
(B)§	50		20	1	......	......	......	......	4	12	0.5	1,660	5	0.03	0.03	0.4	......
Including deep-green and yellow																	
Fruit, citrus‖	100	1 serving	40	......	......	......	......	......	10	18	0.1	140	40	0.05	0.01	0.1	......
Other fruit#		2 servings	80	......	......	......	......	......	20	14	0.8	945	9	0.04	0.06	0.8	......
Subtotal			1,215	82	18	5.4	7.8	2.0	165	915	11.7	5,380	106	1.20	1.84	19.2	260
Fat or oil**																	
"Special" margarine‡‡	5	1 teaspoon	45	......	4	.7–1	1–2	1–1.7	......	......	......	......	......	......	......	......	......
Corn oil	10	2 teaspoons	90	......	10	.7	2.6	5	......	......	......	......	......	......	......	......	......
Total††			1,350	82	32	6.8–7.1	11.4–12.4	8–8.7§§	165	915	11.7	5,380	106	1.20	1.84	19.2	260

* Egg 4 times weekly.

† The average figure was derived from an assumed intake of 175 gm. beef, 70 gm. lamb, 105 gm. pork or ham, 175 gm. fish, 525 gm. poultry, 210 gm. cottage cheese per week.

‡ Commonly used vegetables selected from the vegetable A group of the exchange lists were: tomatoes, snap beans, spinach, asparagus, broccoli, cabbage, lettuce, and cucumber. It was estimated that these vegetables might be used 10 times weekly, averaging 150 gm. daily. Weighting was adapted from Agriculture Handbook No. 215, *Consumption, Trends and Patterns for Vegetables* (U.S. Department of Agriculture, Economic and Statistical Analysis Division, Economic Research Service [July, 1961]).

§ It was assumed that the most commonly used vegetables from the vegetable B group of the exchange lists were peas, carrots, beets, and squash. It was estimated that these vegetables might be used 4 times weekly averaging 50 gm. daily. Weighting was adapted from Agriculture Handbook No. 215, *Consumption Trends and Patterns for Vegetables* (U.S. Department of Agriculture Economic and Statistical Analysis Division, Economic Research Service [July, 1961]).

‖ Fresh orange, fresh grapefruit, canned orange juice, blended grapefruit and orange, and frozen citrus juice were considered to be commonly used citrus fruits or juice. Weighting was adapted from *Consumption of Food in the United States*, Supplement for 1962 to Agriculture Handbook No. 62 (U.S. Department of Agriculture, Agricultural Marketing Service [October, 1963]).

\# Apples, bananas, canned peaches, pineapples, pears, apricots, and plums were considered commonly used. Weighting was adapted from *Consumption of Food in the United States*, Supplement for 1962 to Agriculture Handbook No. 62 (U.S. Department of Agriculture, Agricultural Marketing Service [October, 1963]).

** For additional values on saturated fatty acids, oleic, and linoleic acids, see Tables 16, 36.

†† Meets Recommended Dietary Allowances (Table 3) for adult in good health except for iron level for women.

‡‡ "Special" margarine differs from regular in having a higher polyunsaturated fatty acid content (3).

§§ Polyunsaturated: saturated fatty acids = 8/6.8 or 8.7/7.1 = 1.2, approximately.

‖‖ Values from Table 36, page 154, in text for skim milk, egg, meat, and bread.

\## Values from Agriculture Handbook No. 8, *Composition of Foods, Raw, Processed, Prepared* (U.S. Department of Agriculture, [revised 1963]). Weight of one slice bread may vary from 23 to 30 gm.

TABLE 15A

DESCRIPTION OF DAILY FOOD PLAN: BASIC DIET—20–35 GM. FAT
(80 Gm. Protein; 1,215–1,350 Calories; Derived from Table 15)

Daily Food Plan*	Description
MILK 1 pt. skim	*One pint skim milk* contains 180 calories, 18 gm. protein, and important amounts of calcium, phosphorus, and the B complex vitamins. One pint buttermilk, made from completely skim milk, or $\frac{1}{2}$–$\frac{2}{3}$ cup (depending on brand) of non-fat milk solids is equivalent.
EGG 4 per week	*One egg* contributes approximately 7 gm. protein and 75 calories.
MEAT GROUP	*The fat and fatty acid levels* indicated in Table 15 may be attained by the weekly use of approximately 12 oz. of *lean* beef, pork, or lamb; 18 oz. poultry; 6 oz. low-fat fish and 7 oz. cottage cheese. For methods of preparation, see p. 64.
VEGETABLE AND FRUIT GROUP 5 servings	*A dark-green or deep-yellow vegetable* is important each day for its vitamin A value. Asparagus, green beans, broccoli, carrots, green pepper, winter squash, pumpkin, and other greens make up this group. Carrots, winter squash, and pumpkin may contain about 35 calories per serving. The others will be negligible. *Other vegetables*, such as beets, cabbage, cauliflower, celery, cucumber, eggplant, lettuce, mushrooms, onions, peas, tomatoes, or turnips, contribute various amounts of all nutrients. Beets, onions, peas, or turnips may contribute about 35 calories per $\frac{1}{2}$-cup serving. Others will be negligible. *Citrus fruit* or other fruit rich in vitamin C is important each day. One orange or $\frac{1}{2}$ cup juice or $\frac{1}{2}$ grapefruit or 1 cup tomato juice or 1 cup strawberries or 1 cup red raspberries or $\frac{1}{4}$ cantaloupe or 1 large tangerine contains about 40 calories per serving and important amounts of vitamin C. *Other fruits*, such as 1 apple or 1 peach or 1 pear or 4 halves of apricots or 12 grapes or $\frac{1}{2}$ banana, contribute various amounts of all nutrients and contain about 40 calories per serving. For other fruits see Table 26 in text. If sugar or syrup is included, add between 25 and 50 calories per serving.

* See p. 64 in text for food preparation.

TABLE 15A—*Continued*

Daily Food Plan*	Description
BREAD OR CEREAL 6 or 7 servings POTATO OR SUBSTITUTES 1 serving	*One serving provides approximately 70 calories*, important amounts of the vitamin B complex, and iron: One slice enriched or whole-grain bread, ½ cup white potato, ¼ cup sweet potato, ½ cup cooked macaroni, spaghetti, or noodles, rice, cornmeal, cooked dried peas or beans, ¾ cup flake-type cereal, 2 Graham crackers, or 4 arrowroot cookies.
FAT OR OIL	*One teaspoon "special" margarine and 2 teaspoons oil* will add approximately 135 calories bringing the total diet to 1,350 calories.
SWEETS	*If sugar, jelly, or honey* are included approximately 20 calories must be added for each teaspoon.

For additional values on fatty acid composition see Table 36 in the Appendix. These values have been selected from a more complete listing which appears in *Composition of Foods—Raw, Processed, Prepared* (U.S. Department of Agriculture, Agriculture Handbook No. 8 [December, 1963]).

FOOD PREPARATION

Diet containing 20 gm. fat.—Separated fats and oils must be eliminated entirely; and meat should be well trimmed to eliminate fat. Cooking must be limited to boiling or simmering with bouillon or tomato juice and broiling or roasting without added fat. Seasoning may be done with lemon, vinegar, wines, onion, garlic, salts, spices, and herbs instead of fats and oils. Meat tenderizers may be useful. Wrapping fat-trimmed meat, skinned poultry, or fish in aluminum foil also serves as a convenient method for cooking individual servings which must remain fat-free. In this way meat remains moist and well flavored in addition to being protected from fat, even if placed in the same frying pan with meat for the family.

Salad dressing may be prepared without added oil. Tomato juice or tomato puree may be used as a base, with lemon or vinegar, grated onion, grated celery, garlic, horse-radish, sugar, salt, and pepper added to suit the taste. Other seasoning may be used as desired, but oil must be avoided completely. This dressing may be used to marinate meat or may be served hot as a flavoring for cooked vegetables.

TABLE 15B

MENU PATTERN AND SAMPLE MEALS: BASIC DIET—20–35 GM. FAT
(80 Gm. Protein; 1,215–1,350 Calories;* Derived from Tables 15 and 15A)

DAILY FOOD PLAN†	SAMPLE MENU PATTERN‡	SAMPLE MEALS§
	A.M.	
MILK 1 pt. skim EGG One, 4 times weekly MEAT GROUP 12 oz. (cooked weight of edible portion) *lean* beef, pork, or lamb; 18 oz. poultry; 6 oz. low-fat fish; 7 oz. cottage cheese per week‖	½ cup citrus fruit juice or substitute 1 egg ½ cup cooked enriched or whole-grain cereal or ¾ cup flake-type cereal, and 1 slice enriched or whole-grain toast Coffee or tea if desired Skim milk 1 teaspoon "special" margarine	½ cup orange juice Poached egg Toast—2 slices Coffee or tea Skim milk "Special margarine"#
	Noon	
VEGETABLE AND FRUIT GROUP 5 servings Dark-green or deep-yellow vegetable is important for vitamin A value Citrus fruit or other fruit rich in vitamin C is important daily	3 oz. lean meat, poultry, or fish ½ cup potato, rice, spaghetti, or noodles Green or yellow vegetable Fruit Skim milk 1 slice enriched or whole-grain bread	Baked chicken Potato Frozen greens Honeydew melon Skim milk Bread "Special margarine"#
	P.M.	
BREAD OR CEREAL 6 or 7 servings POTATO OR SUBSTITUTE 1 serving FAT OR OIL# (Without fat or oil, the diet will approximate 1,215 calories. With 3 teaspoons fat or oil the diet becomes 1,350 calories) SUGAR*	3 oz. lean meat, poultry, or fish ½ cup potato, rice, spaghetti, or noodles Vegetable Fruit Skim milk 1 slice enriched or whole-grain bread	Salmon, baked in tomato sauce§ Rice with chives Tossed salad with special dressing§ Baked apple Skim milk Bread "Special margarine"#

* If more calories are needed, the following may be included without significant alteration of fatty acids. 1 teaspoon sugar, jelly, or honey, 20 calories; ½ cup plain gelatin dessert or 1 serving sweetened fruit, 100 calories. 3 teaspoons special margarine will add 135 calories and increased amounts of linoleic acid.

† For variety within each food group see Table 15A for alternates.

‡ For foods to avoid, see p. 66 in text.

§ See p. 64 in text for discussion of food preparation.

‖ The average figure was derived from an assumed intake of 175 gm. beef, 70 gm. lamb, 105 gm. pork or ham, 175 gm. fish, 525 gm. poultry, 210 gm. cottage cheese per week.

See "special margarine," Table 15.

Baked goods must be limited to those prepared without added fat, such as angel-food cake, arrowroot cookies, and Graham crackers. Desserts may include gelatin, fruit, fruit whips made from egg white or gelatin, ices, and puddings or frozen desserts prepared from skim milk. Bread may be spread with jam, jelly, or honey.

Olives, potato chips, popcorn, cheese, gravy, or soups containing fat, avocado, nuts, cream, chocolate, and coconut must be restricted. Labels on canned or processed foods must be examined carefully to note any fat content.

TABLE 16

SELECTED FATTY ACIDS IN COMMON FATS AND OILS
(Per 100 Grams, Edible Portion)*

Food	Total Fat (Gm.)	Total Saturated Fatty Acids (Gm.)	Unsaturated Fatty Acids	
			Oleic (Gm.)	Linoleic (Gm.)
Animal fats:				
Lard	100.0	38	46	10
Butter	81.0	46	27	2
Vegetable oils:				
Corn oil	100.0	10	28	53
Cottonseed oil	100.0	25	21	50
Olive oil	100.0	11	76	7
Peanut oil	100.0	18	47	29
Safflower oil	100.0	8	15	72
Sesame oil	100.0	14	38	42
Soybean oil	100.0	15	20	52
Chocolate, bitter or baking	53.0	30	21	1

* Selected from *Composition of Foods—Raw, Processed, Prepared* (U.S. Department of Agriculture, Agriculture Handbook No. 8 [December, 1963]).

Fatty acid modifications.—If the prescribed levels of saturated or unsaturated fatty acids permit adding fats and oils in the diet, these may be incorporated in cooking, in the salad dressing, as a spread for bread and potatoes, or in a beverage made from the egg and skim milk allotted in the basic diet. Two plans for the use of fat-controlled meals have been prepared by the American Heart Association in co-operation with The American Dietetic Association and the Heart Disease Control Program, U.S. Public Health Service: "Planning Fat-Controlled Meals" for 1,200 and 1,800 calories; and "Planning

Fat-Controlled Meals" for unrestricted calories. These booklets may be obtained through a physician or nutritionist from the American Heart Association, 44 East 23d Street, New York, New York.

Numerous special-purpose cookbooks have also been published. However, the suitability of a recipe depends on the particular level of fat, the percentage of fat calories, or the proportion of saturated and unsaturated fatty acids prescribed in the individual diet. For this reason, the physician, dietitian, or nutritionist should aid in selecting appropriate recipes.

For a description of a daily food plan, a sample menu pattern, and sample meals containing 20–35 gm. fat, see Tables 15, 15A, 15B. Modifications from this basic diet may be made to suit individual needs.

Those who wish to read further may refer to "The Regulation of Dietary Fat," a report of the Council on Foods and Nutrition of the American Medical Association published in J.A.M.A. (August 4, 1962), **181**:411–29.

REFERENCES

1. Household food consumption survey, 1955. (U.S. Department of Agriculture, Agricultural Research Service Reports, Nos. 1–10.) 1957.
2. Stiebeling, Hazel K. (Director, Institute of Home Economics, U.S. Department of Agriculture, Agricultural Research Service). Food and nutrient consumption trends and consumer problems. Talk at the American Institute of Nutrition, Chicago, Illinois, April 17, 1957. (Mimeo.)
3. Composition of certain margarines. A council statement. J.A.M.A. (March 3, 1962) **179**:719.

Chapter 7 | *Protein Modifications*

The normal food allowance may be modified in terms of a prescribed level of protein, the kind and amount of amino acids, or the character of the protein fraction. Other nutrients should remain at a level suitable for nutrient sufficiency.

125-GM. PROTEIN DIET

A level of protein above the normal allowance may be indicated most clearly if it is prescribed in terms of grams of protein per kilogram of desirable weight. For the normal, healthy adult, 1 gm. protein per kilogram of desirable weight has been recommended (Table 3). For children, the level will be correspondingly higher per unit of weight (Table 3). For therapeutic purposes, appropriate increases should be specified.

In evaluating proteins, one considers two general aspects: (*a*) digestibility and (*b*) biologic value. By digestibility is meant the percentage of the consumed protein, measured in terms of nitrogen, that is absorbed. Biologic value means the percentage of absorbed nitrogen that is retained by the body and not excreted in the urine. The body requires a definite combination or pattern of amino acids, each in proper amount, for the formation of tissue proteins. If any essential amino acid is supplied in insufficient amounts, then this amino acid will limit the amount of tissue protein made; other amino acids, regardless of the amount present, can be used only to the extent that is required for this tissue protein, and the remainder will be metabolized and the nitrogen excreted in the urine; therefore, the proteins deficient in essential amino acids will have low biologic values. Although there are exceptions, most vegetable proteins have lower digestibilities and biologic values than do animal proteins. For this reason, most nutritionists and dietitians recommend some source of animal protein in each meal. The dietetic practice of providing half or more of the protein from animal sources permits a wide margin of safety in the normal diet for an adult. In diets for children and in most convalescent diets it is a common practice to provide two-thirds of the protein from animal sources.

As an example of a protein allowance for an adult which has been increased above normal, a diet containing 125 gm. protein and 2,000 calories has been evaluated in Table 17. This daily food plan has been derived from the Normal Diet for an Adult (Tables 2, 2A, and 2B), with the addition of 1–1$\frac{1}{3}$ cups (depending on the brand) of non-fat milk solids to 1 quart of fluid skim milk. The total protein for the day then becomes 125 gm. In this illustration, the increase may be obtained by a high-protein drink. Sugar and flavoring could be added as appropriate. If the non-fat milk solids are more acceptable in other forms than a drink, they may be added as a dry ingredient to cottage cheese, mashed potatoes, cereal, milk soups, macaroni or spaghetti, puddings, cake, or cookies.

The possibilities of using other of the essential food groups to increase the protein content may be noted by reference to the protein values indicated in Table 17. If a therapeutic modification of a high-protein diet is desired, such as a liquid or soft diet, see the respective tables.

AMINO ACIDS

A renewed interest in requirements has come about in part from the recognition of amino acid deficiencies in various parts of the world, particularly as *kwashiorkor* in infants and young children (1). Holt (2) and Albanese (3) have made observations on amino acid requirements of infants; Reynolds (4) of young women; and Rose and his associates (5, 6) have indicated tentative minimum quantities necessary for maintenance of nitrogen equilibrium in young adult males. Tentative minimum requirements for amino acids by young adults appear in Table 45. In addition, a committee of the Food and Agriculture Organization of the United Nations (7) has recently appraised protein requirements.

TABLE 17

Nutrient Evaluation of 125-Gm. Protein Diet
(1,990 Calories)

Daily Food Intake	Quantity		Calories*	Protein			Minerals		Vitamins				
	Weight (Gm.)	Approximate Measure		Protein* (Gm.)	Fat* (Gm.)	Carbohydrate* (Gm.)	Ca (Mg.)	Fe (Mg.)	A (I.U.)	Ascorbic Acid (Mg.)	Thiamine (Mg.)	Riboflavin (Mg.)	Niacin (Mg.)
Milk, skim, fluid§§	970	1 quart	360	36	Tr.	52	1,192	0.4	40	8	0.40	1.76	0.8
Milk, dry, non-fat instant§§	100	1½ cups	360	36	1	52	1,293	0.6	30	7	0.35	1.78	0.9
Egg	50	1 medium	75	7	5		27	1.1	590		0.05	0.15	Tr.
Meat, poultry, fish, cooked†	120	4 oz. E.P.§	300	28	20		16	3.4	35		0.40	0.25	5.9
Bread, whole-grain or enriched white‡	180	6 slices	420	12		90	123	4.6	Tr.		0.46	0.31	4.0
Cereal, whole-grain or enriched	20	½ cup	70	2		15	21	0.7	Tr.		0.07	0.05	0.7
Potato, cooked	100	1 small	70	2		15	5	0.5	Tr.	16	0.09	0.03	1.1
Vegetable (A)‖	150	2 servings					43	1.2	2,180	32	0.10	0.10	0.9
(B)#	50		20	1		4	12	0.5	1,660	5	0.03	0.03	0.4
Including deep-green and yellow													
Citrus fruit**	100	1 serving	40			10	18	0.1	140	40	0.05	0.01	0.1
Other fruit††		2 servings	80			20	14	0.8	945	9	0.04	0.06	0.8
Subtotal			1,795	124	26	258	2,764	13.9	5,620	117	2.04	4.53	15.6
Sugar	15	3 level teaspoons	60			15							
Fats or oils	15	3 level teaspoons	135		15				165				
Total‡‡		‖‖	1,990	124	41	273	2,764	13.9	5,785	117	2.04	4.53	15.6

* Values for calories, carbohydrate, protein, and fat from the Food Exchange Lists, Table 20, have been used to evaluate foods and food groups.

† Weighting was adapted from *Meat Consumption Trends and Patterns* (U.S. Department of Agriculture, Agriculture Handbook No. 187, Agricultural Marketing Service, Agricultural Economics Division [Washington, D.C., July, 1960]). Weekly consumption estimated as 350 gm. beef, 280 gm. pork, 140 gm. poultry, and 70 gm. fish.

‡ 30 gm. (1 oz.) has been the weight assigned to one slice of bread in the exchange lists. It is recognized that variation is common. Adjustments should be made where usage varies.

§ Edible portion.

‖ Commonly used vegetables selected from the vegetable A group of the exchange lists were: tomatoes, snap beans, spinach, asparagus, broccoli, cabbage, lettuce, and cucumber. It was estimated that these vegetables might be used 10 times weekly averaging 150 gm. daily. Weighting was adapted from Agriculture Handbook No. 215, *Consumption, Trends and Patterns for Vegetables* (U.S. Department of Agriculture, Economic and Statistical Analysis Division, Economic Research Service [July, 1961]).

It was assumed that the most commonly used vegetables from the vegetable B group of the exchange lists were peas, carrots, beets, and squash. It was estimated that these vegetables might be used 4 times weekly averaging 50 gm. daily. Weighting was adapted from Agriculture Handbook No. 215, *Consumption Trends and Patterns for Vegetables* (U.S. Department of Agriculture, Economic and Statistical Analysis Division, Economic Research Service [July, 1961]).

** Fresh orange, fresh grapefruit, canned orange juice, blended grapefruit and orange and frozen citrus juice were considered to be commonly used citrus fruits or juice. Weighting was adapted from *Consumption of Food in the United States*, Supplement for 1962 to Agriculture Handbook No. 62 (U.S. Department of Agriculture, Agricultural Marketing Service [October, 1963]).

†† Apples, bananas, canned peaches, pineapples, pears, apricots, and plums were considered commonly used. Weighting was adapted from *Consumption of Food in the United States*, Supplement for 1962 to Agriculture Handbook No. 62 (U.S. Department of Agriculture, Agricultural Marketing Service [October, 1963]).

‡‡ Meets Recommended Dietary Allowances (Table 3) for adult in normal good health except for iron level for women.

§§ Values from Table 36 in text for skim milk and dry milk.

‖‖ Caloric needs should be adjusted to individual requirements. For variations in need, see Tables 3 and 5.

Tryptophan has become the first amino acid for which an allowance has been indicated by the Food and Nutrition Board in *Recommended Dietary Allowances*, Revised, 1968 (Table 3). Its sparing action on the need for niacin has been quantitated in terms of tryptophan where 60 mg. tryptophan represents 1 mg. niacin. Horwitt (8) has discussed the basis for this assumption and its application to the evaluation of dietaries. This may be of particular importance in situations where food patterns have become skewed either for therapeutic reasons or from unusual food habits on the part of the patient.

The term "niacin equivalent" is used to apply to the potential niacin value—that is, to the sum of the preformed niacin and the amount of niacin that could be derived from tryptophan (25). There is a need for tryptophan over and above its use as a precursor of niacin, however, and this need has not been established. The average diet in the United States, provides enough tryptophan to increase the niacin value by approximately a third.

PHENYLALANINE-RESTRICTED DIET

A small but significant number of infants are born without the ability to metabolize phenylalanine properly, as a result of a deficiency of the enzyme phenylalanine hydroxylase. This enzyme normally converts phenylalanine to tyrosine. In its absence the accumulation of phenylalanine and abnormal metabolites interferes with normal brain development. Improvement has been brought about in many instances by reducing the phenylalanine in the diet to the minimal levels necessary to permit normal growth and development. Koch (10) has reviewed this topic briefly. More comprehensive reviews have been made by Centerwall (9), Lyman (13), and the Conference on Phenylketonuria called by the British Medical Research Council (14). Also a recent Statement on Treatment of Phenylketonuria by the Committee of the Handicapped Child of the American Academy of Pediatrics has been published (24). An up-to-date, selected, and annotated bibliography on phenylketonuria is available from the U.S. Department of Health, Education, and Welfare, Children's Bureau (12).

Management of the diet requires a reduction of phenylalanine, which is an essential amino acid, to the point where it is low enough to avoid excessive blood levels but high enough to provide for good growth and development. At the same time other nutrients must remain at a level for nutritive sufficiency. Experience seems to indicate wide variations in nutritional requirements both from one individual to another and from time to time in the same infant or child. For this reason constant surveillance of clinical responses, dietary intake, and the blood levels of phenylalanine and other nutrients are necessary to avoid too rigorous or prolonged restrictions. Present experience (24) seems to indicate that phenylalanine requirements for children with phenylketonuria lie somewhere between 20 and 40 mg. per pound of body weight per day, infants needing the upper values, small children the medium values, and children over 5 the lower values. The initial phenylalanine prescription serves only to assess phenylalanine tolerance. From this point, management must be carefully individualized, frequently monitored, and appropriately readjusted as required.

In planning a phenylalanine-restricted diet particular attention must be given to the protein portion of the diet since natural protein has been assumed to contain between 4 and 6 per cent phenylalanine. The basis for the diet must therefore be a specially prepared food from which most of the phenylalanine has been removed. Such a product is Lofenalac, developed by the Mead Johnson Laboratories (16). Phenylalanine has been removed by the passage of an enzymic hydrolysate of casein through a column of activated charcoal. In this way, the phenylalanine is removed, as well as other aromatic acids. The hydrolysate is then supplemented with DL-methionine, L-tryptophan, L-tyrosine, and minerals and vitamins. The powder contains 0.06 to 0.1 per cent phenylalanine in contrast to approximately 5 per cent in natural food proteins. The amount of this powder commonly prescribed for young infants may roughly approximate one measuring cup (150 gm.) per day depending upon the infant's age and condition. Between one and two years of age approximately one-and-one-half to two cups powder may be used daily. Fluid intake should be equivalent to that of healthy normal infants. The composition of 100 gm. Lofenalac powder is indicated in Table 18.

The physician will establish the amounts of phenylalanine, pro-

TABLE 18

COMPOSITION PER 100 GRAMS OF LOFENALAC POWDER*

Approximate Analysis	
Calories	460
Total nitrogen (equivalent to approximately 15 gm. protein)	2.4
Fat, gm.	18
Carbohydrate, gm.	57
Minerals	
Calcium, gm.	0.65
Phosphorus, gm.	0.5
Iron, gm.	0.01
Sodium, gm.	0.4
Potassium, gm.	1
Chlorine, gm.	0.65
Magnesium, gm.	0.087
Copper, mg.	0.1
Zinc, gm.	0.0005
Phenylalanine content of powder, mg.†	80
Vitamin Content	
A, U.S.P. units	1,080
D, U.S.P. units	286
Ascorbic acid, mg.	22
Thiamine hydrochloride, mg.	0.33
Riboflavin, mg.	1.32
Niacin amide, mg.	2.86
Pyridoxine hydrochloride, mg.	0.35
Calcium D-panthothenate, mg.	2.31
Folic acid, mg.	0.033
Biotin, mg.	0.02
Vitamin E, mg.	3.53
Inositol, mg.	
Choline chloride, mg.	168
Vitamin B_{12}, mcg.	3.3
Vitamin K	
Amino Acids	
L-tyrosine, gm.	0.8
L-tryptophan, gm.	0.2
DL-methionine, gm.	0.2
L-methionine, gm.	0.25
L-arginine, gm.	0.3
L-histidine, gm.	0.25
L-lysine, gm.	1.6
L-leucine, gm.	1.4
L-isoleucine, gm.	0.75
L-threonine, gm.	0.81
L-valine, gm.	1.1

* Dilutions: "Normal dilution" for infant formula (20 calories per fl. oz.) is 1 packed "measure" (9.5 gm.) to each 2 fluid oz. water or 1 level measuring cup (150 gm.) to a quart of water. This dilution supplies about 3.5 mg. phenylalanine per fl. oz. and 0.6 gm. protein. A more concentrated preparation (for children) of 1 cup Lofenalac powder to 2½ cups water supplies about 30 calories, 5 mg. phenylalanine per fl. oz., and 1 gm. protein.

† Range 60–100 mg.

tein, and calories to be used by the patient. Since Lofenalac may constitute 85–100 per cent of the total diet depending upon the age and condition of the child, it is important to recommend additional foods carefully to supplement the diet properly. To facilitate selection, foods have been grouped into equivalents representing 15 mg. phenylalanine (see Table 19). Additional considerations concerning the phenylalanine assay of foods have been reported by Miller (15), however, indicating a need for more precise information on phenylalanine content of foods.

Parents, of course, have many questions and problems relating to the diet. To aid professional persons in counseling patients, a publication entitled *The Low Phenylalanine Diet* has been prepared by the State of California, Department of Public Health, Bureau of Public Health Nutrition, Berkeley 4, California. Suggestions for recipes, meal planning, and recording of the daily food intake are included.

MAPLE-SYRUP URINE DISEASE

Another hereditary metabolic aberration in amino metabolism for which dietary alteration has been attempted has been named "maple syrup urine disease," owing to the maple syrup urine odor that appears within two months after birth. The biochemical manifestations of this disease are attributed to a deficiency in the oxidative decarboxylation of the branched chain amino acids—leucine, iso-leucine, and valine—that results in an accumulation of alpha keto-acids in the urine. Westall (17) and Snyderman (26) have reported on dietary treatment of children with this disease.

Recently, new and less costly methods of assay of the amino acid content of foods have resulted in a substantial accumulation of data. These have been compiled by Orr and Watt (18) for eighteen amino acids in 202 food items in terms of amino acids per gram of total nitrogen and in terms of amino acids in 100 gm. food. A portion of the original table on the average amount of amino acids per 100 gm. food appears in Table 40 (p. 191), including the eight "essential amino acids" that are necessary for maintenance of body tissue plus arginine and histidine, which have been found to be important for growth.

An excellent guide for public health nurses entitled *Feeding Mentally Retarded Children* (U.S. Department of Health, Education,

TABLE 19

FOOD EQUIVALENTS FOR LOW-PHENYLALANINE DIET (11)

FOOD	AMOUNT
List I—Lofenalac: 30 Mg. Phenylalanine—2 Equivalents*	
Lofenalac† (dry)	4 Tbsp.
Lofenalac (reconstituted)	1 c.
List II—Vegetables: 15 Mg. Phenylalanine—1 Equivalent	
Beans, green	
Strained and junior	1½ Tbsp.
Regular	3 Tbsp.
Beets	
Strained	2 Tbsp.
Regular	3 Tbsp.
Cabbage, raw, shredded	4 Tbsp.
Carrots	
Strained and junior	3 Tbsp.
Raw	¼ large
Canned	4 Tbsp.
Celery, raw	1½ small stalks
Cucumber, raw	⅓ medium
Lettuce, head	2 leaves
Spinach, creamed—strained and junior	1½ Tbsp.
Squash	
Winter	
Strained	3 Tbsp.
Junior	6 Tbsp.
Cooked	4 Tbsp.
Summer, cooked	4 Tbsp.
Tomato	
Raw	¼ small
Canned	2 Tbsp.
Juice	2½ Tbsp.
List III—Fruits; 15 Mg. Phenylalanine—1 Equivalent‡	
Banana	4 Tbsp.
Dates, dried	2
Fruit cocktail, canned	2½ Tbsp.
Grapefruit	
Sections	⅓ c.
Juice	⅓ c.
Orange	
Sections	3 Tbsp.
Juice	3 Tbsp.
Grape juice	⅓ c.
Lemon juice	3 Tbsp.

* One equivalent may be defined as providing 15 mg. phenylalanine.

† Mead Johnson Laboratories, Evansville, Indiana.

‡ Newer assays for phenylalanine content of fruits indicate a lower value than the ones used in this report (15).

TABLE 19—*Continued*

List III—*Continued*	
Peaches	
Raw	⅔ medium
Canned in syrup	1½ halves
Strained	5 Tbsp.
Junior	7 Tbsp.
Pears	
Raw	⅓ medium
Canned in syrup	3 halves
Strained and junior	10 Tbsp.
Pears and pineapple, strained and junior	7 Tbsp.
Pineapple	
Raw	⅓ c.
Canned in syrup	1½ small slices
Juice	½ c.
Plums, canned in syrup	1½ medium
Plums with tapioca	
Strained	5 Tbsp.
Junior	7 Tbsp.
Prunes	
Cooked	2 medium
Juice	⅓ c.
Strained	3 Tbsp.
Raisins	1½ Tbsp.
Strawberries	3 large
Tangerine	⅔ small
Watermelon	⅔ c.

List IV—Breads: 30 Mg. Phenylalanine—2 Equivalents	
Barley cereal, Gerber's, dry	2⅓ Tbsp.
Biscuits§	1 small
Cereal food, Gerber's, dry	2 Tbsp.
Cookies, arrowroot	1½
Corn	2 Tbsp.
Cornflakes	⅓ c.
Crackers	
Barnum animal	6
Saltines	3
Cream of Wheat, cooked	2 Tbsp.
Farina, cooked	2½ Tbsp.
Ice cream§‖	
Chocolate	⅓ c.
Pineapple	⅓ c.
Strawberry	⅓ c.
Vanilla	⅓ c.
Mixed cereal, Pablum, dry	1⅔ Tbsp.
Oatmeal	
Gerber's strained	1⅔ Tbsp.
Pablum, dry	1⅔ Tbsp.

§ Special recipe must be used.

‖ Milk is very high in phenylalanine (1 oz. contains 55 mg.), but it may on occasion be ordered to bring phenylalanine blood levels up to normal.

TABLE 19—*Continued*

List IV—*Continued*	
Potatoes, Irish	2½ Tbsp.
Rice Flakes, Quaker	⅓ c.
Rice Krispies, Kellogg's	⅓ c.
Rice, Puffed, Quaker	½ c.
Sugar Crisps	¼ c.
Sweet potatoes or yams	
Cooked	3 Tbsp.
Strained	4 Tbsp.
Wafers, sugar, Nabisco	6
Wheat, Puffed, Quaker	⅓ c.
List V—Fats: 5 Mg. Phenylalanine—⅓ Equivalent	
Butter	1 tsp.
Cream, heavy	1 tsp.
Margarine	1 Tbsp.
Mayonnaise	1½ Tbsp.
Olives, ripe	1 large
List VI—Desserts: 15 Mg. Phenylalanine—1 Equivalent	
Cookies	
Rice-flour (19)	1
Corn starch (19)	1
Ice creams—see List IV, Breads	
Puddings‡	½ c.
Sauce, Hershey syrup	1 Tbsp.
List VII—Free Foods: Little or No Phenylalanine; May Be Used as Desired	
Candy	
Butterscotch	—
Cream mints	—
Fondant	—
Gum drops	—
Hard	—
Jelly beans	—
Lollipops	—
Cornstarch	—
Guava butter	—
Honey	—
Jams, jellies, and marmalades	—
Molasses	—
Oil	—
Sauces	—
Lemon‡	—
White‡	—
Syrups	
Corn	—
Maple	—
Sugar	
Brown	—
White	—
Tapioca	—

TABLE 19—*Continued*

List VIII—Foods to Avoid: High Phenylalanine Content; May Be Used Only Occasionally in Very Small Portions	
Breads, most	—
Cheeses of all kinds	—
Eggs	—
Legumes, dried	—
Meat, poultry, fish	—
Nuts	—
Nut butters	—

and Welfare, Children's Bureau, 1964) is available from the Government Printing Office, Washington, D.C., 20402, at a price of 15 cents per copy. This booklet includes guidance in taking a dietary history, assessment of feeding methods, and techniques and teaching for development of skills by the family and child.

PROTEIN FRACTIONS: GLIADIN RESTRICTION

Various fractions of protein have long been of interest in connection with allergic manifestations. As a result, certain foods have been eliminated, the most common being eggs, milk, and various grain products. This has posed a problem in constructing acceptable recipes for breads, desserts, sauces, and so forth, in which the offending products are avoided. Recipes have been collected and tested for this purpose by committees of the Diet Therapy Section of The American Dietetic Association and are now compiled and available in the booklet entitled *Allergy Recipes* (1957).

More recently the gliadin, or glutamine-bound fraction of protein in wheat, rye, oats, and barley has become of particular interest in the treatment of certain malabsorption syndromes (19–22). In this instance, in which wheat, rye, oats, and barley are omitted, other grains and cereal products must be substituted, leaving corn flour, cornmeal, potato flour, rice flour, soybean flour, wheat-starch flour ("gliadin-free") as the alternates.

The wheat-rye-oat-free diet has been described by Sleisenger, Rynbergen, Pert, and Almy (23). Several recipes are included for corn muffins, corn pone, rice-flour bread, rice-flour muffins, rice-flour sponge cake, and rice-flour brownies. Additional recipes may be found in a new booklet by Margaret Abowd, *Low Gluten Diet with*

Recipes (Ann Arbor: University of Michigan, University Hospital, 1958).

Luncheon with Laurie by Carolyn Busbee Carpenter is also an excellent collection of recipes. It is available from the State Printing Company, Columbia, South Carolina at $1.75 per copy postpaid from 237 Pinewood Lane, Rock Hill, South Carolina.

For additional information on the protein fractions in some of the principal proteins of common foodstuffs, reference may be made to W. H. Peterson and F. M. Strong, *General Biochemistry* (Englewood Cliffs, N.J.: Prentice-Hall, Inc., 1953).

REFERENCES

1. Brock, J. F. Survey of world situation on kwashiorkor, Ann. New York Acad. Sci., **57**:696–713, 1954.
2. Holt, L. E., Jr. "Nutrition in infancy and adolescence," in Modern nutrition in health and disease, eds. M. G. Wohl and R. S. Goodhart. Philadelphia: Lea & Febiger, 1955, chap. 34.
3. Albanese, A. A. Protein and amino acid requirements of infants, Pediatrics, **8**:455–62, 1951.
4. Reynolds, M. S. Amino acid requirements of adults, J. Am. Dietet. A., **33**: 1015–18, 1957.
5. Rose W. C. The amino acid requirements of adult man, Nutrition Abstr. & Rev., **27**:631–47, 1957.
6. Rose, W. C., Wixom, R. L., Lockhart, H. B., and Lambert, G. F. The amino acid requirements of man, J. Biol. Chem., **217**:987–95, 1955.
7. Food and Agriculture Organization of the United Nations. Report of the FAO Committee on Protein Requirements. Rome, 1957.
8. Horwitt, M. K. Niacin tryptophan requirements of man, J. Am. Dietet. A., **34**:914–19, 1958.
9. Centerwall, Willard R. Phenylketonuria-A general review, J. Am. Dietet. A., **36**:201–5, 1960.
10. Koch, R., Acosta, P., Ragsdale, N., and Donnell, G. Nutrition in the treatment of phenylketonuria, J. Am. Dietet. A., **43**:212–5, 1963.
11. Acosta, P. B., and Centerwall, W. R., Phenylketeonuria; Dietary Management Special Low Phenylalanine Recipes, J. Am. Dietet. A., **36**:206–11, 1960.
12. Phenylketonuria—A selected Bibliography. U.S. Department of Health, Education, and Welfare, Children's Bureau, 1963.
13. Lyman, Frank (ed.). Phenylketonuria. Springfield, Ill.: Charles C Thomas, 1963, 318 pp.
14. Report to the Medical Research Council of the Conference on Phenylketonuria. Treatment of Phenylketonuria, Brit. Med. J. (June 29, 1963), 1691–97.
15. Miller, G. T., Williams, V. R., and Moschette, D. S. Phenylalanine content of fruit, J. Am. Dietet. A., **46**:43–45, 1965.

16. MEAD JOHNSON LABORATORIES. Phenylketonuria—Low Phenylalanine Dietary Management with Lofenalac-low Phenylalanine, Food (March, 1965), Evansville, Indiana.
17. WESTALL, R. G. Dietary treatment of a child with maple sugar urine disease (branched-chain-keto-aciduria), Arch. diseases childhood **38**:485–91, 1963.
18. ORR, M. L., and WATT, B. K. Amino acid content of foods, (U.S. Department of Agriculture, "Home Economic Research Reports," No. 4.) 1957.
19. ADLERSBERG, D. Problems of management of idiopathic sprue, New York State J. Med., **55**:3575–82, 1955.
20. DICKE, W. K., WEIJERS, H. A., and VAN DE KAMER, J. H. Coeliac disease. 2. The presence in wheat of a factor having a deleterious effect in cases of coeliac disease, Acta paediat., **42**:34–42, 1953.
21. VAN DE KAMER, J. H., WEIJERS, H. A., and DICKE, W. K. Coeliac disease. 4. An investigation into the injurious constituents of wheat in connection with their action on patients with coeliac disease, Acta paediat., **42**:223–31, 1953.
22. VAN DE KAMER, J. H., and WEIJERS, H. A. Coeliac disease. 5. Some experiments on the cause of the harmful effect of wheat gliadin, Acta paediat., **44**:465–69, 1955.
23. SLEISENGER, M. H., RYNBERGEN, H. J., PERT, J. H., and ALMY, T. P. A. Wheat-rye-and-oat-free diet, J. Am. Dietet. A., **33**:1137–40, 1957.
24. COMMITTEE ON THE HANDICAPPED CHILD, AMERICAN ACADEMY OF PEDIATRICS. Statement on treatment of phenylketonuria, Pediatrics, **35**:501–3, 1965.
25. Composition of Foods—Raw, Processed, Prepared, U.S. Department of Agriculture, Agriculture Handbook No. 8 (December, 1963).
26. SNYDERMAN, S. E., NORTON, P. M., ROITMAN, E., HOLT, L. E., JR. Maple syrup urine disease, with particular reference to diet therapy. Pediatrics, **34**:454–72, 1964.

Chapter 8 | Modifications in Protein-Fat-Carbohydrate[1]

Modifications in protein-fat-carbohydrate have been simplified in three ways: first, by combining foods into six groups comparable in protein-fat-carbohydrate content as well as approximate mineral and vitamin worth; secondly, by describing these groups in commonly measured or purchased units of food; and third, by limiting foods in each group to those in common usage. These food groups were originally developed by the Committee on Diabetic Diet Calculations, The American Dietetic Association working co-operatively with the Committee on Education, American Diabetes Association, and the Diabetes Section, U.S. Public Health Service, and were named "Food Exchange Lists."

Since 1950, when the first report was published, there has been a wide acceptance of the Food Exchange Lists that have brought simplification, flexibility, and standardization into the selection of values and foods used in quantitative diets. The diet for patients with diabetes is a prime example.

Inevitably new data on food composition have accumulated, new food products have appeared on the market, and special considerations relating to ethnic groups and educational programs have arisen. In order that appropriate guidelines for adaptations of the exchange lists can be brought into perspective, the original report,

1. Report of the Committee on Diabetic Diet Calculations, The American Dietetic Association. Prepared co-operatively with the Committee on Education, American Diabetes Association, and the Diabetes Section, U.S. Public Health Service. Compiled by Elizabeth K. Caso.

which appeared in 1950, is reproduced below.

For the purpose of working toward the standardization of values on food composition in the dietary management of diabetes, the American Diabetes Association in 1947 invited The American Dietetic Association to select a committee to work jointly with its Committee on Education. Since the work of the Diabetes Section of the U.S. Public Health Service is so intimately concerned with these matters, it joined in this project to become the third co-operating organization. The objectives of this joint committee were to prepare a set of representative values suitable for use in dietary calculation and to develop a simplified method for planning the diet, including several "exchange lists" of foods of similar food value.

The joint committee was faced with many difficulties due in part to a lack of uniformity in the composition of food occurring as a result of varietal differences, variations in conditions of growth, degree of maturity, and methods of harvesting, storage, or preparation. For example, two different types of peaches may vary as much as 125 per cent in carbohydrate content. The composition of a piece of well-done meat will be roughly 25 per cent higher in protein than a piece which is rare, owing to a difference in water content. The carbohydrate content of bread will fluctuate, depending upon its age and the way it has been stored (1). McCance and Widdowson (2) have pointed out that an appreciable amount of carbohydrate may be lost in the cooking of vegetables. American food tables (3, 4) report "total carbohydrate" values which are considered to contain a varying percentage of unavailable carbohydrate (5). All these factors had to be considered carefully and weighted in preparing figures for calculating diabetic diets.

On the other hand, there is a great variation from day to day in bodily requirements and utilization of food which is dependent on such factors as activity, emotional status, and insulin dosage. In fact, differences in bodily needs far exceed differences in food composition and therefore minimize the problem of the inevitable variation in food content. Thus nothing more than reasonable detail is justifiable in calculating diabetic diets. As a result, foods have been grouped in terms of similarity in composition.

FOOD EXCHANGE LISTS

Recognizing these facts, the joint committee has submitted the food values given in Table 20. As mentioned above, the list is greatly abbreviated by combining foods of similar composition into food exchange lists.

TABLE 20

FOOD VALUES FOR CALCULATING DIABETIC DIETS

Group	Amount	Weight (Gm.)	Carbo-hydrate (Gm.)	Protein (Gm.)	Fat (Gm.)	Energy (Calories)
Milk, whole	½ pt.	240	12	8	10	170
Vegetable, group A	As desired	....	....	....	....	....
Vegetable, group B	½ cup	100	7	2	....	36
Fruit	Varies	....	10	....	....	40
Bread exchanges	Varies	....	15	2	....	68
Meat exchanges	1 oz.	30	....	7	5	73
Fat exchanges	1 teaspoon	5	....	....	5	45

Milk.—In rounded figures, the composition of 1 cup (8 oz.) of whole fresh milk averages 12 gm. carbohydrate, 8 gm. protein, and 10 gm. fat (4). One cup or ½ pt. is purposely used as the unit of measurement, since milk in most sections of this country is purchased by the quart. Thus ½ pt. is relatively easy for the patient to measure, and any multiple of ½ pt. can be figured into the meal plan for the day. This is much simpler than prescribing odd amounts, such as 7 or 14 oz. per day.

Several forms of cow's milk are available, such as evaporated, dried, or skim milk. These types of milk have been combined into one table called "List 1—Milk Exchanges" (Table 21). In the amounts listed, one may be substituted for another, since they are all approximately equal in composition.

Problems of measuring carbohydrate.—Innumerable lists have been prepared which classify vegetables according to the amount of carbohydrate they contain. In some instances, vegetables have been divided into lists containing approximately 3, 6, 9, and 12 per cent carbohydrate. In others, they have been grouped as 5, 10, or 15 per cent vegetables. One author might place a vegetable in the 6 per cent group while another might include it in the 3 per cent list. There has been little uniformity in this matter. In addition, the percentage classification has been difficult for the patient to comprehend and to put into practical use.

TABLE 21

LIST 1—MILK EXCHANGES

(Per Serving: Carbohydrate, 12 Gm.; Protein, 8 Gm.; Fat, 10 Gm.)

Type of Milk	Approximate Measure	Weight (Gm.)
Whole milk (plain or homogenized)...	1 cup (8 oz.)	240
Skim milk*..........................	1 cup	240
Evaporated milk....................	½ cup	120
Powdered whole milk...............	¼ cup	35
Powdered skim milk (nonfat dried milk)*.........................	¼ cup	35
Buttermilk (from whole milk)........	1 cup	240
Buttermilk (from skim milk)*........	1 cup	240

* Since these forms of milk contain no fat, two fat exchanges may be added to the diet when they are used.

In seeking some simpler manner of grouping the vegetables, the committee took into account the controversy regarding "total" and "available" carbohydrate. According to the Department of Agriculture (3), "'total' carbohydrate in the majority of cases is reckoned as carbohydrate by difference, that is, as the difference between 100 per cent and the sum of the percentages of water, protein, fat, and ash. This measure includes starch, dextrin, and sugars, and is to this extent an approximate measure of the total carbohydrate that can be utilized by the body. However, it tends to over-estimate the available carbohydrate since it also includes crude fiber and organic acids, when present, and any undetermined solids." The American Diabetes Association, upon the recommendation of W. H. Olmsted, has defined available carbohydrate as follows (5): "This term includes starch, dextrin, glycogen, glucose, fructose, galactose, sucrose, lactose, and maltose. It represents the portion of the carbohydrate of foods available to the human body for glycogen formation." That organization feels that available carbohydrate is the preferred value for computing diabetic diets.

There is evidence to show that cellulose, hemicellulose, and gums are broken down by bacterial action in the human intestinal tract to form volatile fatty acids (5, 6) which do enter into glycogen formation. However, isotopic studies of the intermediary metabolism of volatile fatty acids (7–10) seem to indicate that they do not cause a *net* increase in the body's supply of glycogen.

The organic acids, chiefly malic and citric, are converted to glucose. In each case, two molecules of citrate or malate form one of glucose. Altogether, the total amount of glucose formed from organic acids is variable. Some workers believe that it is negligible. More studies in this field are needed (5).

These studies of the availability of fractions making up "total-carbohydrate-by-difference" are very complex. Bernice K. Watt, of the Bureau of Human Nutrition and Home Economics, Department of Agriculture, feels that it may be a long time before the ideal in food analysis is reached, with not only quantitative data but data on human utilization available for the separate components of the so-called "carbohydrate-by-difference."

The question then arises as to the advisability of using values for starch and sugar alone as the measure of the carbohydrate content of vegetables and fruits. Dr. Watt has stated, after reviewing data in the bureau files, that, for a fair number of fruits, the analyses for sugar and starch appear to be as representative of the product as were estimates of total carbohydrate. For some fruits and many vegetables this is not the case, since products selected for study of sugar or starch content were not always ordinary products but were often selected for study because of some particular characteristic or condition of growth. The Department of Agriculture is currently accumulating considerable data on the carbohydrate fractions of foods.

Furthermore, McCance and Widdowson (2) report a loss of carbohydrate in the cooking process. Although the analyses were done on English foods and have not been, to any extent, carried out on American foods, at least the findings are significant and would tend to justify the use of lower values for carbohydrate content.

This whole problem resolves itself into the need for some practical basis to use for the calculation of carbohydrate in diabetic diets. After some consideration, the joint committee finally recommended the figures for starch and sugar as representative of available carbohydrate, even though they may be short of the ideal.

Classification of vegetables.—In Table 22 are summarized the data used to arrive at a simplified grouping of the more commonly used vegetables.

The first group of vegetables (group A) contains 3 gm. or less of carbohydrate per 100-gm. serving. Therefore, the committee recommends that these vegetables be grouped in one list (Table 23), and that the negligible amount of carbohydrate which they contain need not be figured in the diet unless more than 200 gm. is used at a meal.

The second group of vegetables in Table 22 contains more carbohydrate. Some of them are more popular than others. Therefore, a weighted average was taken (Table 24), and, based on these data, the committee decided to figure the composition of these vegetables as 7 gm. carbohydrate and 2 gm. protein per 100-gm. serving.

Although the list of group B vegetables is short, it contains some of the more popular vegetables. However, it is not likely that more than one of these vegetables would be eaten in one day. The dietitian who has previously figured three or more vegetables in the diet may now find that she needs to calculate only one group B vegetable and allow the patient other vegetables from group A as desired.

The remainder of the vegetables in Table 22 contains appreciably more carbohydrate. For simplicity they are included in the list of bread exchanges and will be considered later. None of the other lists represents as major a change as this new classification of vegetables (Table 23).

Fruit.—The carbohydrate content of fruit differs with the variety as in vegetables, and fruits have been classified into groups according to their carbohydrate content. To avoid the confusion of having several groups and to simplify dietary instruction for the patient, the practice in the past few years (13, 14) has been to list all fruits together in *amounts* that would supply either 10 or 15 gm. carbohydrate. The committee working on the material was in favor of the list (Table 25) which contained 10 gm. carbohydrate, since it presented the majority of the more common fruits in serving sizes that are easy to purchase, economical to serve, and relatively satisfying in amount. The carbohydrate values of the fruits are based on the starch and sugar analyses of the Department of Agriculture (3). For practicality the figures were rounded.

TABLE 22

CARBOHYDRATE CONTENT OF VEGETABLES PER 100-GM. SERVING

Food	Source of Reference		
	U.S. Dept. of Agriculture (3) (Sugar and Starch) (Gm/100 Gm)	McCance and Widdowson (2) (Gm/100 Gm)	Williams *et al.* (11) (Gm/100 Gm)
	List 2, Group A—Vegetable Exchanges		
Asparagus	1.7	1.1	...
Beans, string, young	2.6	2.9	5.8
Beet greens	0.5	...	...
Broccoli	1.9	0.4 (tops)	1.1
Brussels sprouts	...	1.7	2.6
Cabbage	3.5	3.0	2.5
Cauliflower	2.6	1.2	1.0
Celery	1.2	1.3	...
Chard	0.8	...	...
Chicory	0.2	...	...
Cucumber	2.6	1.8	...
Dandelion greens	0.9	...	...
Eggplant	...	3.1	...
Kale	1.4	...	...
Lettuce	1.6	1.8	1.4
Mushrooms	0	0	...
Mustard greens	0.4	0.9	...
Radishes	3.4	2.8	...
Spinach	0.3	1.4	0.7
Squash, summer	1.2	...	...
Tomatoes	3.4	2.8	1.6
	List 2, Group B—Vegetable Exchanges		
Beets	9.6 (total CHO)	9.9	7.3
Carrots	7.5	5.4	6.0
Onions	7.2	5.2	...
Peas, greens	9.0	10.6	8.3
Pumpkin	5.1	3.4	...
Rutabaga	6.7	...	...
Squash, winter	4.9	...	...
Turnip	4.6	3.8	3.5
	List 4—Bread Exchanges		
Beans, baked	18.8	17.3	...
Beans, dried	62.1 (total CHO)	...	...
Beans, Lima	23.5	...	...
Corn	18.9	...	14.8
Parsnips	11.9	11.3	...
Peas, dried	45.1	50.0 (raw) 19.1 (cooked)	...
Potato, white	15.6	18.3	16.4
Potato, sweet	25.6	20.1	23.7

TABLE 23

LIST 2—VEGETABLE EXCHANGES

Group A

Negligible Carbohydrate, Protein, and Calories if 1 Cup (200 Gm.) or Less Is Used

Asparagus	Eggplant	Lettuce
Beans, string, young	Greens*	Mushrooms
Broccoli*	Beet	Okra
Brussels sprouts	Chard, Swiss*	Pepper*
Cabbage	Collard	Radish
Cauliflower	Dandelion	Sauerkraut
Celery	Kale	Squash, summer
Chicory*	Mustard	Tomatoes*
Cucumbers	Spinach	Watercress*
Escarole*	Turnip	

Group B

Per Serving: Carbohydrate, 7 Gm.; Protein, 2 Gm. (1 Serving = ½ Cup = 100 Gm.)

Beets	Peas, green	Squash, winter*
Carrots*	Pumpkin*	Turnip
Onions	Rutabaga	

* These vegetables have high vitamin A value. At least one serving should be included in the diet each day.

TABLE 24

DATA USED TO CALCULATE THE COMPOSITION OF VEGETABLES, GROUP B

Food	Carbohydrate Content (Starch and Sugar)* (Gm/100 Gm)	Weighting (Based on Usual Rate of Consumption)†
Beets	8.0	3
Carrots	7.5	4
Onions	7.2	1
Peas, green (medium)	9.0	4
Pumpkin	5.1	....
Rutabaga	6.7	½
Squash, winter	4.9	2
Turnip	4.6	1

* U.S. Department of Agriculture figures (3).

† From *Family Food Consumption in the United States, Spring, 1942* (18) and *Consumption of Food in the United States, 1909–48* (12).

In Table 26 the fruits have been listed in household measurements. Since each fruit in the amount listed contains approximately 10 gm. carbohydrate, one may be exchanged for the other. There is some variation between measured and weighed portions of fruit. Every so-called "small" apple will not weigh exactly 80 gm. Here again, however, the variation seems reasonable on the basis of the difference in actual carbohydrate content of each food.

Bread, cereals, and vegetables of high carbohydrate content.—Again, it was obvious that if many foods of high carbohydrate content could be included in the one list of bread exchanges, it would be much easier for all those concerned with the planning of diabetic diets. Many lists of this sort have been prepared by other groups. The joint committee agreed upon the list given in Table 27, which includes several types of breadstuffs, a number of cereals, different varieties of crackers, and the vegetables with the highest carbohydrate content, as shown in Table 22.

Although the average slice of bread may weigh 25 gm. and contain approximately 13 gm. carbohydrate, it was decided that it would be preferable to list all the foods in this group in amounts that contain approximately 15 gm. carbohydrate. A ½-cup serving of many of these foods, which is an easy quantity to measure, yields this amount of carbohydrate. During the course of a day, an individual who is allowed six bread exchanges, for example, is likely to select several different foods from List 4, such as potato, cereal, or crackers. The average typical day's consumption of bread exchanges is therefore approximately 15 gm. carbohydrate per serving.

Meat, fish, poultry, eggs, and cheese.—The foods which are high in protein have been listed in amounts that are equal in protein and fat content to approximately 1 oz. meat. It was noted that the method or preparation or the cut of the meat (rib or rump) will influence the protein and fat content. Also, some forms of cheese are higher in fat than others as a result of the type of milk (whole or skim) used in their preparation. Some varieties of fish (cod versus mackerel) contain more fat than others. In a mixed diet, these differences become minimized. After reviewing the dietary analyses of these foods, the committee recommended the list of meat exchanges given in Table 28 and the figures of 7 gm. protein and 5 gm. fat per unit of exchange.

TABLE 25

Amount of Fruit Supplying 10 Gm. Carbohydrate

Food	Source of Reference: U.S. Dept. of Agriculture (3) (Gm.)	Source of Reference: Joint Committee's Recommendations (Gm.)
Apple	97	80
Applesauce	126	100
Apricots, fresh	96	100
Apricots, dried	22	20
Banana	52	50
Blackberries	164	150
Blueberries	103	100
Canteloupe	238	200
Cherries	75	75
Dates	16	15
Figs, fresh	62	50
Figs, dried	18	15
Grape juice	60	60
Grapefruit	154	125
Grapefruit juice	118	100
Grapes	67–87	75
Honeydew melon	143	150
Mango	73	70
Orange	113	100
Orange juice	111	100
Papaya	111	100
Peach	114	100
Pear	112	100
Pineapple	84	80
Pineapple juice	83	80
Plums	120	100
Prunes, dried	24	25
Raisins	16	15
Raspberries	139	150
Strawberries	189	150
Tangerines	115	100
Watermelon	167	175

TABLE 26

List 3—Fruit Exchanges*
(Carbohydrate—10 Gm. per Serving)

Food	Approximate Measure
Apple (2-in. diameter)	1
Applesauce	½ cup
Apricots	
Fresh	2 medium
Dried	4 halves
Banana	½ small
Blackberries	1 cup
Blueberries	⅔ cup
Cantaloupe (6-in. diameter)†	¼
Cherries	10 large
Dates	2
Figs, fresh	2 large
Figs, dried	2
Grape juice	¼ cup
Grapefruit†	½ small
Grapefruit juice†	½ cup
Grapes	12
Honeydew melon (7-in. diameter)	⅛
Mango	½ small
Orange†	1 small
Orange juice†	½ cup
Papaya	⅓ medium
Peach	1 medium
Pear	1 small
Pineapple	½ cup
Pineapple juice	⅓ cup
Plums	2 medium
Prunes, dried	2 medium
Raisins	2 tablespoons
Raspberries	1 cup
Strawberries†	1 cup
Tangerine	1 large
Watermelon	1 cup

* Unsweetened canned fruits may be used in the same amount as listed for the fresh fruit.

† These fruits are rich sources of ascorbic acid. At least one serving should be included in the diet each day.

TABLE 27

LIST 4—BREAD EXCHANGES
(Per Serving: Carbohydrate, 15 Gm.; Protein, 2 Gm.)

Food	Approximate Measure	Weight (Gm.)
Bread:	1 slice	25
biscuit, roll (2-in. diameter)	1	35
muffin (2-in. diameter)	1	35
cornbread (1½-in. cube)	1	35
Flour	2½ tablespoons	30
Cereal:		
cooked	½ cup	100
dry (flake and puffed)	¾ cup	20
rice and grits, cooked	½ cup	100
Spaghetti and noodles, cooked	½ cup	100
Crackers:		
graham (2½-in. square)	2	20
oysterettes	20 (½ cup)	20
saltines (2-in. square)	5	20
soda (2½-in. square)	3	20
round, thin (1½-in. diameter)	6–8	20
Vegetables:		
beans and peas, dried, cooked (Lima, navy, split pea, cowpeas)	½ cup	100
beans, Lima, fresh	½ cup	100
beans, baked, no pork	¼ cup	50
corn, sweet	⅓ cup	80
corn, popped	1 cup	20
parsnips	⅔ cup	125
potatoes, white—baked or boiled (2-in. diameter)	1	100
potatoes, white—mashed	½ cup	100
potatoes, sweet or yams	¼ cup	60
Sponge cake, plain (1½-in. cube)	1	25
Ice cream (omit 2 fat exchanges)	½ cup	70

Diets which include odd amounts of meat, such as 75 or 105 gm., are difficult to measure. Servings of 1, 2, or 3 oz., for example, are more practical for the patient, since the food is usually purchased in these amounts. This factor was taken into consideration in preparing this list.

Fats.—The problem of arriving at a figure for the composition of

TABLE 28

LIST 5—MEAT EXCHANGES
(Per Serving: Protein, 7 Gm.; Fat, 5 Gm.)

Food	Approximate Measure	Weight (Gm.)
Meat and poultry, medium fat (beef, lamb, pork, liver, chicken)	1 oz.	30
Cold cuts (4½ in. square, ⅛ in. thick)	1 slice	45
Frankfurter (8 or 9 per lb.)	1	50
Fish:		
cod, mackerel	1 oz.	30
salmon, tuna, crab	¼ cup	30
oysters, shrimp, clams	5 small	45
sardines	3 medium	30
Cheese:		
Cheddar or American	1 oz.	30
cottage	¼ cup	45
Eggs	1	50
Peanut butter*	2 tablespoons	30

* Limit use or adjust carbohydrate (deduct 5 gm. carbohydrate per serving when used in excess of one exchange).

fats was relatively simple, since there are fewer variable factors involved. The joint committee accepted the value of 5 gm. fat per fat exchange. The list (Table 29) contains foods that are approximately equal in fat content.

These six exchange lists (Tables 21, 23, 26, 27, 28, and 29) will allow the patient great variety in his diet and permit him to select foods from the different groups that may suit his income and food habits. The lists should also help to establish some uniformity in dietary instruction and counteract a practice that has no scientific basis, that of excluding various foods, such as potato, certain fruits, and some other foods, from the diet.

TABLE 29

LIST 6—FAT EXCHANGES
(Fat—5 Gm. per Serving)

Food	Approximate Measure	Weight (Gm.)
Butter or margarine	1 teaspoon	5
Bacon, crisp	1 slice	10
Cream:		
light, 20%	2 tablespoons	30
heavy, 40%	1 tablespoon	15
Cream cheese	1 tablespoon	15
French dressing	1 tablespoon	15
Mayonnaise	1 teaspoon	5
Oil or cooking fat	1 teaspoon	5
Nuts	6 small	10
Olives	5 small	50
Avocado (4-in. diameter)	1/8	25

Special considerations.—The following foods contain negligible amounts of carbohydrate, protein, and fat and may therefore be used as desired in the diet:

Coffee
Tea
Clear broth
Bouillon
Gelatin, unsweetened
Rennet tablets
Cranberries
Lemon
Rhubarb
Mustard
Pickles, sour
Pickles, dill—unsweetened
Saccharin
Pepper
Spices
Vinegar

"Specialty" foods for diabetic patients are not recommended. They are expensive, the information on the package is often misleading, and the patient can usually eat all the natural foods (breads, cereals, unsweetened fruits, vegetables) in the amount specified in his diet outline.

CALCULATION OF THE DIABETIC DIET

By using the short list of food values given in Table 20, it will be possible to calculate diet prescriptions with considerable ease and simplicity, taking into account the amount of each of these food groups which the patient should eat. This simplicity in calculating a diet will result in the saving of time for both the physician and the dietitian. The patient will also benefit immeasurably by a diet that is made to suit his food habits. Variety in the diet will be achieved by using the food exchange lists (Tables 21, 23, 26, 27, 28, and 29).

The nutritive adequacy of the diet will be assured by including the same *basic foods* that are recommended for the normal individual. These include the following:

Milk	1 pt. for adults; 1 qt. for children
Meat, fish, poultry, eggs, and cheese	4–5 oz.
Whole-grain or enriched cereal or bread	To meet caloric needs
Fruit—one a citrus fruit or tomato	2 servings
Vegetables—one green or yellow	2 servings
Fat or oil	To meet caloric needs

The actual calculation of the diet can be reduced to a simple formula, as shown in the tabulation on p. 83. To determine the number of servings of bread, meat, and fat exchanges required to complete the diet prescription, it is necessary only to:

a) Subtract the number of grams of carbohydrate (61 in the example in the table) furnished by the other sources of carbohydrate from the amount prescribed (180) and divide the result by 15, the number of grams of carbohydrate in one serving of bread exchange, as noted in List 4.

b) Adjust the amount of protein in the diet to the prescription by subtracting the number of grams of protein (34 in the example) supplied by milk, vegetables, and bread exchanges from the amount prescribed (80) and dividing the remainder by 7, the amount of protein in each meat exchange.

c) Follow the same procedure with regard to fat, except to divide the result by 5, the number of grams of fat in one serving, as noted in List 6.

The diet is figured to coincide as closely as possible with the prescription. However, it is not practical to split bread or meat exchanges into halves or to add extra fruits and vegetables if the patient does not care for larger amounts. Therefore, the carbohydrate may vary as much as 7 gm. from the amount ordered, and the protein may differ by 3 gm. The fat will agree closely with the prescription, since the figures for fat are all in multiples of 5.

DIVISION OF FOOD INTO MEALS

Division of the total amount of food prescribed into meals should be worked out with the patient. In doing this, several factors must be considered:

a) Present meal patterns, which are usually related to such factors as occupation, working hours, and place of eating.

PROCEDURE FOR CALCULATING A DIABETIC DIET (15)

Sample Prescription

Carbohydrate	180 gm.
Protein	80 gm.
Fat	70 gm.
Calories	1,700

	Amount	Carbohydrate (Gm.)	Protein (Gm.)	Fat (Gm.)
Milk, whole (List 1)	1 pt.	24	16	20
Vegetables (List 2, Group A)	As desired	...	..	..
Vegetables (List 2, Group B)	1 serving	7	2	..
Fruit (List 3)	3 servings	30	..	..
Total carbohydrate from sources other than bread exchanges	....	61		
180 gm. carbohydrate in prescription − 61 gm. from sources other than bread exchanges 119÷15=8 bread exchanges				
Bread exchanges (List 4)	8 servings	120	16	
Total protein from sources other than meat exchanges	....	...	34	
80 gm. protein in prescription −34 gm. from sources other than meat exchanges 46 gm.÷7=7 meat exchanges				
Meat exchanges (List 5)	7 servings		49	35
Total fat from sources other than fat exchanges	....	...	..	55
70 gm. fat in prescription −55 gm. from sources other than fat exchanges 15 gm.÷5=3 fat exchanges				
Fat exchanges (List 6)	3 servings			15
		181	83	70

b) Diabetic condition, i.e., tendency to excrete more or less sugar at varying times during the day.

c) Type of insulin—regular, protamine zinc, globin, or Lente.

The carbohydrate content of the diet should be divided between the meals, avoiding too large a proportion of the total at any one meal. When protamine insulin is used, nourishment at bedtime (perhaps one-seventh of the day's allowance of carbohydrate) should be recommended. When globin insulin is used, also give an afternoon lunch (approximately one-seventh) and reduce the carbohydrate of the breakfast to about the same amount.

A good source of protein should be included at each meal (milk, eggs, meat, fish, or cheese). The fat is apt to divide itself naturally with fairly even distribution throughout the meals.

SAMPLE MEAL PLANS

The simplified method of calculating a diabetic diet just described is recommended, since it is the procedure most likely to make certain that the diet is adjusted to the food preferences of the individual. "Diet lists" prepared in advance can be used for convenience, provided that they are modified to suit the special needs of the individual. For this reason nine sample meal plans (Tables 30 and 31) were prepared by the committee to fit various needs.

Each of these nine diets has been outlined and illustrated with sample menus in small leaflets which may be distributed to patients. It is expected that these will be used in conjunction with the booklet *Meal Planning with Exchange Lists* which has also been prepared for the use of patients. In addition, two other leaflets for patients have been prepared in one of which appropriate changes in the exchange lists have been made to fit the need for modifications in sodium content. The other leaflet indicates adaptations of the exchange lists to fit those who may need to use bland-flavored foods.

For the physician, a special leaflet has been prepared, containing the carbohydrate, protein, fat, and caloric content of each food exchange, tables of prescriptions for various levels of dietary intake, desirable weights for men and women, and notes regarding the selection of diet prescriptions for adults and children.

The twelve leaflets and the *Meal Planning with Exchange Lists* are available from The American Dietetic Association, 620 North Michigan Avenue, Chicago 11, Illinois.

CONSIDERATIONS IN ADAPTING THE FOOD EXCHANGE LISTS

New data on food composition.—Since 1950 new values for some food items now included in the exchange lists have been reported in *Composition of Foods—Raw, Processed, Prepared* (U.S. Department of Agriculture, Agriculture Handbook No. 8 [December, 1963]). In

TABLE 30

CALORIC LEVELS OF SAMPLE MEALS FOR DIABETICS

Meal Plan	Carbo-hydrate (Gm.)	Protein (Gm.)	Fat (Gm.)	Energy (Calories)
1	125	60	50	1,200
2	150	70	70	1,500
3	180	80	80	1,800
4	220	90	100	2,200
5*	180	80	80	1,800
6*	250	100	130	2,600
7*	370	140	165	3,500
8	250	115	130	2,600
9	300	120	145	3,000

* Planned particularly for children.

TABLE 31

SAMPLE MEAL PLANS FOR DIABETICS

Diet	Milk	Veg. A	Veg. B	Fruits	Bread Exchange	Meat Exchange	Fat Exchange
1	1 pt.	As desired	1	3	4	5	1
2	1 pt.	As desired	1	3	6	6	4
3	1 pt.	As desired	1	3	8	7	5
4	1 pt.	As desired	1	4	10	8	8
5*	1 qt.	As desired	1	3	6	5	3
6*	1 qt.	As desired	1	4	10	7	11
7*	1 qt.	As desired	1	6	17	10	15
8	1 pt.	As desired	1	4	12	10	12
9	1 pt.	As desired	1	4	15	10	15

* These diets contain more milk and are especially suitable for children.

most instances, however, the change has been small and when related to the usual frequency of consumption of the varied items in an exchange list, no real impact is made on the representative value for carbohydrate, protein, and fat now assigned.

An exception may occur, however, if the frequency of use of certain items is altered. For example, in certain areas of the country, more lean cuts of meat are available on the market, reflecting in part a demand for lower calories and less saturated fat. If this increased consumption of lean meat were coupled with increased use of fish and poultry and a concomitant reduction in the use of items higher in fat such as bologna, frankfurters, peanut butter, and most cheeses, the present value of the meat exchange might be closer to 8 gm. protein and 2 gm. fat than the present value of 7 gm. protein and 5 gm. fat. These considerations have been pointed up by Parente *et al.* (19) in "Adaptation of Exchange Lists—Use in Planning Metabolic Ward Diets."

Various ratios of polyunsaturated to saturated fats, percentages of fats, and reduced levels of cholesterol may easily be incorporated for therapeutic purposes. For an assessment of a basic diet that may be used for this purpose, see Table 15.

Some variations are also known to occur from state to state in the fat content of milk. In addition, convenience foods and numerous special purpose foods vary from market to market and from time to time in the same market, necessitating continuous alertness on the part of the dietitian and special compilations of data on food composition representing foods available in the local market.

Total nutrient worth.—Since the integrity of the total diet depends upon the nutrient merit of the component food groups, a critical appraisal by the dietitian not only of carbohydrate, protein, and fat, but also of minerals and vitamins is in order. With these criteria alone, the frequent substitution, for example, of a candy bar for a glass of milk, or of a soft drink for orange juice would be unjustified —in spite of any "equivalence" in carbohydrate, protein, or fat. For a gross comparison of the nutrient worth of a food item not on the exchange list, reference may be made to Tables 2 and 36.

Frequency of use.—If a wide variety of the food items enumerated in any one food group is consumed, and if this food intake represents some proximity to the proportions indicated in the per capita consumption of foods reported by the U.S. Department of Agriculture (20), the present values for carbohydrate, protein, and fat in the exchange lists will be approximated. If the patient narrows his food intake to one or two items, however, or if intentional changes are recommended, a reassessment of the selection should be made to determine the effect of the bias introduced on the nutrient quality of the diet as a whole.

Ethnic food habits.—Some adaptations of the exchange list may be advisable in those situations where nationality, religious, or regional food preferences represent foods not now included in the exchange lists. Many of these items may be of equal or superior nutrient merit. Information on nutrient content, methods of food preparation, and appropriateness for therapeutic use should be determined in conference with the physician.

Sweets and alcohol.—Concentrated sweets and alcohol will reduce the total nutrient merit of the diet and in some cases alter the utilization of medication. The inclusion of either in the diet should be determined in conference with the physician.

EDUCATIONAL PROGRAM

Stone (21) has directed an excellent paper to the dietitian entitled "A Rational Approach to Diet and Diabetes in 1964." He defines a rational diet as one that has been made to fit the individual patient with the first step being a careful assessment of the diet history. From this point, the dietitian can plan appropriate meals from familiar foods, from foods within the income of the patient, and in line with the therapeutic goals established by the physician. In counseling the patient, factors of motivation, educational level, and appropriate materials become of major concern.

The expanding range of responsibilities of the dietitian for patient care is described by Kaufman (see chap. 13). More sophisticated means are now available to present information needed by the patient. After an appropriate diet history has been obtained and an individual meal plan has been discussed with him by the dietitian, programmed instruction in book form or teaching machines serve to amplify in effective detail the basic background information needed by every patient and his family. For individual or group instruction, film strips or slide sets in color together with sound recordings are also available and serve as another sophisticated medium for hospital and community service (22, 23). Information regarding available materials of this nature may be obtained from the U.S. Public Health Service, Diabetes and Arthritis Program, Division of Chronic Diseases, Washington, D.C. The series covers practical presentations of the Food Exchange Lists, as well as the other aspects of patient care.

For professional reference, an up-to-date volume entitled *Dia-*

betes Mellitus Diagnosis and Treatment has been published by the American Diabetes Association, Inc. 18 East 48th Street, New York, New York 10017.

Nutritional evaluation.—An appraisal of the various nutrient, mineral, and vitamin contents of the diet may be made simply by comparison with the normal dietary plans. As previously stated, an evaluation of the vitamin A and the carotene content of various diets has been made by a committee of the Diet Therapy Section (17). It was found that low-caloric and low-fat diets frequently served to diabetics contained between 91 and 2,600 I.U. of vitamin A when liver was not served once a week. These same diets were high in carotene, however, owing to the large amount of fruits and vegetables present. These facts become of importance where there is a dysfunction in the assimilation and metabolism of carotene, as frequently occurs in diabetes and liver damage. In these cases it will be desirable to use liver one or more times per week or to add vitamin A supplements.

THE GALACTOSE-FREE DIET

A review of the current concepts of the basic defects in galactosemia has been presented by Koch *et al.*, and a method of monitoring dietary control is suggested (25). The chief dietary modification involves the elimination of milk, of galactose-storing organ meats such as liver, pancreas, and brain, and possibly of the oligosaccharides, raffinose, and stachyose that occur in legumes and beets. A list of foods to include, those to exclude, and galactose-free recipes are reported.

The Children's Bureau, U.S. Department of Health, Education, and Welfare has prepared a selected and annotated bibliography entitled *Galactosemia, A Selected Bibliography*, 1963. This may be obtained from the Government Printing Office for 30 cents a copy.

Also, an excellent guide to the feeding of mentally retarded children has been prepared by the Children's Bureau, U.S. Department of Health, Education, and Welfare, Washington, D.C. This booklet includes guidance in taking a dietary history, assessment of feeding methods, and techniques and teaching for development of skills by the family and child. The booklet entitled, *Feeding Mentally Retarded Children*, 1964, may be obtained from the Government Printing Office, Washington, D.C. for 15 cents.

REFERENCES

1. Calculation of diabetic diets, J. Am. Dietet. A., **24**:218–19, 1948.
2. McCance, R. A., and Widdowson, E. M. Chemical composition of foods. 2d ed. Brooklyn, N.Y.: Chemical Publishing Co., 1947.
3. Chatfield, C., and Adams, G. Proximate composition of American food materials. (U.S. Department of Agriculture Circular No. 549.) 1940.
4. Bureau of Human Nutrition and Home Economics in co-operation with the National Research Council. Tables of food composition in terms of eleven nutrients. ("U.S. Department of Agriculture Miscellaneous Publications," No. 572.) 1945.
5. Olmsted, W. H. The available carbohydrate of fruits and vegetables, Proc. Am. Diabetes A., **9**:385–406, 1950.
6. Hummel, F. C., Shepherd, M. L., and Macy, I. G. Disappearance of cellulose and hemicellulose from the digestive tracts of children, J. Nutrition, **25**:59–70, 1943.
7. Buchanan, J. M., and Hastings, A. B. The use of isotopically marked carbon in the study of intermediary metabolism, Physiol. Rev., **26**:120–55, 1946.
8. Bloch, K. The metabolism of acetic acid in animal tissues, Physiol. Rev., **27**:574–620, 1947.
9. Wood, H. G. The fixation of carbon dioxide and the inter-relationships of the tricarboxylic acid cycle, Physiol. Rev., **26**:198–246, 1946.
10. Stadie, W. C. The intermediary metabolism of fatty acids, Physiol. Rev., **25**:395–441, 1945.
11. Williams, R. D., Wicks, L., Bierman, H. R., and Olmsted, W. H. Carbohydrate values of fruits and vegetables, J. Nutrition, **19**:593–604, 1940.
12. Bureau of Human Nutrition and Home Economics. Consumption of food in the United States, 1909–48. ("U.S. Department of Agriculture Miscellaneous Publications," No. 691.) 1949.
13. Stern, F. Applied dietetics. 3d ed. Baltimore: Williams & Wilkins Co., 1949.
14. Turner, D. Handbook of diet therapy. 1st ed. Chicago: University of Chicago Press, 1946.
15. Caso, E. K., and Stare, F. J. Simplified method for calculating diabetic diets, J.A.M.A., **133**:169–71, 1947.
16. Revised tables of food values, Proc. Am. Diabetes A., **9**: 403–6, 1950.
17. Johnson, D. Vitamin A versus carotene content of low-fat diets in obesity, cholecystitis, and liver disease, J. Am. Dietet. A., **25**:873–74, 1942.
18. Bureau of Human Nutrition and Home Economics. Family food consumption in the United States, spring, 1942. ("U.S. Department of Agriculture Miscellaneous Publications," No. 550.) 1944.
19. Parente, B. P., Gaffield, B. E., Hill, R. B., and Ohlson, M. A. Adaptation of Exchange Lists—Use in Planning Ward Diets, J. Am. Dietet. A., **46**:267–75, 1965.
20. Economic Research Service. Consumption of Food in the United States, Supplement for 1961. (U.S. Department of Agriculture, Agriculture Handbook No. 62.) 1962.

21. STONE, DANIEL B. A. rational approach to diet and diabetes in 1964, J. Am. Dietet. A., **46**:30–35, 1965.
22. KAUFMAN, M. Programmed instruction materials on diabetes J. Am. Dietet. A., **46**:36–38, 1965.
23. DOWNING, C. B. What is programmed instruction? J. Am. Dietet. A., **46**:39–42, 1965.
24. Composition of Foods—Raw, Processed, Prepared. (U.S. Department of Agriculture, Agriculture Handbook No. 8 [December, 1963].)
25. KOCH, R., ACOSTA, P., RAGSDALE, N., and DONNELL, G. N. Nutrition in the treatment of galactosemia. J. Am. Dietet. A., **43**:216–22, 1963.

Chapter 9 | The Sodium-restricted Diet

The sodium-restricted diet is an allowance of food and drink in which the sodium content is restricted to a prescribed level. Other nutrients remain as nearly as possible on a level satisfactory for nutritive sufficiency.

Sodium restriction is most often prescribed in the control of edema accompanying congestive heart failure, and has been shown also to be of benefit in the treatment of some cases of hypertension, cirrhosis of the liver, toxemias of pregnancy, and certain kidney diseases.

Physicians vary in their use of sodium-restricted diets and the levels prescribed. Some prescribe them in conjunction with drug therapy, such as diuretics, thereby making it possible to use a less restricted level of sodium. Certain patients experience toxic reactions or other complications with drug therapy; and for these, dietary restriction of sodium remains the safest treatment.

Since it is the sodium ion that is significant in sodium-restricted therapy such terms as "low salt," "salt poor," and "salt free" are inadequate. A prescribed level of dietary sodium should be indicated and with due consideration for the sodium content of drinking water and medications.

The person on an unrestricted diet may consume ordinarily between 5 and 10 gm. sodium daily. Water varies in sodium content from source to source and from time to time depending in part upon the water softeners added at the treatment plant or at home. Foods in their natural state contain widely differing amounts of sodium; and the amount of sodium added in food preparation and in commercial processing is significant. Bills *et al.* (2) have pointed out:

Many manufactured food products which are not intentionally salted contain somewhat more sodium than the natural foods from which they are prepared. The source of this sodium is found in the numerous special uses of sodium compounds in the food industry. Sodium chloride is employed for many purposes besides seasoning, preserving, pickling, and koshering. As brine it is used (*a*) in the flotation process of sorting green peas from hardened peas and heavy extraneous matter, (*b*) for preventing enzymic discoloring of freshly sliced apples and pears which are to be canned, (*c*) as a heat transfer and blanching agent in freezing foods, and (*d*) for regenerating base-exchange water softeners (the sodium appears in the softened water as bicarbonate, and water thus treated is used in canning to prevent toughening of vegetables).

Sodium alginate is employed as a stabilizer for ice cream and chocolate milk drinks. Sodium aluminum sulphate is the alum of baking powders. Sodium benzoate is used as a preservative in fruit juice concentrates, confectionery, margarine, and so on. Sodium bicarbonate is the gas source in baking powders and self-rising flours. It is also used with cocoa in the "Dutching" process, for tenderizing vegetables, and for neutralizing. Sodium carbonate is used for Dutching, neutralizing, and water softening. It has a special use in removing hop resins from brewers' yeast in the debittering process. Sodium citrate is used as a stabilizing agent in evaporated milk and jellies. Sodium glutamate is an important flavoring adjunct. Sodium hydroxide is used for Dutching cocoa, neutralizing corn syrup, debittering ripe olives, and hulling corn in the old lye process of hominy manufacture. It is also widely used in peeling apricots, peaches, grapefruit segments, carrots, and sweet potatoes, for canning, and for dipping fruits prior to drying. Sodium acid phosphate is used as an acidulating agent. The secondary phosphate is used for emulsifying process cheese, for stabilizing evaporated milk, and as the quickening agent in quick-cooking farina. Sodium acid sulphite is employed for sulphuring fruits prior to drying. These few examples may serve to explain the almost ubiquitous occurrence in processed foods of sodium in amounts greater than are present in the corresponding natural products.

In planning a regimen, reference should be made to sodium since equal weights of different sodium compounds do not contain equal weights of sodium. With respect to sodium chloride, 58.5 gm. or one gram-molecule is composed of 23 gm. sodium (one gram-atom) and 35.5 gm. chlorine (one gram-atom). To convert a specified weight of sodium chloride to sodium, multiply by 0.393; thus 10 gm. of sodium chloride contains 3.93 gm. of sodium.

The millimolecular weight (mmole) and milliequivalent weight (mEq.) are one thousandth of the gram molecular weight and the equivalent gram-atomic weight, respectively.

$$1 \text{ mEq. of sodium} = 23 \text{ mg.}$$

To derive the sodium content in mEq. divide the weight of sodium in mg. by 23. For example, if the sodium content of milk is 50 mg. per

100 gm. or approximately 500 mg. per liter, the mEq. weight is $\frac{500}{23}$ or about 22 mEq. per liter. The following conversions may be useful (6):

1,000 mg. (1 gm.) of sodium = 43.5 mEq.
100 mg. of sodium = 4.35 mEq.
10 mg. of sodium = 0.44 mEq.
1 mg. of sodium = 0.04 mEq.
100 mEq. of sodium = 2,300 mg. (2.3 gm.)
10 mEq. of sodium = 230 mg.
1 mEq. of sodium = 23 mg.

10 gm. of sodium chloride = $\frac{10{,}000}{58.5}$ = 171 mEq. of sodium chloride, sodium, or chloride.

1 gm. of sodium chloride = 17.1 mEq. of sodium chloride, sodium, or chloride.

Selected values for sodium and potassium content of foods appear in Table 41, pages 209–20. A more extensive list of values may be found in *Composition of Foods* (U.S. Department of Agriculture, Agricultural Research Service, Agriculture Handbook No. 8), 1963.

NUTRIENT CONTENT

Since the level of sodium prescribed for therapy may vary from 200 mg. daily to 2,000 mg. or more, depending upon the needs of the individual patient, it becomes desirable to have a basic plan in which protein, mineral, and vitamin needs may be at a level for nutritive sufficiency but from which modifications may be made to suit the level of sodium prescribed. For this reason, adaptations of the plans of normal diet described, are recommended as the basic pattern of diet. For example, if the patient is an adult, the appropriate basic pattern (Table 2) may be used for making modifications. If the patient is a pregnant woman, the respective plan of diet (Table 7) should be used. In the case of an adolescent or a child, normal patterns of diet (Tables 8 and 9) should be used as a basis for the sodium modifications. In planning a 500-mg. sodium diet for an adult, an illustration of the kind and amount of the food groups which might be used are described in Table 32A. The meal pattern and sample menus appear in Table 32B.

TABLE 32

500-MG. SODIUM DIET FOR AN ADULT
(70 Gm. Protein; 1,500 Calories; Adapted from Normal Diet, Table 2)

Daily Food Plan	Sodium† (Mg.)	Protein (Gm.)	Calories
MILK GROUP*			
1 pt. whole	244	16	340
MEAT AND EGG GROUP			
1 egg	60	7	75
4 oz. cooked meat, poultry or fish (edible portion), *no sodium added*	70	28	300
VEGETABLE AND FRUIT GROUP			
5 servings (*no sodium added*)			
Dark-green or yellow (1 serving)	9	....	....
Other vegetable (1 serving)	4	....	35
Citrus fruit or other fruit rich in vitamin C (1 serving)	1	....	40
Other fruit (2 servings)	5	....	80
BREAD CEREAL POTATO LEGUME GROUP			
8 servings (*no sodium added*)			
Bread, 6 slices (*no sodium added*)	54	12	420
Potato, ½ cup, or ½ cup cooked rice, white or red beans, cornmeal, noodles, spaghetti, ⅓ cup corn or ¼ cup sweet potato (*no sodium added*)	5	2	70
Cereals, cooked, ½ cup, such as farina, rolled oats, rolled wheat cereal (*no sodium added*)	5	2	70
FATS AND SWEETS‡			
1 teaspoon butter or margarine (*no sodium added*)	1	....	15
1 teaspoon sugar, jelly, or jam	1	....	20
WATER†			
Total	459†	67	1,495‡

* During pregnancy, adolescence, and childhood, 1 quart of milk may be used, thus increasing calories to 1,800, protein to 83 gm., and sodium to 700 mg. If less sodium is desired, low-sodium milk may be used.

† For additional values on sodium (and potassium) content of foods, see Table 41. Sodium content of water should be added to the total. Local health department should be contacted for information on current sodium content of municipal water supplies.

‡ For substitutions or additions to suit caloric needs see Table 36. For a sample menu pattern and sample meals see Table 32B.

Modification for 250-mg. sodium diet.—The use of low-sodium milk may reduce the sodium content by about 90 per cent. This change alone will reduce the diet to about 250 mg. sodium.

Modification for 1,000-mg. sodium diet.—Numerous choices are possible in making substitutions where an additional amount of sodium is permitted on the 500-mg. sodium diet. One slice of ordinary salted bread may contain approximately 180 mg. sodium; and 1 teaspoon of ordinary salted butter or margarine may provide approximately 50 mg. sodium; thus totaling 230 mg. sodium per one slice of ordinary bread and butter or margarine. If ordinary canned vegetables are an item of choice, approximately 250 mg. sodium per one-half cup serving may be expected if no salt is added at the table. These and other items may be substituted for items in the 500-mg. sodium diet by reference to the values for sodium content of foods in Table 41.

Modification for 2,000–2,500-mg. sodium diet.—If the eight servings of the bread group were from ordinary salted bread, approximately 1,500 mg. sodium would be added, making the diet 2,000 mg. sodium. If 8 teaspoons ordinary salted butter or margarine were used with the bread, 400 more mg. sodium would be added, making the total sodium approximately 2,400 mg. Alternates, sample menu patterns, and sample meals appear in Tables 32, 32A, and 32B.

TABLE 32A

DAILY FOOD PLAN OF DIET CONTAINING 500 MG. SODIUM
(70 Gm. Protein; 1,500 Calories; Derived from Table 32)

Daily Food Plan	Description
MILK GROUP	
1 pt.	*One pint of whole milk* contains approximately 16 gm. protein, 340 calories, and 244 mg. sodium. It is also an important source of minerals and vitamins of the B complex. One pint skim milk may contain approximately 180 calories and similar protein and sodium to whole milk.
	Palatable milks prepared by an ion-exchange process are available in some areas. Sodium is reduced by 90 per cent; thiamine, niacin, and vitamin B_{12} by about 50 per cent; and calcium and vitamin B_6 by about 75 per cent. Potassium may be increased to about twice ordinary milk.
MEAT AND EGG GROUP	
1 egg	*One egg* will contain approximately 60 mg. sodium, 7 gm. protein, and 75 calories.
4 oz. cooked meat, poultry, or fish	*One ounce (edible portion) of cooked beef, veal, lamb, pork, poultry or fish (no sodium added)* contains about 18 mg. sodium, 7 gm. protein, and 75 calories. Meat, poultry, or fish salted at any stage of processing will not be suitable for use; therefore, ordinary canned or smoked and seasoned meat and cheese should be omitted. All products must be specially canned or prepared without added sodium, to be suitable for this diet. Four ounces meat contain approximately 70 mg. sodium.
VEGETABLE AND FRUIT GROUP	
5 servings A dark-green or yellow vegetable is important daily for vitamin A value	*A dark-green or yellow vegetable* is important each day for vitamin A value. This group includes asparagus, green beans, peppers, yellow squash, pumpkin. Each serving may be estimated at 9 mg. sodium. Carrots, kale, beet greens, chard, and spinach have been excluded. One-half cup squash and pumpkin may contain 35 calories. Others are negligible.
	Other vegetables to which no sodium has been added may be used, such as cauliflower, cucumber, eggplant, onion, radishes, summer squash, and tomatoes. Each serving will contain about 4 mg. sodium. Calories are negligible. Beets, celery, and white turnips have been excluded.
A citrus fruit or other fruit rich in vitamin C daily	*One orange or ½ grapefruit or 1 large tangerine or ½ cup citrus juice* is considered one serving of citrus fruit. One cup strawberries, or 1 cup red raspberries, or ¼ cantaloupe is a satisfactory substitute. Sodium content of fruit is approximately 1 mg. per serving and 40 calories per serving.
Other fruit, 2 servings	*Will contribute 5 mg. sodium and 80 calories for 2 servings.*

TABLE 32A—*Continued*

Daily Food Plan	Description
BREAD-CEREAL-POTATO-LEGUME GROUP (no sodium added)	
8 servings	*One slice of bread* or substitute (*no sodium added*) contains about 70 calories and 9 mg. sodium or less; i.e., $\frac{1}{2}$ cup cooked potato, rice, dried beans, cornmeal, noodles, spaghetti, $\frac{1}{3}$ cup corn, or $\frac{1}{4}$ cup sweet potato will contain less than 5 mg. sodium. Certain cooked cereals, such as farina, rolled oats, rolled wheat cereal, and wheat meals are low in sodium (avoid "quick-cooking" cereals to which a sodium salt has been added). Certain prepared cereals which have no sodium added are Puffed Rice, Puffed Wheat, and Shredded Wheat. Avoid any prepared cereals with sodium added.
FATS AND SWEETS	
	If 1 teaspoon sugar, jelly, or honey is included, approximately 20 calories are added. No sodium need be estimated for this.
	If 1 teaspoon fat or oil is included, approximately 45 calories are added. Oils are not ordinarily salted. Bacon, ham fat, salt pork, sausage fat, margarine, and butter will have considerable amounts of sodium. Two teaspoons ordinary, salted butter or margarine contain about 100 mg. sodium. Unsalted butter and margarine to which no sodium has been added will be a negligible source of sodium.
SALT SUBSTITUTES	
	Salt substitutes should be used only upon recommendation of a physician.
ARTIFICIAL SWEETENERS	
	Sodium cyclamate or saccharin may be significant sources of sodium.
IODINE	*A source of iodine* may become necessary, since iodized sodium chloride cannot be used.
WATER	*Drinking water* may be an important source of sodium. Check with local health department regarding sodium content of municipal water supplies.

TABLE 32B

500-MG. SODIUM DIET—MENU PATTERN AND SAMPLE MEALS FOR AN ADULT
(70 Gm. Protein; 1,500 Calories; Derived from Table 32A)

DAILY FOOD PLAN*	SAMPLE MENU PATTERN‡	SAMPLE MEALS‡
	A.M.	
MILK GROUP 1 pt. MEAT AND EGG GROUP 1 egg and 4 oz. (edible portion) meat, poultry, or fish *No sodium added*	1 citrus fruit or $\frac{1}{2}$ cup juice 1 egg $\frac{1}{2}$ cup low-sodium cooked cereal or $\frac{3}{4}$ cup flake-type with milk* 1 slice low-sodium, enriched, or whole-grain bread or toast Spread† Coffee or tea if desired Sugar	Sliced tangerine 1 egg Oatmeal with milk and sugar† Toast with spread† Coffee Sugar
	Noon	
VEGETABLE AND FRUIT GROUP 5 servings A dark-green or deep-yellow vegetable daily Citrus fruit or other fruit rich in vitamin C daily *No sodium added*	2 oz. (edible portion) meat, poultry, or fish 3 servings of the bread-potato-cereal group* Fresh or cooked vegetable Fruit Milk Tea or coffee if desired	Club sandwich: Sliced chicken Sliced tomato Lettuce Spread† Fresh mixed fruits Milk
BREAD-CEREAL-POTATO-GROUP	P.M.	
8 servings *No sodium added* FATS AND SWEETS† *No sodium added* (Without this group the diet contains 1,500 calories)	2 oz. (edible portion) meat, poultry, or fish 3 servings from potato-bread-cereal group* Dark-green or deep-yellow vegetable Other vegetable Fruit Milk	Roast pork Sweet potato Frozen green beans Baked apple Hot roll (*no sodium added*) Spread† Milk

* See Table 32A for alternates or substitutes in each food group.

† If 1 teaspoon fat or oil is included in addition to the basic diet of 1,500 calories, 45 calories per teaspoon should be added. This may be used on bread or in cooking.

If 1 teaspoon sugar, jelly, or honey is included in addition to the basic diet, approximately 20 calories should be added. These may be added in amounts suitable to meet caloric needs of individual patients.

‡ For discussion of food preparation see pp. 111–12.

FOOD PREPARATION

Meat, poultry, and fish may be enhanced in flavor by using fruit combinations. Cranberry sauce with poultry, applesauce with pork, mint jelly with lamb, and lemon with fish are standbys. For those who like meat or fish cooked in tomato sauce, unsalted canned tomatoes, juice, or puree may be combined with garlic, onion, green pepper, and mushrooms and flavored with such herbs as oregano if desired. Meat and fish may be simmered or baked in this sauce. Low-sodium wines, French-type dressings, lemon, and vinegar provide excellent marination for meat.

Some additional flavor combinations are as follows:

Beef—dry mustard, marjoram, nutmeg, onion, sage, thyme, pepper, bay leaf, grape jelly
Lamb—mint, garlic, rosemary, curry, broiled pineapple rings, lemon juice, and oregano
Veal—bay leaf, ginger, marjoram, curry, currant jelly, spiced apricots
Chicken—paprika, mushroom, thyme, sage, parsley, cranberry sauce
Fish—dry mustard, paprika, curry, bay leaf, lemon juice, mushrooms, and sherry
Eggs—pepper, green pepper, mushrooms, dry mustard, paprika, curry, jelly, or pineapple omelet

Vegetables may be flavored with a sweet-sour sauce (diluted vinegar and sugar, seasoned with grated onion, spices, and herbs as desired) or with hot low-sodium salad dressing made as follows: canned tomatoes, tomato juice, or puree (no sodium added) may be flavored with lemon or vinegar, sugar, grated horse-radish root, onion, garlic, spices, and herbs as desired. Calories will be negligible. Other possible flavor combinations are as follows:

Asparagus—lemon juice
Beans, green—marjoram, lemon juice, nutmeg, dill seed
Broccoli—lemon juice
Cabbage—mustard dressing, dill seed, unsalted butter with lemon and sugar
Cauliflower—nutmeg
Corn—green pepper, tomatoes
Peas—mint, mushroom, parsley, onion
Potatoes—parsley, unsalted butter, mace, chopped green pepper, chives, onion
Squash—ginger, mace
Sweet potatoes—candied, or glazed with cinnamon or nutmeg, or escalloped with apples
Tomatoes—basil, oregano

Vegetable aspics may be concocted with plain gelatin, tomato juice (no sodium added), and lemon, grated cabbage, cucumber, and green pepper. Low-sodium dressing or mayonnaise with no added sodium may be used. Vegetables canned without added sodium are available. Frozen Lima beans or peas may have sodium added. Labels should be carefully read, and information sought from commercial firms.

Baked goods pose a special problem because usual products may contain added salt, salted shortening, baking powder, or soda. Such products might exceed 300 mg. sodium per 100 gram. This can be reduced greatly by preparation with unsalted shortening and with a low-sodium baking powder, possibly as low as 20 to 40 mg. sodium per 100 gm. On the other hand, the potassium content of products made with the low-sodium baking powder may increase by one-and-a-half to three-and-a-half times more than if sodium aluminum sulfate baking powder were used.

Low-sodium products may be prepared from combinations of foods permitted on the diet. Unsalted fats and oils are available. Leavening may be obtained from yeasts or sodium-free baking powder. The following formula for sodium-free baking powder may be obtained from a pharmacist:

Potassium bicarbonate	39.8 gm.
Cornstarch	28.0 gm.
Tartaric acid	7.5 gm.
Potassium bitartrate	56.1 gm.

Bread and rolls also pose special problems. Ordinary bread might contain approximately 600 mg. per 100 gm. In low-sodium bread, the sodium content might be reduced to approximately 60 mg. per 100 gm. of product. Ranges are wide, however, and it is important to read the labels of commercial products purported to be low in sodium to assess the mg. of sodium per 100 gm. of product. The same admonition applies to cereal products, since such items as puffed wheat, and shredded wheat, for example, appear in both the salted and unsalted form.

Low-sodium milk is available. In many parts of the country a palatable product has been obtained by passing fluid milk through an ion-exchange resin at 35°–40° F. The result is the replacement of sodium with an equivalent amount of potassium. The taste and flavor of the milk are only slightly affected. However, this product contains only about 50 per cent of the thiamine, niacin, and vitamin B_{12} of the original milk and about 75 per cent of the calcium and vitamin B_6. The potassium is doubled but is still within the normal physiologic intake of 3–5 gm. for adults. The Council on Foods and Nutrition of the American Medical Association (3) recommends the following levels per quart:

Sodium, less than	50	mg.
Potassium, less than	2.5	gm.
Thiamine, at least	0.15	mg.
Riboflavin, at least	1.0	mg.
Niacin, at least	0.4	mg.
Vitamin B_6, at least	300	μg.
Vitamin B_{12}, at least	3	μg.

Dried, low-sodium milk products are also available.

Other low-sodium dietetic foods are available. Such foods as vegetables canned without added salt, specially processed cheeses and meat add variety, save time, and increase the acceptance of the diet by the patient. Two federal regulations relating to labeling provide protection and information to persons on sodium-restricted therapy. One regulation requires that all labels on low-sodium, dietetic foods must indicate the sodium content in milligrams of sodium per 100 grams of food as well as in an average serving of food. The other regulation relates to frozen vegetables. If salt has been used either directly or indirectly during processing, the label must state that salt has been added or is present.

SUPPLEMENTARY MATERIALS

Numerous special cookbooks have been prepared for patients on low-sodium diets. However, the value of any recipe depends upon an accurate estimate of the sodium content per serving and the proper substitution within each individual diet. This usually requires guidance from a dietitian, nutritionist, or physician. A critical review of low-sodium cookbooks, booklets, and materials on meal planning has been prepared at the request of the Nutrition Committee, American Heart Association, and published in the *Journal of the American Dietetic Association* (5).

Three booklets (4) for patients have been prepared by a Subcommittee on Sodium Restricted Diets, American Heart Association. Whys and wherefores of a sodium-restricted diet are discussed; diet plans limited in sodium and calories are described; and questions regarding food preparation are answered. The plans are limited to 500 mg., 1,000 mg., and 2,400–4,500 mg. sodium diets, since it was felt that prescriptions between these levels are usually unnecessary for therapeutic purposes. These booklets are available from the American Heart Association, 44 East Twenty-third Street, New York, New York, to physicians, dietitians, nutritionists, and nurses without charge. Simplified leaflets have been derived from the booklets as well as a recipe booklet for the patient.

The Food You Eat and Heart Disease (Public Health Service Publication No. 537), revised 1963, is a 12-page pamphlet for the layman on the importance of diet as specific therapy in some forms of heart disease. It counteracts the popular misconception of diet as a cure-all or preventive of cardiac diseases. Single copies are available without charge from the U.S. Department of Health, Education, and Welfare, Washington, D.C., 20402. Up to 50 copies may be obtained free by professional persons.

For professional persons, the publication entitled *Sodium Restricted Diets: The Rationale, Complications, and Practical Aspects of Their Use* ("Food and Nutrition Board–National Research Council Publications," No. 325 [1954]) continues to provide an excellent reference on the normal physiology of sodium metabolism, the use of sodium-restricted diets in congestive cardiac failure, hypertension, renal disease, cirrhosis of the liver, toxemias of pregnancy, Ménière's disease, and hormone therapy, as well as contra-indications for the use of low-sodium diets and salt substitutes.

Since sodium is closely related to other extra- and intra-cellular ions, particularly potassium, a limited number of values for both potassium and sodium have been included in Table 41, page 209. A more complete listing of sodium and potassium values appears in *Composition of Food—Raw, Processed, Prepared* (U.S. Department of Agriculture, Agricultural Research Service, Agriculture Handbook No. 8), 1963. Additional mineral elements (1) appear in Table 42.

REFERENCES

1. Peterson, W. H., Skinner, J. T., and Strong, F. M. Elements of food biochemistry. New York: Prentice-Hall, Inc., 1953, pp. 262–65.
2. Bills, C. E., McDonald, F. G., Niedermeier, W., and Schwartz, M. C. Sodium and potassium in foods and water, J. Am. Dietet. A., **25**:304–14, 1949.
3. Council on Foods and Nutrition. Low sodium milk, J.A.M.A., **163**:739, 1957.
4. Heap, B., and Robinson, C. New diet booklets for cardiac patients and sodium restriction, J. Am. Dietet. A., **34**:277–79, 1958.
5. Reimer, A., Johnson, D., and Robinson, C. Sodium restricted diets, J. Am. Dietet. A., **33**:104–7, 1957.
6. Sodium Restricted Diets: The Rationale, Complications, and Practical Aspects of Their Use. (Food and Nutrition Board–National Research Council Publications, No. 325.) 1954.

Chapter 10 | *The Low-Purine Diet*

The low-purine diet is a food allowance in which sources of purines, such as glandular organs, dried legumes and lentils, and meat extractives are eliminated, and other meat and fish are restricted to 4 oz. weekly, thus reducing the daily intake of uric acid equivalent to approximately 35 mg. If a high-carbohydrate, low-fat regimen is imposed in addition, as has been suggested by Bartels (1), further modifications may be made as outlined in the discussion of the low-fat diet (p. 60).

The following discussion of the purine content of foods and the outline for the low-purine diet is taken from a report of a committee of the Diet Therapy Section of The American Dietetic Association (2):

> A review of the available literature regarding the purine content . . . of foods revealed a distressing paucity of usable figures and consistent values. The committee felt itself incompetent to evaluate the data inasmuch as the sources used and methods of analyses could not be satisfactorily compared.
>
> In an attempt to obtain the most recent figures available, aid was solicited from outstanding authorities throughout the United States. It was found that none were using purine calculations or could add to the common list of references, or would attempt to evaluate comparatively the tables given in current texts.

An outline has been prepared by this committee as a guide for practical use in planning a low-purine diet. When protein-rich foods have been omitted because of their relatively high purine content, increases have been made in milk, eggs, and cheese to maintain normal protein levels.

BREAKFAST

Fruit—citrus fruit or tomato juice
Cereal (except oatmeal), with cream or milk and sugar
Eggs—2
Toast (whole-grain or enriched white), with butter or enriched margarine. Jelly, jam, honey, or marmalade if desired
Beverages—decaffeinated coffee or cereal coffee with cream and sugar

LUNCH AND DINNER

Soup—milk soups made with any vegetables except those forbidden (see special instructions below)
Meat, fish, or fowl—only 2-oz. portion twice weekly, omitting glandular meats entirely; 2-oz. portion of cheese daily on days meat is not served
Vegetables—potato daily if desired; 2–4 additional vegetables (any except those on forbidden list)
Bread—whole-grain or enriched, with butter or enriched margarine
Dessert—fruit, puddings, cake, ice cream, gelatin desserts, or pie
Beverage—milk or buttermilk and decaffeinated coffee or cereal coffee

SPECIAL INSTRUCTIONS

1. Avoid liver, sweetbreads, brains, and kidney. A 2-oz. portion of any other meat, fish, or fowl may be served twice weekly.
2. Serve cheese and eggs as meat substitutes. Fish roe and caviar may be used as desired.
3. Use 1–2 pt. of milk daily to meet the protein need.
4. Omit all meat extracts, broth soups, and gravies.
5. Eliminate the following vegetables entirely from the diet: dried beans, lentils, dried peas, spinach.
6. Avoid coffee, tea, chocolate, and cocoa. Use decaffeinated coffee or a cereal coffee if desired. (There is some question as to whether or not caffeine can be converted into uric acid in the body.)
7. Omit alcoholic beverages of all kinds.
8. Allow fruits of all kinds—fresh, canned, and dried.
9. Allow cereals of all kinds except oatmeal.
10. Serve sugar as desired with amounts adjusted to caloric needs. Cream and butter may be restricted when a low-caloric allowance is needed or when a low-fat regimen is desired.

TABLE 33

PURINE CONTENT OF FOODS PER 100 GM.

Group I (0–15 Mg.)	Group II (50–150 Mg.)	Group III (150–800 Mg.)
Vegetables	Meats	Sweetbreads
Fruits	Fish	Anchovies
Milk	Sea food	Sardines
Cheese	Beans, dry	Liver
Eggs	Peas, dry	Kidney
Cereals	Lentils	Meat extracts
	Spinach	

TABLE 34

EVALUATION OF A BASIC PLAN FOR A LOW-PURINE DIET
(1,885 Calories; 70 Gm. Protein)

DAILY FOOD INTAKE	QUANTITY		CALORIES*	FOODSTUFFS			MINERALS		VITAMINS				
	Weight (Gm.)	Approximate Measure		Protein* (Gm.)	Fat* (Gm.)	Carbohydrate* (Gm.)	Ca (Mg.)	Fe (Mg.)	A (I.U.)	Ascorbic Acid (Mg.)	Thiamine (Mg.)	Riboflavin (Mg.)	Niacin (Mg.)
Milk, whole	976	1 quart	680	32	40	48	1,152	0.4	1,400	8	0.32	1.68	0.4
Egg	50	1 medium	75	7	5	...	27	1.1	590	...	0.05	0.15	Tr.
Cheese, cheddar	60	2 oz.	240	15	20	2	450	0.6	785	...	0.02	0.28	0.1
Bread, whole-grain or enriched white†	150	5 slices	350	10	...	75	102	3.9	Tr.	...	0.38	0.26	3.3
Cereal, whole-grain or enriched	20	½ cup, cooked	70	2	...	15	21	0.7	Tr.	...	0.07	0.05	0.7
Potato, cooked	100	1 small	70	2	...	15	5	0.5	Tr.	16	0.09	0.03	1.1
Vegetable (A)‡	150	2 servings	...	...	...	...	43	1.2	2,180	32	0.10	0.10	0.9
(B)§	50		20	1	...	4	12	0.5	1,660	5	0.03	0.03	0.4
Including deep green or yellow													
Fruit, citrus‖	100	1 serving	40	...	...	10	18	0.1	140	40	0.05	0.01	0.1
Other fruit#	...	2 servings	80	...	...	20	14	0.8	945	9	0.04	0.06	0.8
Subtotal	...	...	1,625	69	65	189	1,844	9.8	7,700	110	1.15	2.65	7.8
Sugar	20	4 teaspoons	80	...	...	20	...	...	...	...	...	...	...
Butter, fortified margarine or oil	20	4 teaspoons	180	...	20	...	...	...	660	...	...	...	...
Total**	...	...	1,885††	69	85	209	1,844	9.8	8,360	110	1.15	2.65	7.8

* Values for calories, carbohydrate, protein, and fat from the Food Exchange Lists, Table 20, have been used to evaluate foods and food groups.

† 30 gm. (1 oz.) has been the weight assigned to one slice of bread in the exchange lists. It is recognized that variation is common. Adjustments should be made where usage varies.

‡ Commonly used vegetables selected from the vegetable A group of the exchange lists were tomatoes, snap beans, asparagus, broccoli, cabbage, lettuce, and cucumber. It was estimated that these vegetables might be used 10 times weekly averaging 150 gm. daily. Weighting was adapted from Agriculture Handbook No. 215, *Consumption Trends and Patterns for Vegetables* ((U.S. Department of Agriculture, Economic and Statistical Analysis Division, Economic Research Service [July, 1961]).

§ It was assumed that the most commonly used vegetables from the vegetable B group of the exchange lists were peas, carrots, beets, and squash. It was estimated that these vegetables might be used 4 times weekly averaging 50 gm. daily. Weighting was adapted from Agriculture Handbook No. 215, *Consumption Trends and Patterns for Vegetables.*

‖ Fresh orange, fresh grapefruit, canned orange juice, blended grapefruit and orange and frozen citrus juice were considered to be commonly used citrus fruits or juice. Weighting was adapted from *Consumption of Food in the United States*, Supplement for 1962 to Agriculture Handbook No. 62 (U.S. Department of Agriculture, Agricultural Marketing Service [October, 1963]).

\# Apples, bananas, canned peaches, pineapples, pears, apricots, and plums were considered commonly used. Weighting was adapted from *Consumption of Food in the United States*, Supplement for 1962 to Agriculture Handbook No. 62.

** Meets Recommended Dietary Allowance (Table 3) for adult in good health except for iron.

†† Caloric needs should be adjusted to individual requirements. For variations in need, see Tables 3 and 5.

The approximate content of the above diet is 11 mg. of purine nitrogen or 34 mg. of uric acid. The normal diet plan as outlined in Table 2 contains approximately 132 mg. of purine nitrogen or 265 mg. of uric acid.

Table 33, adapted from Stare and Thorn (3), gives a rough approximation of the purine content of foods. Table 34 contains an enumeration and evaluation of the mineral, vitamin, carbohydrate, protein, and fat content of a low-purine diet. Modifications may be made to meet the needs of individual patients by making adjustments in any of the components of the diet.

REFERENCES

1. BARTELS, E. C. Successful treatment of gout, Ann. Int. Med., **18**:21–28, 1943.
2. DUCKLES, D. Purine and cholesterol content of foods, J. Am. Dietet. A., **15**:772–74, 1939.
3. STARE, F. J., and THORN, G. W. Protein nutrition in problems of medical interest, J.A.M.A., **127**:1120–27, 1945.

Chapter 11 | *Miscellaneous Modifications*

KETOGENIC DIETS

A ketogenic diet is one in which the proportion of carbohydrate, protein, and fat is regulated so that the ratio of the ketogenic to the antiketogenic values equals 2 or more or until it is sufficiently high to produce a ketosis (see Glossary).

Ketogenesis.—The production of the ketone bodies, that is, acetone, aceto-acetic acid, and beta-oxybutyric acid, is known as ketogenesis. The precursors of the ketone bodies are the fatty acids and certain of the amino acids such as phenylalanine, tyrosine, leucine, and histidine; these are known as "ketogenic substances." For clinical purposes the ketogenic portion of the diet may be estimated as 90 per cent of the weight of the fat and 50 per cent of the protein.

Antiketogenesis.—Carbohydrate and the amino acids, such as alanine and glycine which are convertible to glucose in the body, tend to prevent the accumulation of ketone bodies and are said to be "antiketogenic." Approximately 10 per cent of the weight of the fat in the diet, 50 per cent of the protein, and 100 per cent of the carbohydrate may be estimated as the antiketogenic portion. When the supply of carbohydrate is inadequate, ketogenesis becomes predominant.

Plan of daily food intake.—If the basic plan of normal diet contains carbohydrate, 150 gm.; protein, 70 gm.; and fat, 70 gm., the ketogenic to antiketogenic ratio is 1:2. To reverse this ratio and produce a ketosis, it is necessary to reduce the carbohydrate and change the proportions approximately to carbohydrate, 20 gm.; protein, 70 gm.;

and fat, 125 gm. When a higher caloric intake is desired, the carbohydrate may be slightly increased. Thus, for a 1,860-calorie diet (Table 35), the distribution could be carbohydrate, 35 gm.; protein, 70 gm.; and fat, 160 gm.

Preparation.—This diet is likely to be unpalatable, expensive, and difficult to follow. Some degree of acceptability may be obtained, however, by the following measures:

Cream of high fat content may be used in ice cream, custards, and other desserts, as well as in salad dressings and soups. Saccharin may be used for sweetening.

The fruits and vegetables used should be those of minimum carbohydrate content and may be served in salads with oil dressings or hot in cream soups. Gelatin sweetened with saccharin may be used for desserts.

Washed-bran wafers may be offered as a bread substitute. Soybean muffins offer a low-carbohydrate bread substitute.

ACIDIC AND BASIC ELEMENTS IN THE DIET

The major mineral elements which are evaluated when an estimate is made of the acid ash residue or the alkaline ash residue of the diet are sodium, potassium, calcium, magnesium, phosphorus, sulfur, and chlorine.

In evaluating the acid ash residue, the inorganic constituents—chlorine, sulfur, and phosphorus, which form acid ions (anions) in the body, namely, chloride, sulfate, and phosphate—are measured as the amount of tenth-normal alkali required for neutralization. In appraising the alkaline ash residue, the inorganic constituents—sodium, potassium, calcium, and magnesium, which form basic ions (cations) in the body—are measured as the amount of tenth-normal acid required for neutralization.

An acid-forming (acidogenic) diet is an allowance of foods having a total anion-forming ash content that is equivalent to 10–20 cc. of tenth-normal acid in excess of the total cation-forming ash, which will be equivalent to 30–35 cc. of tenth-normal alkali when milk, fruits, and vegetables are included as in the normal diet; proteins, minerals, and vitamins remain at levels necessary for nutritive sufficiency (see Glossary).

An alkali-forming (alkalinogenic) diet is an allowance of foods

TABLE 35

EVALUATION OF A BASIC PLAN FOR A KETOGENIC DIET
(Carbohydrate 35 Gm.; Protein 70 Gm.; Fat 160 Gm.; Calories 1,860)

DAILY FOOD INTAKE	QUANTITY		CALORIES	FOODSTUFFS			MINERALS		VITAMINS				
	Weight (Gm.)	Approximate Measure		Protein (Gm.)	Fat (Gm.)	Carbohydrate (Gm.)	Ca (Mg.)	Fe (Mg.)	A (I.U.)	Ascorbic Acid (Mg.)	Thiamine (Mg.)	Riboflavin (Mg.)	Niacin (Mg.)
Milk, whole*	100	3/8 cup	65	3	4	5	118	Tr.	140	1	0.03	0.17	0.1
Cream, 20 per cent*	100	3/8 cup	210	3	20	4	102	Tr.	840	1	0.03	0.15	0.1
Eggs†	100	2 medium	150	14	10	...	54	2.2	1,180	...	0.10	0.30	Tr.
Meat, poultry, or fish*	180	6 oz. E.P.	450	42	30	...	24	5.1	50	...	0.60	0.38	8.9
Bacon*	32	4 strips	210	8	20	...	4	1.0	...	...	0.15	0.10	1.6
Vegetable (A)†	150	2 servings	...	...	...	...	43	1.2	2,180	32	0.10	0.10	0.9
(B)†	50		20	1	...	4	12	0.5	1,660	5	0.03	0.03	0.4
Including deep-green or yellow													
Fruit, citrus†	100	1 serving	40	...	...	10	18	0.1	140	40	0.05	0.01	0.1
Other fruit†	...	1 serving	40	...	...	10	7	0.4	475	5	0.02	0.03	0.4
Butter, fortified margarine or oil†	75	1/3 cup	675	...	75	...	...	...	2,100	...	...	...	...
Total‡	...	...	1,860	71	159	33	382	10.5	8,765	84	1.11	1.27	12.5

* Values for nutrients from Table 36.

† Values for carbohydrate, protein, fat from Exchange Lists (Tables 21–29).

‡ Meets Recommended Dietary Allowances (Table 3) for adult in good health except for calcium, iron, thiamine, and riboflavin.

having a total cation-forming ash content that is equivalent to 20 cc. or more of tenth-normal alkali in excess of the total anion-forming ash, which will be equivalent to 25 cc. or less of tenth-normal acid; proteins, minerals, and vitamins remain at levels necessary for nutritive sufficiency.

In general, it can be said that vegetable and fruits are predominantly basic, whereas cereals, meats, poultry, and fish are predominanantly acidic in residue. Most fruits, in spite of their acidity, exert a basic effect on the body, since a number of organic acid radicals, such as citrate and malate, may be oxidized completely to carbon dioxide and water, leaving the salts to contribute to the supply of basic elements in the residue. A few organic acids such as benzoic and quinic acids, however, are not so oxidized, and hence contribute to the total acidity. Cranberries, plums, and prunes are examples of such fruits. Exceptions have been found, however, in certain varieties of prunes and plums (1). Foods which exert no acidic or basic effect are refined sugar, butter, lard, oil, cornstarch, and tapioca. Molasses is strongly basic in residue, with an excess of 59.4 cc. of tenth-normal base per 190 gm. Information relating to the excess acid and base values may be found in Table 42, taken from Bridges and Mattice (2).

REFERENCES

1. TURNER, D., and PARSONS, H. Not all plums and prunes acid-forming when used in human diet. In: Annual report of the director, 1930–31. Madison: Agricultural Experiment Station, University of Wisconsin, 1932 (Bull. 421), p. 121.
2. MATTICE, M. R. Bridges' food and beverage analyses, 3d revised ed. Philadelphia: Lea & Febiger, 1950, pp. 201–32.

SECTION III | INTERVIEWING THE PATIENT

Chapter 12 Interviewing the Patient[1]

by Margaret Mead

Formerly
Executive Secretary, Committee on Food Habits, National Research Council, Washington, D.C.

The modern trend in therapy is to consider the patient as a whole personality in a social setting[2] and to regard as significant and important every therapeutic contact with the physician, with medical or family caseworker, and with the dietitian. It is realized that, to obtain the best results, specialists must, in addition to performing their special tasks, co-operate in a common therapeutic task—the work and skill of one complementing that of the others. The increased emphasis upon the importance of the patient's whole personality makes new demands upon the dietitian as increased knowledge shows the many ways in which specific food behavior, as well as disease pictures requiring special diets, are themselves concomitants of deep-seated personality distortions and overemphasis.[3]

1. This discussion draws upon materials contributed by the large group of members of The American Dietetic Association who co-operated in the project of the Diet Therapy Section on Food and Emotions during 1942–44, which was undertaken in co-operation with the Committee on Food Habits, National Research Council; and the case histories were analyzed by Dr. Margaret Mead, executive secretary of that committee. Received for publication, February 5, 1945. From *Journal of The American Dietetic Association*, Vol. 21, No. 7, July–August, 1945.

2. H. B. Richardson, *Patients Have Families* (New York: Commonwealth Fund, 1944); also G. C. Robinson, *The Patient as a Person* (New York: Commonwealth Fund, 1939).

3. F. Alexander, The influence of psychologic factors upon gastro-intestinal disturbances: a symposium: a report upon research carried on at the University of Chicago Institute for Psychoanalysis. I. General principles, objectives, and preliminary results. Summarized in Psychosom. Med., 1:429, 1939. See also the following: H. Bruch, *Ad-*

Just as at an earlier period in the development of dietetic practice the dietitian learned to understand the extent to which aspects of the patient's behavior in the dietetic interview might be referred to a need for attention, to a desire to show off, or to the gratification of long-denied needs for a relationship with another human being who appeared to take an interest in one's health and fate, now there is a need to integrate into dietetic practice the new findings based upon the work of psychiatrists exploring the new field of psychosomatic medicine. If this integration is to keep pace with the growing discoveries in this field, it must take place not only in the professional schools as new students enter dietetics and in the training for internships of recent graduates but also in the established practice within the hospital and food clinic. In the professional schools young dietitians can profit by instruction from psychiatrists; in the operating clinical situation the new methods can spread best by self-aware teamwork in which the dietitian re-evaluates her current procedures in the light of increasing knowledge of the patient's whole personality and takes it upon herself to communicate to her colleagues—the physician, the psychiatrist, the medical caseworker, and the nurse—just what the possibilities of a dietetic interview are in terms of an all-round therapy designed to meet the needs of the patient as a whole personality who emerges from the hospital to live in a real social situation.

One of the ways in which this increased awareness on the part of the dietitian may be developed is by a consideration of the different roles in which the dietitian sees herself, in which the patient sees her, and in which her professional colleagues in related professions see her. The role of the dietitian is subject to great variation in scope, from that of someone who merely works out a list of foods based

---

justment to Dietary Changes in Various Somatic Disorders, in the Problem of Changing Food Habits (Committee on Food Habits, National Research Council Bull. 108 [Washington, 1943]), p. 66; H. Bruch and G. Touraine, Obesity in childhood. V. The family frame of obese children, Psychosom. Med., **2**:141–206, 1940; H. Bruch, Food and emotional security, in *The Nervous Child,* **3**:165. Also M. Mead, Dietary patterns and food habits, J. Am. Dietet. A., **19**:1, 1943; L. Rahman, H. B. Richardson, and H. S. Ripley, Anorexia nervosa with psychiatric observations, Psychosom. Med., **1**:335, 1939; J. V. Waller, R. M. Kaufman, and F. Deutsch, Anorexia nervosa, a psychosomatic entity, Psychosom. Med., Vol. **2**, No. 1, 1940; B. Mittelmann, H. G. Wolff, and M. P. Scharf, Emotions and gastroduodenal function: experimental studies on patients with gastritis, duodenitis, and peptic ulcer, Psychosom. Med., **4**:5–61, 1942.

upon a physician's prescription and the age and body weight and degree of activity of the patient, through to the concepts of the worker in a food clinic (*a*) as a specialist who can *translate* for the patient-client a *regime* prescribed by the physician into exact amounts and kinds of foods prepared in specific ways; (*b*) as a specialist in the relationship between food and bodily needs who can *guide* the patient-client in making a selection of foods which will produce changes or maintain a given bodily state; (*c*) as a specialist in all the *problems of adjustment* which an individual faces in one facet of his or her existence—the consumption of food, including budgetary problems, conditions of preparation, etc.; and (*d*) as a *member of a team* of therapists—including the physician, psychiatrist, caseworker, public health nurse—in which case the specific type of help and instruction which the dietitian gives must be keyed to the treatment being given by the whole team and oriented not only to the physical needs of the patient-client but to his whole personality.

Each of these roles, or any combination of them, has to be clear to the dietitian and to the patient; and, if the referral from physician or caseworker has not indicated to the patient what role the dietitian plays, it is necessary for her to indicate it herself. This can usually be done best if the dietitian takes a minute to discover what the patient has been led to expect and then elaborates upon and corrects that impression. But a clear definition of why the dietitian is there, what the referring specialist has asked her to do, and what the patient may and may not expect is very important if the dietetic interview is to have its fullest usefulness. Roles *a* and *b* are discussed in the preceding sections. This present section is concerned primarily with roles *c* and *d*.

As growing interest and research amplify the scope of the dietitian's work and bring into it an increasing knowledge of social conditions, of personality dynamics, and of the process of therapy as an interpersonal relationship, it is important that these new emphases should not obscure the dietitian's distinctive role as a specialist in the adjustment between bodily needs and eating habits. It is important that she should include in the interview as many as possible of the insights and procedures which make for a good interview, whether conducted by physician, caseworker, or any other specialist in human relations. But it is also necessary that she do definite and concrete teaching about foods, the nature of the particular diet, how it may be calculated, and how the recommended amounts and proportions may be obtained within the framework of the patient's habit patterns. While it is true that, in the past, physicians and caseworkers have underestimated the general therapeutic implications of the dietetic interview and regarded the dietitian as an automatic source of information upon which the patient would inevitably act, it would easily be possible to err in the other direction and demand so much caseworking skill from the dietitian that her necessary and distinctive teaching function would be obscured.

This distinctive character of the dietetic interview imposes definite limitations upon its form. The dietitian must teach concrete, precise material. She must, whenever possible, also convey to the patient some sense of the principles upon which her concrete teaching is based, and in practically every instance she has to persuade the patient to do something which is painful, that is, to attend, from a new point of view, to the details of diet. This is painful because in our society the conscious application of thought—especially of measuring, counting, calculating, estimating—to an aspect of life which is ordinarily associated with gratification of the senses is regarded as reducing pleasure. Reduction in pleasure is likely to be resisted, except by those patients whose peculiar character formation makes them enjoy deprivation, and such patients will present other problems equally difficult to the therapist. However, attempts to make the following of a diet meaningful can be highly successful. The dietitian may expect the patient to feel that her advice is definitely useful if she makes the diet prescription intelligible and easier to follow, makes the goal of loss or gain in weight or a very altered pattern of intake possible of attainment, and makes the diet itself reasonably related to the patient's own bodily state and not an arbitrary set of rules. But the dietitian *cannot* expect to make the following of a diet a pleasure-giving experience, and efforts to clothe the interview in such terms are likely to be disappointing. Many instances have been reported where the patient has developed a tie to the dietitian and improved in health and functioning because someone was taking an interest in him, but this usually means that the dietitian has had to overstep her role and engage in casework for which she may not have been specially trained and at the expense of giving other patients specific dietary help.

The dietetic interview remains an interview between a specialist-in-food-adjustments and a patient-who-needs-to-learn-something-about-his-diet, and all improvements in procedure must necessarily take this core into account.

EXTENSION OF THE DIETITIAN'S SKILL IN HELPING THE PATIENT ADJUST HIS FOOD HABITS

Recognition of the importance of treating the patient as a whole personality, with a specific cultural background and real life-situation, leads to the inclusion in the dietetic interview of an attempt to get some understanding of the patient's personality, what his reaction is to the diagnosis which has brought him there, what motives may be invoked in teaching new food patterns, and what special resistances have to be overcome. This preliminary exploration of the patient's personality can take place within the framework of the dietetic interview itself and need not wander to wider topics. The more knowledge the dietitian has of the human personality, the better. She needs to be aware of such special problems of childhood as the conflict between dependence upon the mother and the need to be independent, which is likely to express itself strongly in the field of eating, or of the adolescent desire to be like other young people, as illustrated in the following:

EXTRACT FROM AN INTERVIEW WITH A THIRTEEN-YEAR-OLD DIABETIC GIRL

Patient had come in crying, after a two-month absence, and her tests showed sugar.

DIETITIAN: Why K, what seems to be the trouble? You've always had such a nice smile.

PATIENT: Oh, I've been hungry since school started and have eaten more than I should have—even candy sometimes. I just can't help it when all the others can have everything. I *hate* school.

D: What would you like to have to eat? We should be able to get together on this and plan your meals the way you want them.

P: Oh, *could* you? I'd love to have more bread, dessert once in a while, a little gum and candy.

D: Have you ever tried D-Zerta or candy or gum sweetened with saccharin? D-Zerta is a gelatin dessert and can be used in many ways, such as with whipped cream or with fruit. [*D. conferred with doctor.*] If you like, we might increase the amount of insulin and your food allowance to include another slice of bread and a couple of pieces of candy.

P: Why, that will make my meals practically the same as all the other girls! That's swell!

The patient came in once a month from then on. She was happy, felt well, liked school, and tests were good.

The foregoing illustrates the methods of a dietitian who responded sensitively to the evidences of distress and placed them in context against the patient's previous behavior. She estimated carefully the importance—to an adolescent—of behaving like the other girls and so evaluated correctly the phrase, "I *hate* school," treated the dietary prescriptions as flexible and capable of adjustment to a genuine need on the part of the patient, and succeeded in establishing the patient in an adequate adjustment.

Each age, each sex, has its special problems. For old age it is important to realize that the patient needs to be treated with the respect due to age and experience of life, yet protected, by written advice for instance, from a growing forgetfulness. Thus increased understanding of different regularities of this sort provides a background for a better understanding of personality.

Knowledge of the patient's cultural background—whether from a rural American home; from a foreign-born family's home; from a minority group, which almost inevitably means poor housing and limited household equipment; from a home where religious usages are observed; or from a type of home where no traditional practices may be relied upon, as when mountain people of the South are transplanted to a northern or western area where all the ways of living are unfamiliar—helps the dietitian to make her teaching realistic and relevant. The more she knows of these differences in dietary practice from one socioeconomic group to another and from one nationality background to another, the surer will be her understanding of the patient's questions or probable confusions, misunderstandings, or embarrassments.

A skilled dietitian will also take into account the patient's social situation in terms of status, occupation, income, and living arrangements—making specific allowance for the difficulties of the patient who lives in a cheap club for girls, the bus driver, or the elevator operator; the domestic servant, who is likely to nibble; the underprivileged mother of young children, who is likely to skimp her own diet to feed them better; the housewife, who must shop on a hand-to-mouth basis or who works and must leave the shopping to a small child; the three-shift household with its irregular meals; and the family in an overcrowded district that has only restricted kitchen privileges. Imaginative inclusion within the dietetic interview of the reality situation of the patient goes a long way toward insuring its success and has high general therapeutic value in increasing the patients' sense that the dietitian is someone who is treating them as they really are—people with ten minutes for lunch, people who have iceboxes but cannot afford to run them, people who are too poor to shop in chain stores where cash must be paid and who depend instead on credit.[4]

A knowledge of current prices, scarcities, and abundances, of current food fads among young people, and of the trend of radio advertising—especially for children—is also important in helping the dietitian to make it seem possible for the patient to follow her instructions easily. While every physician and every nurse should understand the basic principles of nutrition, it devolves upon the dietitian to translate this knowledge into everyday practice in terms of the needs, the intelligence, the emotional attitudes, and the actual situation of each patient.

THE DIETITIAN AS A MEMBER OF A THERAPEUTIC TEAM

The dietitian's functioning in the therapeutic team in hospital or clinic may be considered from three points of view: (1) referral to the dietitian; (2) the dietetic interview or series of interviews; (3) referral from the dietitian, or case report to some other member of the team.

Referral to the dietitian.—At present, referral to the dietitian comes usually from the physician if the need is a medical one and from the caseworker if it is a matter of home management. The physician tends to limit himself to such phrases as "reducing diet," "low-fat diet," "high-caloric diet," "high-vitamin diet," "bland diet," and to omit any information on the patient's personality, capacity to

4. Background materials for the inclusion in dietetic practice of cultural and socio-economic factors may be found among the materials developed at the Boston Dispensary Food Clinic by Frances Stern; at the Community Service Society, New York, by Lucy Gillett; and materials currently issued by the Massachusetts Department of Health and the Committee on Food Habits, National Research Council.

follow directions, the role that the patient's illness plays in the patient's life, etc. Upon the hospital dietitian devolves the task of developing such a working relationship with the physician that, instead of saying, "Stop in and see Miss Jones, the dietitian, and she'll give you your diet," the physician will realize the importance of an interpretative referral and say: "Now Miss X, you will need some help in planning the diet which I have prescribed for you. You'll find that Miss Y, our dietitian who specializes in helping people adjust their meals to their particular health needs, will help you work out the details." With increasingly good working relationships between other therapists and the dietitian, the physician and the caseworker also come to appreciate the importance of giving the dietitian clues about the personality of the patient, namely, summaries of what otherwise would often demand many hours of contact with the patient and experience with the way he responds to different types of suggestions; warnings about ways in which the patient will try to use a relationship; and diagnosis of the role that eating plays in the patient's life—as the only available form of sense gratification, as a reaction to mood, as a method of punishing other people or the self, etc. The interested dietitian can accustom physicians to including such suggestions in their referrals. Thus the dietetic interview will get off to a quick start, the patient will be better oriented in what to expect, and the dietitian already alert to some of the patient's most conspicuous characteristics.

The dietetic interview.—The extent to which the dietetic interview itself becomes an integral part of the treatment of a patient who, in addition to being cured of a specific disease condition or taught to keep the disease under control, is also being adjusted as a whole to a life-situation, depends not only on the dietitian's knowledge of personality but on the knowledge of other members of the therapeutic team concerning the character of dietetic interviews in that particular dietetic department of their own hospital or clinic. Too often physicians, caseworkers, and nurses include in their planning for patients their picture of a dietetic interview, experienced or witnessed twenty years ago, in quite another setting. They may actually seek to prepare the patient for, or seek to adjust subsequent treatment to, a dietetic interview very different from that which the patient actually experiences. This ever present danger can be guarded against by the dietitian's assuming responsibility for seeing that the other members of the therapeutic team actually know what her practice and that of her staff are, what types of alternatives are recognized in adjusting different kinds of patients to the same general dietary prescription, how much detailed instruction is actually involved, and what sorts of aids, written schedules, models, scales, slides, charts, etc., she uses. Adequate exposure of physicians and caseworkers to the procedure of a dietetic department will result in their raising questions about the possibilities inherent in the situation, which in turn will assist the dietitian in orienting her practice to their premises and deepen her knowledge of the emotional factors with which she has to deal.

Referral from the dietitian and case reports.—As the dietitian works more in a team, the other members of which know what her special skills actually are, both she and they will recognize ways in which material gleaned in the dietetic interview may be used as an indicator of the patient's problems or progress. A series of dietetic interviews is sometimes an excellent device for maintaining contact with a patient, especially if the dietitian is alert to signs of improvement or deterioration, of indications of developing conditions—as when a problem which at first looked like simple malnutrition begins to show signs of anorexia nervosa. Attempts to fit the dietetic interview into an integrated pattern of treatment are an excellent device for focusing more attention upon the whole personality of the patient, thereby making the treatment more effective.

REFERENCES

1. ALDRICH, C. K. Prescribing a diet is not enough, J. Am. Dietet. A., **33**: 785–87, 1957.
2. BABCOCK, CHARLOTTE G. Psychologically significant factors in the nutrition interview, J. Am. Dietet. A., **23**:8–12, 1947.
3. ———. Food and its emotional significance, *ibid.*, **24**:390–93, 1948.
4. ———. Problems in sustaining the nutritional care of the patient, *ibid.*, **28**:222–27, 1952.
5. ———. Comments on human interrelations, *ibid.*, **33**:871–79, 1957.
6. BAYLES, S., and EBAUGH, F. G. Emotional factors in eating and obesity, J. Am. Dietet. A., **26**:430–34, 1950.
7. BERGEVIN, P. Telling vs. teaching—learning by participation, J. Am. Dietet. A., **33**:781–84, 1957.
8. BRENER, R. Dietitian and patient: evaluation of an interpersonal relationship, J. Am. Dietet. A., **28**:515–19, 1952.

9. BRUCH, HILDE. The importance of overweight. New York: W. W. Norton & Co., Inc., 1957.
10. COWING, A. G. Readable writing, J. Am. Dietet. A., **23**:1036–40, 1947.
11. ———. Writing that sells good diet, *ibid.*, **24**:592–94, 1948.
12. DONAHUE, W. T. Psychologic aspects of feeding the aged, J. Am. Dietet. A., **27**:461–66, 1951.
13. ENGLISH, O. SPURGEON. Psychosomatic medicine and dietetics, J. Am. Dietet. A., **27**:721–25, 1951.
14. EPPRIGHT, E. S. Factors influencing food acceptance, J. Am. Dietet. A., **23**:579–87, 1947.
15. FLESCH, R. The art of plain talk. New York: Harper & Bros., 1946.
16. ———. The art of readable writing. New York: Harper & Bros., 1949.
17. GALDSTON, IAGO. Motivation in health education, J. Am. Dietet. A., **25**: 745–51, 1949.
18. ———. Nutrition from the psychiatric viewpoint, *ibid.*, **28**:405–9, 1952.
19. GARRETT, ANNETTE. Interviewing: its principles and methods. New York: Family Service Association of America, 1950.
20. GEBHARD, B. Exhibit planning and analysis, J. Am. Dietet. A., **24**:394–98, 1948.
21. HALL, DOROTHY. The dietetic interview as a tool in changing food habits, J. Am. Dietet. A., **22**:999–1002, 1946.
22. HAMBURGER, W. W. The psychology of weight reduction: the initial nutritional interview; the nutritionist-patient relationship; and complications of weight reduction, J. Am. Dietet. A., **34**:17–22, 1958.
23. HOULE, C. O. The dietitian as a teacher of adults, J. Am. Dietet. A., **24**: 837–40, 1948.
24. HYMES, J. L. Significance of feeding from the viewpoint of child development, J. Am. Dietet. A., **25**:611–12, 1949.
25. ILG, F. L. The child's idea of what and how to eat, J. Am. Dietet. A., **24**: 658–60, 1948.
26. KREITLOW, B. W. Teaching adults democratically, J. Am. Dietet. A., **33**: 788–92, 1957.
27. LEACH, J. M. Motivating people to use educational material, J. Am. Dietet. A., **29**:245–47, 1953.
28. MEAD, MARGARET. Cultural patterning of nutritionally relevant behavior J. Am. Dietet. A., **25**:677–80, 1949.
29. MILLER, C. D. Food and food habits in the Hawaiian Islands, J. Am. Dietet. A., **27**:461–66, 1951.
30. MITCHELL, HELEN S., and JOFFE, NATALIE F. Food patterns of some European countries: background for study programs and guidance of relief workers, J. Am. Dietet. A., **24**:676–87, 1944.
31. POSZ, A. C. Do you irritate others when you listen? J. Am. Dietet. A., **34**: 730–32, 1958.
32. PRAGOFF, HALE. Areas of cooperation between medical social workers and dietitians, J. Am. Dietet. A., **24**:485–90, 1948.
33. RABINOVITCH, R. D., and FISCHHOFF, J. Feeding in childhood to meet emotional needs: a survey of the psychologic implications of eating, J. Am. Dietet. A., **28**:614–21, 1952.
34. RADKE, MARIAN, and CASO, E. K. Experiments in changing food habits, J. Am. Dietet. A., **23**:403–9, 1947.

35. ———. Lecture and discussion—decision as method of influencing food habits, *ibid.*, **24**:23–31, 1948.
36. SPENCER, M. E. An educator talks about motivating people, J. Am. Dietet. A., **25**:209–12, 1949.
37. TOWLE, C. Common human needs. ("Public Assistance Reports," No. 8.) Washington: Federal Security Agency, 1945.
38. TRULSON, M., WALSH, E. D., and CASO, E. K. A study of obese patients in a nutrition clinic, J. Am. Dietet. A., **23**:941–46, 1947.
39. WALSH, ETHEL. Nutritionists and social workers cooperate on mutual problems, J. Am. Dietet. A., **25**:681–83, 1949.
40. WHITE, G. The patient as the focus of attention, J. Am. Dietet. A., **30**:25–28, 1954.
41. DEPARTMENT OF PEDIATRICS, UNIVERSITY OF CHICAGO. Liberal infant feeding, J. Am. Dietet. A., **22**:622–24, 1946.
42. Motivation in health education. (The 1947 Health Education Conference of the New York Academy of Medicine.) New York: Columbia University Press, 1948.
43. MARGARET MEAD. Food Habits Research: Problems of the 1960's. NAS-NRC Publication 1225, Washington, D.C. 1964.
44. The Problem of Changing Food Habits (1943), Bull. 108.
45. Manual for the Study of Food Habits (1945), Bull. 111 from Printing and Publishing Office, NAS, Washington, D.C. 20418.

SECTION IV | EXPANDING OPPORTUNITIES IN THE PRACTICE OF DIET THERAPY

Chapter 13 Expanding Opportunities in the Practice of Diet Therapy

by Mildred Kaufman

Nutrition Consultant, Diabetes and Arthritis Branch, Division of Chronic Diseases, Public Health Service, Washington, D.C.

It is the responsibility of the dietitian and public health nutritionist to assist patients to apply in their daily lives the current scientific knowledge of nutrition and diet therapy. As their contribution to medical care, the dietitian and nutritionist should be expected to assess the patient's dietary needs, interpret these to the physician and other members of the health team, and implement this aspect of care with the patient.

It has recently been pointed out that

> to meet the changing health needs of our changing population a new concept of patient care is developing. It envisions a wide spectrum of medical and health service facilities—coordinated on a community-wide basis for both in-patient and out-patient care. It is designed to provide continuity of care in line with the patient's need and current medical knowledge (1).

This suggests that if the dietitian or public health nutritionist is to move with this trend, each must widen her horizons to encompass the entire continuum of medical care. Each must define her responsibilities to the in-patient cared for in the hospital, nursing home, or rehabilitation center; to the ambulatory patient seen in the doctor's office, out-patient clinic, or health center; and to the patient cared for in his own home. The dietitian or public health nutritionist must deepen her background in the basic sciences, the science of nutrition and therapeutic dietetics to fully develop her role as a consultant to her professional colleagues. And she must sharpen her understanding of the behavioral sciences and skills in educational methodology to be an effective counselor to patients and their families. It is a challenge to the dietitian or nutritionist to clearly state her contributions to patient care and delineate her functions. She must interpret to administrators and fellow workers that the job of modifying patterns of eating to improve dietary practices or as a part of therapy demands not only knowledge and skills, but the time, patience, and the ability to work with each individual at his own pace. In Chapter 12 on "Interviewing the Patient," Margaret Mead pictures the scope of responsibility of the dietitian and nutritionist in changing food habits, and suggests the perceptiveness that must be cultivated to counsel patients effectively.

A constructive diet therapy program requires the interaction of the dietitian or nutritionist with the physician, nurse, and social worker, along with the most important member of the team, the patient. With the trend toward enlarging the skills applied in health care this involvement can be extended to include the psychiatrist, dentist, health educator, physical, occupational, and speech therapist, and others. Auxiliary workers, such as the aide in the hospital or homemaker in home care, also assume responsibilities related to diet and become part of the team. Shorter periods of hospitalization and the increasing use of nursing home and home care services put stress on planning for continuity of care between the hospital, nursing home, and the home. The dietitian, with other staff in the hospital and out-patient clinic, must coordinate her efforts with those of the public health nutritionist and related health workers in the community who provide services to patients in their homes. Without coordination the only result can be confusion and frustration for the patient and his family.

To mobilize all of the resources, coordinate the variety of efforts, and provide meaningful dietary counseling, it is necessary for the dietitian and nutritionist to use every available channel of communication. To fully meet her responsibilities in patient care the dietitian or nutritionist must be able to communicate easily with (1) the patient and his family, (2) her professional co-workers, and (3) the staff of other community agencies.

COMMUNICATION WITH THE PATIENT

Learning about the patient's food intake.—Through the process of dietary counseling the dietitian or nutritionist seeks to guide the patient to make those changes in his eating pattern that are necessary to improve his health. Since it is difficult for most patients to change firmly-rooted food habits, it is imperative that changes not be suggested unless they are necessary. Those changes which are recommended should be consistent with the patient's age, cultural background, financial situation, religious observances, present living situation, daily routine, and individual food preferences. The dietitian or nutritionist takes a giant stride toward the successful practice of diet therapy by identifying and understanding the distinguishing characteristics and variety of needs displayed by each individual she sees.

The basic tool for learning about the patient and his diet is a diet history or a record of past eating patterns. A written record from the patient of his current food practices provides the means for the diet counselor to become acquainted with the patient, and for the patient to develop an awareness of his own food intake. The food record provides the basis for assessment of the patient's diet and for developing an appropriate plan to meet his food needs. The nutrient analysis of dietary practices with which the dietitian or nutritionist can provide the physician can help him interpret some of the laboratory and clinical findings. An assessment of the patient's food habits further serves as a guide to the physician in prescribing the most appropriate and acceptable diet for the patient. For the dietitian or nutritionist the record of past eating practices serves importantly as the starting point for counseling about diet.

The tool for obtaining dietary information should be designed by the dietitian or nutritionist in collaboration with the physician and other interested co-workers. Guiding considerations in developing the device should be (*a*) the kind and amount of dietary information required, how it is to be evaluated and used, (*b*) the characteristics of the patient population—educational level, degree of physical, mental, and emotional incapacity, whether the patient is being seen in the hospital, the out-patient clinic, the office, or the home, and (*c*) the characteristics of the staff using the tool—the amount of time they can devote to obtaining the dietary information and their skill in interviewing.

Two distinct methods of collecting food intake information have been identified. Both of these methods which have been used in research are also applicable to planning for the dietary aspects of patient care. One of these methods is based upon record of food intake or diary in which meal by meal notes are kept of all food eaten during a stated period of time. The other approach to the diet history is based upon a detailed verbal statement of food consumed during the recent past. This may be for the past day, or two days, or a description of the "usual" food pattern. (2)

The record of food intake should be kept by the patient or those who care for him either at home, in the hospital, or in the nursing home. The format for record keeping at home can be simple, including sufficient space to write down all food eaten at each meal and between meals in estimated or measured amounts, and to describe the method of preparation. Such a record has the advantage of showing the actual food eaten and the variations from day to day. In the hospital the food consumed should be accurately observed, assessed, and recorded as part of the medical record. Recognizing the importance of food on the patient's progress in the hospital, the Joint Commission on Accreditation of Hospitals now asks whether notes on the patient's food intake are being included in the medical record. (3) In using and interpreting the patient's food intake while he is in the hospital, it should be remembered that for many reasons the kind and amount of food the individual eats in the hospital may be different from what he eats at home.

A food record is also needed from patients in a nursing home, under home care, or for those who are being seen regularly in the office or out-patient clinic. For patients at home, the record usually covers a stated period of time, a minimum of three days being desirable. Obvious disadvantages of the food record kept by the patient are that he may omit items, describe amounts incorrectly, or he may make some changes in his habits during the period recorded. However, many patients find the discipline of keeping a food record helpful in modifying their eating habits and the changes they make can indicate their knowledge about diet. For patients at home who have writing or language difficulties, someone else in the home may be able to keep the record.

An interview is commonly used to "recall" food intake information, particularly in the out-patient clinic, office, or home. Obtaining a detailed diet history is a time-consuming procedure which cannot be hurried. When good rapport is achieved and the dietitian is relaxed and an educated listener, the conference provides many additional, useful insights into the abilities, attitudes, and personality of the patient. Frequently an outline or interview form is used to structure the discussion. However, in designing such a form, a conversational approach should be preserved. Open-ended statements such as, "Tell me what you usually eat for breakfast," are more productive than leading questions like, "Do you drink orange juice for breakfast?" Questions leading to a "Yes" or "No" reply should be used only after the patient has had an uninterrupted opportunity to describe his eating practices in his own words. The meal pattern can be identified by asking the respondent to recall all of the food eaten during the previous 24 to 48 hours, or by asking him to describe his "usual" meals and snacks. The risk in recalling the previous day is that the day cited may not be typical. On the other hand, if the individual has erratic ways of eating, the "usual" meals may be difficult for him to describe and his replies may be misleading. With perceptive use, a cross-check for both of these methods should be possible by determining the frequency with which a wide variety of individual food items are eaten. Desserts, sweets, soft drinks, and alcoholic beverages must be included on the check list along with a wide variety of the basic food items—milk, eggs, cheeses, meats, fats, breads, cereals, fruits, vegetables. Although the check list should be constructed to include all the foods most commonly used locally, the interviewer should be alert to any additional items eaten which may not be on the list. While asking about frequency of consumption of each specific food item, it also is helpful to ask the patient to indicate his like or dislike for it.

Other ways of obtaining information about eating patterns may be possible with persons who express themselves easily in writing. For example, a food preference questionnaire requires only a short form with questions stated simply and clearly so that patients can complete the form themselves with little or no assistance. Questions must be appropriately worded to elicit the desired information. To gain the patient's cooperation, the worker using the form should take a few minutes to explain the purpose and use of the questionnaire and to give instructions on the degree of detail expected in the responses. This approach has the advantage of taking less time for the dietitian who is unable to spend the longer period required for the detailed diet-history interview. Meanwhile the patient is free to give considered responses and to take the time he needs to write the answers to the questionnaire thoughtfully. The form should be given to the patient to complete at a time when he will not be distracted or under pressure. Upon its completion the form must be reviewed by the dietitian with the patient to give them an opportunity to discuss and amplify responses. Those patients who are unable or unwilling to complete the questionnaire should not be urged to use it. In fact, unwillingness may be a significant clue concerning attitudes toward diagnosis, dietary restriction, or the authority of those involved in the dietary treatment. For such patients the more personal approach to the dietary interview is preferable. The food preference questionnaire appears to be particularly useful for hospitalized patients, but it can be used with patients seen in the office, clinic, or at home.

Learning about the patient's needs and problems.—In addition to the information about the meal pattern, some additional questions must be asked to learn how the patient feels about the dietary changes to be recommended, and to determine his ability and motivation to change his food habits. For these purposes answers must be obtained to the following:

What does the patient know about his present health problem and about its dietary treatment?

What past experiences has this patient had with a diet prescribed by a physician?

What feelings does the patient have about his ability to change his present eating pattern or about the suggested dietary treatment?

What foods are particularly important to this individual and would be most difficult for him to do without?

What foods can he not eat because of allergy, intolerance, or dislike?

Where are meals and snacks usually eaten, and at what hours?

What kinds of meals or refreshments are part of the patient's usual business, social, or recreational activities?

Who prepares the patient's meals? If meals are prepared at home, what are the facilities for food storage and preparation? If meals are eaten away from home, such as in a restaurant or school lunch, what choices are available?

Does the patient eat alone or with others? If alone, does this limit his food choices and methods of preparation? If with others, how does this limit the kinds and amount of food available to him?

Is the individual or family budget adequate and will it cover any possible additional costs for the modified diet? If it is not adequate, are there any resources such as public assistance, food stamp plan, or commodities?

What physical, emotional, intellectual, or social incapacities does this patient have that should be considered in giving him dietary guidance?

What kinds of educational programs and materials would be most suitable for this patient and what other resources are available to him for additional or continuing dietary guidance?

For guidance in the actual preparation and design of tools to obtain a diet history, some of the pertinent references are listed at the end of this chapter. It may also be helpful to learn about procedures and forms used by other dietitians and public health nutritionists in the geographical area.

Assessing the patient's food intake.—Having obtained the food intake information, an assessment or appraisal of the patient's dietary needs and needs for counseling can be made. The early chapters of this handbook provide the basic principles for evaluation of the patient's food intake, using the requirements for a "normal diet" or a diet modified for specific therapy as the criteria. When working with the physician to develop procedures for the dietary assessment, it should be decided whether an appraisal of the food intake by food groups is appropriate, or a more detailed calculation of specific nutrients is preferred. Calculations of nutrients should be viewed as important indicators of the nutrient quality of the dietary pattern, not as absolute values. A short method of calculation is generally used in the clinical situation. In the near future the use of computers for calculating nutrients may streamline the mechanical aspects of dietary assessment (5).

In interpreting the information obtained, it should be made clear that it is based on a dietary appraisal. A *nutrition history* and appraisal to describe nutritional status is a much more comprehensive procedure including extensive laboratory and clinical observations in addition to dietary studies and is beyond the scope of this handbook.

Planning and implementing the patient's dietary care and counseling.—Using the background information from the food record and the dietary assessment, the physician can prescribe the diet and the plan for dietary care of the patient that can reflect the strengths of the individual's own eating pattern. Thus, past eating habits can be modified to meet therapeutic needs (4). Where drastic changes must be made these changes should be explained, and the patient involved in the decision about how best to handle them. For the in-patient, the food served can demonstrate how dietary changes can be made and the selective menu or patient cafeteria used for teaching. In addition to discussions with the patient about his diet, individualized written plans should be provided. In preparing written materials and selecting supplementary printed teaching materials, the language skills and reading level of the patient and his family should be considered.

Group counseling or classes can supplement individual counseling for patients having a similar condition. Such classes have proved useful in motivating members in the group, and in helping them to share problems and their solutions. In addition, a larger patient audience can be reached when professional time is limited. Films, filmstrips, slides, and other audio-visual aids prepared on diabetes, heart disease, arthritis, weight control, and other subjects can be useful in presenting basic information to such groups. Programmed instruction also has been found to be an effective method to provide basic information to patients with diabetes. This is a new technique which has possibilities in other areas of health education. As new teaching tools become available, the dietitian and public health nutritionist should participate in testing their potentialities to develop more effective methods of patient education (6).

The dietary plan, once made and introduced, must be reviewed and adjusted periodically for the patient in the hospital or at home. Patients require continuing encouragement and support to continue to adhere to the modified dietary pattern. The record of food intake is needed for follow-up purposes to determine the patient's understanding of the diet and his ability to cope with the new way of eating. When the dietitian talks with the patient in the hospital or clinic, or the public health nurse or nutritionist sees him at home, some plan must be made to provide continuing dietary guidance. This might be offered either by the dietitian or nutritionist who initiates the counseling or by others with whom she coordinates her efforts.

COMMUNICATION WITH PROFESSIONAL CO-WORKERS

The medical record.—To best serve the patient, the dietitian or nutritionist must coordinate her efforts with those of other health workers providing care. The medical record is the basic means of communication between professional staff within the hospital, nursing home, or out-patient clinic. Here will be found recorded information such as the patient's medical history, the physician's physical findings, diagnostic impressions, prognosis and orders, laboratory reports, height and weight, and progress notes. Social service reports usually include financial data, and some description of the patient's family, home situation, and occupation. This information may reveal some of the problems in daily living which the individual faces and which may hinder his adherence to a planned dietary routine. Reports and notes from any consultants, other staff, or from cooperating community agencies provide additional insights into the patient's over-all problems and needs.

As the first step in planning for the patient's dietary care program, it is essential to read the medical record carefully. Further, the dietitian or nutritionist should note in this record the findings of the dietary assessment, the dietary care plan, counseling provided to the patient, and any pertinent impressions of the patient's ability to cope with the recommended diet modification. She can thereby share her experiences with other staff members and record her contribution to patient care as part of the total picture.

Conferences and ward rounds.—Participation in ward rounds and conferences with other staff giving service to the patient can help fill in details not found in the record. The dietitian or nutritionist should particularly confer with the physician in the early stages of patient care so that the dietary appraisal can be available to him and plans can be made for appropriately individualized dietary care. Conferences should also be sought with other staff on behalf of any patient having a special problem which might be resolved by cooperative planning. Case conferences are often used in both in-patient facilities and in home care services for cooperative planning and evaluation of care to selected patients. The dietitian or nutritionist should seek the opportunity to participate in such conferences, since joint planning to meet patient needs can often pay dividends both in improved patient care and saving of professional time. Unrecognized dietary needs can be identified as can problems interfering with the patient's dietary adherence.

COMMUNICATION WITH STAFF OF OTHER COMMUNITY AGENCIES

Knowing community resources.—For effective coordination and cooperation between the in-patient facilities and other health and social agencies it is increasingly necessary for dietitians and public health nutritionists to be well informed about the many resources available in their communities, and the channels for referral. Since, at home, total responsibility for diet is placed upon the patient and his family, they frequently need diet counseling even when they have received considerable guidance in the hospital. At home the situation is constantly changing and new needs become apparent. Diet counseling for the patient at home may be available through the public health nursing agency, the public health nutritionist, a diet counseling service, or as a service of a coordinated home care program. Some patients may have no one at home to prepare meals, and if unable to do so themselves, can benefit from homemaker services or a home-delivered-meal service (7).

To provide for continuity of care, many communities have developed an information and referral service and/or an interagency referral system. These mechanisms provide formalized channels by which information about the patient and his family can be exchanged between agencies. The information and referral service lists services available in the community and helps families to locate the best ones to meet their needs.

The interagency referral system.—With an interagency referral system, a referral may be initiated by any member of the health team in the hospital or community who recognizes a need which can be met by another agency. A standard form is usually developed for the community by an interagency committee and is the basis for the referral system. The form is used to supply complete information about the patient including identifying data, reason for referral, diagnosis and prognosis, physician's orders and instructions. Space is provided for instructions and comments by hospital or clinic personnel (physician, nurse, medical social worker, dietitian, physical therapist, occupational therapist, and others) and by the public health nurse or other community workers. Included as attachments are copies of any written dietary plans given to the patient for home use. The form is initiated in the agency making the referral and directed through the appropriate channels to the agency providing the needed services. With this kind of referral system the dietitian and public health nutritionist have the opportunity to exchange information with all other workers offering service to the patient. Using this procedure each worker benefits from the experience each has with the patient, and can relate his own efforts to the total patient care plan. Moreover, the referral form serves as a permanent record of these services. It also serves as a way of measuring patient progress and identifying the contributions of the various services (8).

By using all these formal, established channels, as well as the informal channels of communication available to her, the dietitian and public health nutritionist can improve and extend services to patients and better fulfill her role on the health team.

REFERENCES

1. WALSH, HELEN E. The changing nature of public health, J. Am. Dietet. A., **46**:93–95, 1965.
2. BECKER, BERYL G., BEEUWKES, ADELIA M., and INDEK, BERNARD B. Dietary intake methodologies. A review. Ann Arbor, Mich.: Office of Research Administration, November, 1960.
3. Hospital Dietitians: Do you chart? J. Am. Dietet. A., **44**:361, 1964.
4. STONE, DANIEL B. A rational approach to diet and diabetes, J. Am. Dietet. A., **46**:30–35, 1965.
5. THOMPSON, ETHEL M., and TUCKER, HENRY. Computers in dietary studies, J. Am. Dietet. A., **40**:308, 1962.
6. KAUFMAN, MILDRED. Programmed instruction materials on diabetes, J. Am. Dietet. A., **46**:36–38, 1965.
7. PIPER, GERALDINE M. Planning new community nutrition services, J. Am. Dietet. A., **44**:461, 1964.
8. NEW YORK STATE DEPARTMENT OF HEALTH. Interagency referral form and instructions for interagency referral form. Albany.

ADDITIONAL SELECTED REFERENCES ON METHODS FOR OBTAINING FOOD INTAKE INFORMATION

ADELSON, S. F. Some problems in collecting dietary data from individuals, J. Am. Dietet. A., **36**:453, 1960.

ANDERSON, L., and BROWE, J. Nutrition and family service. Philadelphia: W. B. Saunders Company, 1960, chapter 7.

*BLECHA, E. E. Dietary study methods. IV. The dietary history for use in diet therapy, J. Am. Dietet. A., **27**:968–69, 1951.

*BURKE, B. S. The dietary history as a tool in research, J. Am. Dietet. A., **23**: 1041–46, 1946.

HAYES, O. B., ABRAHAM, S., and CACERES, C. A. Computers in epidemiologic dietary studies, J. Am. Dietet. A., **44**:456, 1964.

HUNSCHER, H. A., and MACY, I. G. Dietary study methods. I. Uses and abuses of dietary study methods, J. Am. Dietet. A., **27**:558–63, 1951.

INTERDEPARTMENTAL COMMITTEE ON NUTRITION FOR NATIONAL DEFENSE. Manual for Nutrition Surveys, 2d edition, 1963.

* Includes forms being used.

*ROSENTHAL, H., BAKER, P. C., and MCVEY, W. A. Stern's applied dietetics. Baltimore: The Williams and Wilkins Co., 1949, pp. 8–12, 35.

TRULSON, MARTHA F. Assessment of dietary study methods. I. Comparison of methods for obtaining data for clinical work, J. Am. Dietet. A., **30**:991, 1954.

*TURNER, D. The estimation of the patient's home dietary intake, J. Am. Dietet. A., **16**:875–81, 1940.

YOUNG, C. M. Diet therapy—interviewing the patient, Am. J. Clin. Nutr., **8**: 523, 1960.

———. The interview itself, J. Am. Dietet. A., **35**:677–81, 1959.

YOUNG, C. M., and MUSGRAVE, K. Dietary study methods. II. Uses of dietary score cards, J. Am. Dietet. A., **27**:745–48, 1951.

YOUNG, C. M., and TRULSON, M. Methodology for dietary surveys in epidemiological surveys. II. Strengths and weaknesses of existing methods, Am. J. Pub. H., **50**:803, 1960.

APPENDIXES

APPENDIX 1

Food Values in Common Portions

The 1964 revision of *Nutritive Value of Foods* (U.S. Department of Agriculture, Home and Garden Bulletin No. 72) provides a compact table on food composition of nearly 500 food items commonly used in this country. Edible portions are indicated in both weights and measures thereby providing a quick and convenient unit for assessing the nutrient content of diets.

The values are based on data in *Composition of Foods—Raw, Processed, Prepared* (U.S. Department of Agriculture, Agriculture Handbook No. 8 [December, 1963]). Data on more than 2,500 food items appear in this handbook, which is prepared by the Agricultural Research Service of United States Department of Agriculture.

NIACIN AND NIACIN EQUIVALENT

The term niacin, used in Table 36, is a less inclusive term than niacin equivalent used in Table 3. Nearly all foods contain some tryptophan, an amino acid found in protein, which the body can convert to niacin. Niacin equivalent is the composite of the niacin already in the food and that which may be formed from tryptophan. Among the better sources of tryptophan are milk, meats, eggs, legumes, and nuts.

The average diet in the United States, which contains a generous amount of protein, provides enough tryptophan to increase the niacin value by about a third.

TABLE 36A

Yield of Cooked Meat per Pound of Raw Meat

Meat as Purchased	Meat after Cooking (less Drippings)	
	Parts weighed	Approximate weight of cooked parts per pound of raw meat purchased
		Ounces
Chops or steaks for broiling or frying:		
With bone and relatively large amount of fat, such as pork or lamb chops; beef rib, sirloin, or porterhouse steaks.	Lean, bone, fat	10–12
	Lean and fat	7–10
	Lean only	5–7
Without bone and with very little fat, such as round of beef, veal steaks	Lean and fat	12–13
	Lean only	9–12
Ground meat for broiling or frying, such as hamburger, lamb, or pork patties	Patties	9–13
Roasts for oven cooking (no liquid added):		
With bone and relatively large amount of fat, such as beef rib, loin, chuck; lamb shoulder, leg; pork, fresh or cured.	Lean, bone, fat	10–12
	Lean and fat	8–10
	Lean only	6–9
Without bone	Lean and fat	10–12
	Lean only	7–10
Cuts for pot-roasting, simmering, braising, stewing:		
With bone and relatively large amount of fat, such as beef chuck, pork shoulder	Lean, bone, fat	10–11
	Lean and fat	8–9
	Lean only	6–8
Without bone and with relatively small amount of fat, such as trimmed beef, veal	Lean with adhering fat	9–11

TABLE 36—NUTRITIVE VALUES OF THE EDIBLE PART OF FOODS

Reprinted from *Nutritive Value of Foods* (U.S. Department of Agriculture, Home and Garden Bulletin No. 72).

[Dashes show that no basis could be found for imputing a value although there was some reason to believe that a measurable amount of the constituent might be present]

Food, Approximate Measure, and Weight (in Grams)			Food Energy	Protein	Fat (Total Lipid)	Fatty acids: Saturated (Total)	Fatty acids: Unsaturated: Oleic	Fatty acids: Unsaturated: Linoleic	Carbohydrate	Calcium	Iron	Vitamin A Value	Thiamine	Riboflavin	Niacin	Ascorbic Acid
		Grams	(Calories)	(Gm.)	(Gm.)	(Gm.)	(Gm.)	(Gm.)	(Gm.)	(Mg.)	(Mg.)	(I.U.)	(Mg.)	(Mg.)	(Mg.)	(Mg.)
MILK, CREAM, CHEESE; RELATED PRODUCTS																
Milk, cow's:																
Fluid, whole (3.5% fat).	1 cup	244	160	9	9	5	3	Trace	12	238	0.1	350	0.08	0.42	0.1	2
Fluid, nonfat (skim)	1 cup	246	90	9	Trace	------	------	------	13	298	.1	10	.10	.44	.2	2
Buttermilk, cultured, from skim milk.	1 cup	246	90	9	Trace	------	------	------	13	298	.1	10	.09	.44	.2	2
Evaporated, unsweetened, undiluted.	1 cup	252	345	18	20	11	7	1	24	635	.3	820	.10	.84	.5	3
Condensed, sweetened, undiluted.	1 cup	306	980	25	27	15	9	1	166	802	.3	1,090	.23	1.17	.5	3
Dry, whole	1 cup	103	515	27	28	16	9	1	39	936	.5	1,160	.30	1.50	.7	6
Dry, nonfat, instant	1 cup	70	250	25	Trace	------	------	------	36	905	.4	20	.24	1.25	.6	5
Milk, goat's:																
Fluid, whole	1 cup	244	165	8	10	6	2	Trace	11	315	.2	390	.10	.27	.7	2
Cream:																
Half-and-half (cream and milk).	1 cup	242	325	8	28	16	9	1	11	261	.1	1,160	.08	.38	.1	2
	1 tablespoon	15	20	Trace	2	1	1	Trace	1	16	Trace	70	Trace	.02	Trace	Trace
Light, coffee or table	1 cup	240	505	7	49	27	16	1	10	245	.1	2,030	.07	.36	.1	2
	1 tablespoon	15	30	Trace	3	2	1	Trace	1	15	Trace	130	Trace	.02	Trace	Trace
Whipping, unwhipped (volume about double when whipped):																
Light	1 cup	239	715	6	75	41	25	2	9	203	.1	3,070	.06	.30	.1	2
	1 tablespoon	15	45	Trace	5	3	2	Trace	1	13	Trace	190	Trace	.02	Trace	Trace
Heavy	1 cup	238	840	5	89	49	29	3	7	178	.1	3,670	.05	.26	.1	2
	1 tablespoon	15	55	Trace	6	3	2	Trace	Trace	11	Trace	230	Trace	.02	Trace	Trace
Cheese:																
Blue or Roquefort type	1 ounce	28	105	6	9	5	3	Trace	1	89	.1	350	.01	.17	.1	0
Cheddar or American:																
Ungrated	1 inch cube	17	70	4	5	3	2	Trace	Trace	128	.2	220	Trace	.08	Trace	0
Grated	1 cup	112	445	28	36	20	12	1	2	840	1.1	1,470	.03	.51	.1	0
	1 tablespoon	7	30	2	2	1	1	Trace	Trace	52	.1	90	Trace	.03	Trace	0
Cheddar, process	1 ounce	28	105	7	9	5	3	Trace	1	219	.3	350	Trace	.12	Trace	0
Cheese foods, Cheddar	1 ounce	28	90	6	7	4	2	Trace	2	162	.2	280	.01	.16	Trace	0

TABLE 36—*Continued*

Food, Approximate Measure, and Weight (in Grams)			Food Energy	Protein	Fat (Total Lipid)	Fatty acids: Saturated (Total)	Fatty acids: Unsaturated: Oleic	Fatty acids: Unsaturated: Linoleic	Carbohydrate	Calcium	Iron	Vitamin A Value	Thiamine	Riboflavin	Niacin	Ascorbic Acid
MILK, CREAM, CHEESE; RELATED PRODUCTS—Continued																
Cheese—Continued			(Calories)	(Gm.)	(Gm.)	(Gm.)	(Gm.)	(Gm.)	(Gm.)	(Mg.)	(Mg.)	(I.U.)	(Mg.)	(Mg.)	(Mg.)	(Mg.)
Cottage cheese, from skim milk:		*Grams*														
Creamed	1 cup	225	240	31	9	5	3	Trace	7	212	0.7	380	0.07	0.56	0.2	0
	1 ounce	28	30	4	1	1	Trace	Trace	1	27	.1	50	.01	.07	Trace	0
Uncreamed	1 cup	225	195	38	1	Trace	Trace	Trace	6	202	.9	20	.07	.63	.2	0
	1 ounce	28	25	5	Trace	-------	-------	-------	1	26	.1	Trace	.01	.08	Trace	0
Cream cheese	1 ounce	28	105	2	11	6	4	Trace	1	18	.1	440	Trace	.07	Trace	0
	1 tablespoon	15	55	1	6	3	2	Trace	Trace	9	Trace	230	Trace	.04	Trace	0
Swiss (domestic)	1 ounce	28	105	8	8	4	3	Trace	1	262	.3	320	Trace	.11	Trace	0
Milk beverages:																
Cocoa	1 cup	242	235	9	11	6	4	Trace	26	286	.9	390	.09	.45	.4	2
Chocolate-flavored milk drink (made with skim milk).	1 cup	250	190	8	6	3	2	Trace	27	270	.4	210	.09	.41	.2	2
Malted milk	1 cup	270	280	13	12	-------	-------	-------	32	364	.8	670	.17	.56	.2	2
Milk desserts:																
Cornstarch pudding, plain (blanc mange).	1 cup	248	275	9	10	5	3	Trace	39	290	.1	390	.07	.40	.1	2
Custard, baked	1 cup	248	285	13	14	6	5	1	28	278	1.0	870	.10	.47	.2	1
Ice cream, plain, factory packed:																
Slice or cut brick, ⅛ of quart brick.	1 slice or cut brick.	71	145	3	9	5	3	Trace	15	87	.1	370	.03	.13	.1	1
Container	3½ fluid ounces.	62	130	2	8	4	3	Trace	13	76	.1	320	.03	.12	.1	1
Container	8 fluid ounces.	142	295	6	18	10	6	1	29	175	.1	740	.06	.27	.1	1
Ice milk	1 cup	187	285	9	10	6	3	Trace	42	292	.2	390	.09	.41	.2	2
Yoghurt, from partially skimmed milk.	1 cup	246	120	8	4	2	1	Trace	13	295	.1	170	.09	.43	.2	2
EGGS																
Eggs, large, 24 ounces per dozen:																
Raw:																
Whole, without shell	1 egg	50	80	6	6	2	3	Trace	Trace	27	1.1	590	.05	.15	Trace	0

Yolk of egg	1 yolk	17	60	3	5	2	2	Trace	Trace	24	.9	580	.04	.07	Trace	0
Cooked:																
Boiled, shell removed	2 eggs	100	160	13	12	4	5	1	1	54	2.3	1,180	.09	.28	.1	0
Scrambled, with milk and fat.	1 egg	64	110	7	8	3	3	Trace	1	51	1.1	690	.05	.18	Trace	0
MEAT, POULTRY, FISH, SHELLFISH; RELATED PRODUCTS																
Bacon, broiled or fried, crisp.	2 slices	16	100	5	8	3	4	1	1	2	.5	0	.08	.05	.8	------
Beef, trimmed to retail basis,[1] cooked:																
Cuts braised, simmered, or pot-roasted:																
Lean and fat	3 ounces	85	245	23	16	8	7	Trace	0	10	2.9	30	.04	.18	3.5	------
Lean only	2.5 ounces	72	140	22	5	2	2	Trace	0	10	2.7	10	.04	.16	3.3	------
Hamburger (ground beef), broiled:																
Lean	3 ounces	85	185	23	10	5	4	Trace	0	10	3.0	20	.08	.20	5.1	------
Regular	3 ounces	85	245	21	17	8	8	Trace	0	9	2.7	30	.07	.18	4.6	------
Roast, oven-cooked, no liquid added:																
Relatively fat, such as rib:																
Lean and fat	3 ounces	85	375	17	34	16	15	[illegible]	0	8	2.2	70	.05	.13	3.1	------
Lean only	1.8 ounces	51	125	14	7	3	3	Trace	0	6	1.8	10	.04	.11	2.6	------
Relatively lean, such as heel of round:																
Lean and fat	3 ounces	85	165	25	7	3	3	Trace	0	11	3.2	10	.06	.19	4.5	------
Lean only	2.7 ounces	78	125	24	3	1	1	Trace	0	10	3.0	Trace	.06	.18	4.3	------
Steak, broiled:																
Relatively fat, such as sirloin:																
Lean and fat	3 ounces	85	330	20	27	13	12	1	0	9	2.5	50	.05	.16	4.0	------
Lean only	2.0 ounces	56	115	18	4	2	2	Trace	0	7	2.2	10	.05	.14	3.6	------
Relatively lean, such as round:																
Lean and fat	3 ounces	85	220	24	13	6	6	Trace	0	10	3.0	20	.07	.19	4.8	------
Lean only	2.4 ounces	68	130	21	4	2	2	Trace	0	9	2.5	10	.06	.16	4.1	------
Beef, canned:																
Corned beef	3 ounces	85	185	22	10	5	4	Trace	0	17	3.7	20	.01	.20	2.9	------
Corned beef hash	3 ounces	85	155	7	10	5	4	Trace	9	11	1.7	------	.01	.08	1.8	------
Beef, dried or chipped	2 ounces	57	115	19	4	2	2	Trace	0	11	2.9	------	.04	.18	2.2	------
Beef and vegetable stew	1 cup	235	210	15	10	5	4	Trace	15	28	2.8	2,310	.13	.17	4.4	15
Beef potpie, baked: Individual pie, 4¼-inch diameter, weight before baking about 8 ounces.	1 pie	227	560	23	33	9	20	2	43	32	4.1	1,860	.25	.27	4.5	7

[1] Outer layer of fat on the cut was removed to within approximately ½ inch of the lean. Deposits of fat within the cut were not removed.

TABLE 36—*Continued*

Food, Approximate Measure, and Weight (in Grams)			Food Energy	Protein	Fat (Total Lipid)	Fatty acids: Saturated (Total)	Fatty acids: Unsaturated: Oleic	Fatty acids: Unsaturated: Linoleic	Carbohydrate	Calcium	Iron	Vitamin A Value	Thiamine	Riboflavin	Niacin	Ascorbic Acid
MEAT, POULTRY, FISH, SHELLFISH; RELATED PRODUCTS—Continued																
		Grams	(Calories)	(Gm.)	(Gm.)	(Gm.)	(Gm.)	(Gm.)	(Gm.)	(Mg.)	(Mg.)	(I.U.)	(Mg.)	(Mg.)	(Mg.)	(Mg.)
Chicken, cooked:																
Flesh only, broiled	3 ounces	85	115	20	3	1	1	1	0	8	1.4	80	0.05	0.16	7.4	------
Breast, fried, ½ breast:																
With bone	3.3 ounces	94	155	25	5	1	2	1	1	9	1.3	70	.04	.17	11.2	------
Flesh and skin only	2.7 ounces	76	155	25	5	1	2	1	1	9	1.3	70	.04	.17	11.2	------
Drumstick, fried:																
With bone	2.1 ounces	59	90	12	4	1	2	1	Trace	6	.9	50	.03	.15	2.7	------
Flesh and skin only	1.3 ounces	38	90	12	4	1	2	1	Trace	6	.9	50	.03	.15	2.7	------
Chicken, canned, boneless	3 ounces	85	170	18	10	3	4	2	0	18	1.3	200	.03	.11	3.7	3
Chicken potpie. *See* Poultry potpie.																
Chile con carne, canned:																
With beans	1 cup	250	335	19	15	7	7	Trace	30	80	4.2	150	.08	.18	3.2	------
Without beans	1 cup	255	510	26	38	18	17	1	15	97	3.6	380	.05	.31	5.6	------
Heart, beef, lean, braised	3 ounces	85	160	27	5	------	------	------	1	5	5.0	20	.21	1.04	6.5	1
Lamb, trimmed to retail basis,[1] cooked:																
Chop, thick, with bone, broiled.	1 chop, 4.8 ounces.	137	400	25	33	18	12	1	0	10	1.5	------	.14	.25	5.6	------
Lean and fat	4.0 ounces	112	400	25	33	18	12	1	0	10	1.5	------	.14	.25	5.6	------
Lean only	2.6 ounces	74	140	21	6	3	2	Trace	0	9	1.5	------	.11	.20	4.5	------
Leg, roasted:																
Lean and fat	3 ounces	85	235	22	16	9	6	Trace	0	9	1.4	------	.13	.23	4.7	------
Lean only	2.5 ounces	71	130	20	5	3	2	Trace	0	9	1.4	------	.12	.21	4.4	------
Shoulder, roasted:																
Lean and fat	3 ounces	85	285	18	23	13	8	1	0	9	1.0	------	.11	.20	4.0	------
Lean only	2.3 ounces	64	130	17	6	3	2	Trace	0	8	1.0	------	.10	.18	3.7	------
Liver, beef, fried	2 ounces	57	130	15	6	------	------	------	3	6	5.0	30,280	.15	2.37	9.4	15
Pork, cured, cooked:																
Ham, light cure, lean	3 ounces	85	245	18	19	7	8	2	0	8	2.2	0	.40	.16	3.1	------

Luncheon meat:																
Boiled ham, sliced	2 ounces	57	135	11	10	4	4	1	0	6	1.6	0	.25	.09	1.5	-----
Canned, spiced or unspiced.	2 ounces	57	165	8	14	5	6	1	1	5	1.2	0	.18	.12	1.6	-----
Pork, fresh, trimmed to retail basis,[1] cooked:																
Chop, thick, with bone	1 chop, 3.5 ounces.	98	260	16	21	8	9	2	0	8	2.2	0	.63	.18	3.8	-----
Lean and fat	2.3 ounces	66	260	16	21	8	9	2	0	8	2.2	0	.63	.18	3.8	-----
Lean only	1.7 ounces	48	130	15	7	2	3	1	0	7	1.9	0	.54	.16	3.3	-----
Roast, oven-cooked, no liquid added:																
Lean and fat	3 ounces	85	310	21	24	9	10	2	0	9	2.7	0	.78	.22	4.7	-----
Lean only	2.4 ounces	68	175	20	10	3	4	1	0	9	2.6	0	.73	.21	4.4	-----
Cuts, simmered:																
Lean and fat	3 ounces	85	320	20	26	9	11	2	0	8	2.5	0	.46	.21	4.1	-----
Lean only	2.2 ounces	63	135	18	6	2	3	1	0	8	2.3	0	.42	.19	3.7	-----
Poultry potpie (based on chicken potpie). Individual pie, 4¼-inch diameter, weigh before baking about ounces.	1 pie	227	535	23	31	10	15	3	42	68	3.0	3,020	.25	.26	4.1	5
Sausage:																
Bologna, slice, 4.1 by 0.1 inch.	8 slices	227	690	27	62	-----	-----	-----	2	16	4.1	-----	.36	.49	6.0	-----
Frankfurter, cooked	1 frankfurter	51	155	6	14	-----	-----	-----	1	3	.8	-----	.08	.10	1.3	-----
Pork, links or patty, cooked.	4 ounces	113	540	21	50	18	21	5	Trace	8	2.7	0	.89	.39	4.2	-----
Tongue, beef, braised	3 ounces	85	210	18	14	-----	-----	-----	Trace	6	1.9	-----	.04	.25	3.0	-----
Turkey potpie. *See* Poultry potpie.																
Veal, cooked:																
Cutlet, without bone, broiled.	3 ounces	85	185	23	9	5	4	Trace	-----	9	2.7	-----	.06	.21	4.6	-----
Roast, medium fat, medium done; lean and fat.	3 ounces	85	230	23	14	7	6	Trace	0	10	2.9	-----	.11	.26	6.6	-----
Fish and shellfish:																
Bluefish, baked or broiled.	3 ounces	85	135	22	4	-----	-----	-----	0	25	.6	40	.09	.08	1.6	-----
Clams:																
Raw, meat only	3 ounces	85	65	11	1	-----	-----	-----	2	59	5.2	90	.08	.15	1.1	8
Canned, solids and liquid.	3 ounces	85	45	7	1	-----	-----	-----	2	47	3.5	-----	.01	.09	.9	-----
Crabmeat, canned	3 ounces	85	85	15	2	-----	-----	-----	1	38	.7	-----	.07	.07	1.6	-----
Fish sticks, breaded, cooked, frozen; stick, 3.8 by 1.0 by 0.5 inch.	10 sticks or 8-ounce package.	227	400	38	20	5	4	10	15	25	.9	-----	.09	.16	3.6	-----

[1] Outer layer of fat on the cut was removed to within approximately ½ inch of the lean. Deposits of fat within the cut were not removed.

TABLE 36—*Continued*

Food, Approximate Measure, and Weight (in Grams)			Food Energy	Protein	Fat (Total Lipid)	Fatty acids: Saturated (Total)	Fatty acids: Unsaturated: Oleic	Fatty acids: Unsaturated: Linoleic	Carbohydrate	Calcium	Iron	Vitamin A Value	Thiamine	Riboflavin	Niacin	Ascorbic Acid
MEAT, POULTRY, FISH, SHELLFISH; RELATED PRODUCTS—Continued																
Fish and shellfish—Continued		*Grams*	(Calories)	(Gm.)	(Gm.)	(Gm.)	(Gm.)	(Gm.)	(Gm.)	(Mg.)	(Mg.)	(I.U.)	(Mg.)	(Mg.)	(Mg.)	(Mg.)
Haddock, fried	3 ounces	85	140	17	5	1	3		5	34	1.0	------	0.03	0.06	2.7	2
Mackerel:																
Broiled, Atlantic	3 ounces	85	200	19	13	------	------	------	0	5	1.0	450	.13	.23	6.5	------
Canned, Pacific, solids and liquid.[2]	3 ounces	85	155	18	9	------	------	------	0	221	1.9	20	.02	.28	7.4	------
Ocean perch, breaded (egg and breadcrumbs), fried.	3 ounces	85	195	16	11	------	------	------	6	28	1.1	------	.08	.09	1.5	------
Oysters, meat only: Raw, 13–19 medium selects.	1 cup	240	160	20	4	------	------	------	8	226	13.2	740	.33	.43	6.0	------
Oyster stew, 1 part oysters to 3 parts milk by volume, 3–4 oysters.	1 cup	230	200	11	12	------	------	------	11	269	3.3	640	.13	.41	1.6	------
Salmon, pink, canned	3 ounces	85	120	17	5	1	1	Trace	0	[3] 167	.7	60	.03	.16	6.8	------
Sardines, Atlantic, canned in oil, drained solids.	3 ounces	85	175	20	9	------	------	------	0	372	2.5	190	.02	.17	4.6	------
Shad, baked	3 ounces	85	170	20	10	------	------	------	0	20	.5	20	.11	.22	7.3	------
Shrimp, canned, meat only.	3 ounces	85	100	21	1	------	------	------	1	98	2.6	50	.01	.03	1.5	------
Swordfish, broiled with butter or margarine.	3 ounces	85	150	24	5	------	------	------	0	23	1.1	1,750	.03	.04	9.3	------
Tuna, canned in oil, drained solids.	3 ounces	85	170	24	7	------	------	------	0	7	1.6	70	.04	.10	10.1	------
MATURE DRY BEANS AND PEAS, NUTS, PEANUTS; RELATED PRODUCTS																
[illegible]	[illegible]	[illegible]	850	26	77	6	52	15	28	332	6.7	0	.34	1.31	5.0	Trace

Food	Measure	Weight	Food energy	Protein	Fat	?	?	?	Carbohydrate	Calcium	Iron	Vitamin A	Thiamine	Riboflavin	Niacin	Ascorbic acid
Beans, dry:																
Common varieties, such as Great Northern, navy, and others, canned:																
Red	1 cup	256	230	15	1				42	74	4.6	Trace	.13	.10	1.5	
White, with tomato sauce:																
With pork	1 cup	261	320	16	7	3	3	[illegible]	50	141	4.7	340	.20	.08	1.5	5
Without pork	1 cup	261	310	16	1				50	177	5.2	160	.18	.09	1.5	5
Lima, cooked	1 cup	192	260	16	1				48	56	5.6	Trace	.26	.12	1.3	Trace
Brazil nuts	1 cup	140	915	20	94	19	45	2[illegible]	15	260	4.8	Trace	1.34	.17	2.2	
Cashew nuts, roasted	1 cup	135	760	23	62	10	43	[illegible]	40	51	5.1	140	.58	.33	2.4	
Coconut:																
Fresh, shredded	1 cup	97	335	3	34	29	2	Trace	9	13	1.6	0	.05	.02	.5	3
Dried, shredded, sweetened.	1 cup	62	340	2	24	21	2	Trace	33	10	1.2	0	.02	.02	.2	0
Cowpeas or blackeye peas, dry, cooked.	1 cup	248	190	13	1				34	42	3.2	20	.41	.11	1.1	Trace
Peanuts, roasted, salted:																
Halves	1 cup	144	840	37	72	16	31	2[illegible]	27	107	3.0		.46	.19	24.7	0
Chopped	1 tablespoon	9	55	2	4	1	2	[illegible]	2	7	.2		.03	.01	1.5	0
Peanut butter	1 tablespoon	16	95	4	8	2	4	[illegible]	3	9	.3		.02	.02	2.4	0
Peas, split, dry, cooked	1 cup	250	290	20	1				52	28	4.2	100	.37	.22	2.2	
Pecans:																
Halves	1 cup	108	740	10	77	5	48	1[illegible]	16	79	2.6	140	.93	.14	1.0	2
Chopped	1 tablespoon	7.5	50	1	5	Trace	3	[illegible]	1	5	.2	10	.06	.01	.1	Trace
Walnuts, shelled:																
Black or native, chopped.	1 cup	126	790	26	75	4	26	3[illegible]	19	Trace	7.6	380	.28	.14	.9	
English or Persian:																
Halves	1 cup	100	650	15	64	4	10	4[illegible]	16	99	3.1	30	.33	.13	.9	3
Chopped	1 tablespoon	8	50	1	5	Trace	1	[illegible]	1	8	.2	Trace	.03	.01	.1	Trace
VEGETABLES AND VEGETABLE PRODUCTS																
Asparagus:																
Cooked, cut spears	1 cup	175	35	4	Trace				6	37	1.0	1,580	.27	.32	2.4	46
Canned spears, medium:																
Green	6 spears	96	20	2	Trace				3	18	1.8	770	.06	.10	.8	14
Bleached	6 spears	96	20	2	Trace				4	15	1.0	80	.05	.06	.7	14
Beans:																
Lima, immature, cooked	1 cup	160	180	12	1				32	75	4.0	450	.29	.16	2.0	28
Snap, green:																
Cooked:																
In small amount of water, short time.	1 cup	125	30	2	Trace				7	62	.8	680	.08	.11	.6	16

[2] Vitamin values based on drained solids.

[3] Based on total contents of can. If bones are discarded, value will be greatly reduced

TABLE 36—*Continued*

Food, Approximate Measure, and Weight (in Grams)			Food Energy	Protein	Fat (Total Lipid)	Fatty acids: Saturated (Total)	Fatty acids: Unsaturated: Oleic	Fatty acids: Unsaturated: Linoleic	Carbohydrate	Calcium	Iron	Vitamin A Value	Thiamine	Riboflavin	Niacin	Ascorbic Acid
VEGETABLES AND VEGETABLE PRODUCTS—Continued																
Beans—Continued																
Snap, green—Continued																
Cooked—Continued		*Grams*	(Calories)	(Gm.)	(Gm.)	(Gm.)	(Gm.)	(Gm.)	(Gm.)	(Mg.)	(Mg.)	(I.U.)	(Mg.)	(Mg.)	(Mg.)	(Mg.)
In large amount of water, long time.	1 cup	125	30	2	Trace	----	----	----	7	62	0.8	680	0.07	0.10	0.4	13
Canned:																
Solids and liquid	1 cup	239	45	2	Trace	----	----	----	10	81	2.9	690	.08	.10	.7	9
Strained or chopped (baby food).	1 ounce	28	5	Trace	Trace	----	----	----	1	9	.3	110	.01	.02	.1	Trace
Bean sprouts. *See* Sprouts.																
Beets, cooked, diced	1 cup	165	50	2	Trace	----	----	----	12	23	.8	40	.04	.07	.5	11
Broccoli spears, cooked	1 cup	150	40	5	Trace	----	----	----	7	132	1.2	3,750	.14	.29	1.2	135
Brussels sprouts, cooked	1 cup	130	45	5	1	----	----	----	8	42	1.4	680	.10	.18	1.1	113
Cabbage:																
Raw:																
Finely shredded	1 cup	100	25	1	Trace	----	----	----	5	49	.4	130	.05	.05	.3	47
Coleslaw	1 cup	120	120	1	9	2	2	5	9	52	.5	180	.06	.06	.3	35
Cooked:																
In small amount of water, short time.	1 cup	170	35	2	Trace	----	----	----	7	75	.5	220	.07	.07	.5	56
In large amount of water, long time.	1 cup	170	30	2	Trace	----	----	----	7	71	.5	200	.04	.04	.2	40
Cabbage, celery or Chinese:																
Raw, leaves and stalk, 1-inch pieces.	1 cup	100	15	1	Trace	----	----	----	3	43	.6	150	.05	.04	.6	25
Cabbage, spoon (or pakchoy), cooked.	1 cup	150	20	2	Trace	----	----	----	4	222	.9	4,650	.07	.12	1.1	23
Carrots:																
Raw:																
Whole, 5½ by 1 inch, (25 thin strips).	1 carrot	50	20	1	Trace	----	----	----	5	18	.4	5,500	.03	.03	.3	4

Cooked, diced	1 cup	145	45	1	Trace	-	-	-	10	48	.9	15,220	.08	.07	.7	9
Canned, strained or chopped (baby food).	1 ounce	28	10	Trace	Trace	-	-	-	2	7	.1	3,690	.01	.01	.1	1
Cauliflower, cooked, flowerbuds.	1 cup	120	25	3	Trace	-	-	-	5	25	.8	70	.11	.10	.7	66
Celery, raw:																
Stalk, large outer, 8 by about 1½ inches, at root end.	1 stalk	40	5	Trace	Trace	-	-	-	2	16	.1	100	.01	.01	.1	4
Pieces, diced	1 cup	100	15	1	Trace	-	-	-	4	39	.3	240	.03	.03	.3	9
Collards, cooked	1 cup	190	55	5	1	-	-	-	9	289	1.1	10,260	.27	.37	2.4	87
Corn, sweet:																
Cooked, ear 5 by 1¾ inches.[4]	1 ear	140	70	3	1	-	-	-	16	2	.5	[5] 310	.09	.08	1.0	7
Canned, solids and liquid.	1 cup	256	170	5	2	-	-	-	40	10	1.0	[5] 690	.07	.12	2.3	13
Cowpeas, cooked, immature seeds.	1 cup	160	175	13	1	-	-	-	29	38	3.4	560	.49	.18	2.3	28
Cucumbers, 10-ounce; 7½ by about 2 inches:																
Raw, pared	1 cucumber	207	30	1	Trace	-	-	-	7	35	.6	Trace	.07	.09	.4	23
Raw, pared, center slice ⅛-inch thick.	6 slices	50	5	Trace	Trace	-	-	-	2	8	.2	Trace	.02	.02	.1	6
Dandelion greens, cooked.	1 cup	180	60	4	1	-	-	-	12	252	3.2	21,060	.24	.29	-	32
Endive, curly (including escarole).	2 ounces	57	10	1	Trace	-	-	-	2	46	1.0	1,870	.04	.08	.3	6
Kale, leaves including stems, cooked.	1 cup	110	30	4	1	-	-	-	4	147	1.3	8,140	-	-	-	68
Lettuce, raw:																
Butterhead, as Boston types; head, 4-inch diameter.	1 head	220	30	3	Trace	-	-	-	6	77	4.4	2,130	.14	.13	.6	18
Crisphead, as Iceberg; head, 4¾-inch diameter.	1 head	454	60	4	Trace	-	-	-	13	91	2.3	1,500	.29	.27	1.3	29
Looseleaf, or bunching varieties, leaves.	2 large	50	10	1	Trace	-	-	-	2	34	.7	950	.03	.04	.2	9
Mushrooms, canned, solids and liquid.	1 cup	244	40	5	Trace	-	-	-	6	15	1.2	Trace	.04	.60	4.8	4
Mustard greens, cooked	1 cup	140	35	3	1	-	-	-	6	193	2.5	8,120	.11	.19	.9	68
Okra, cooked, pod 3 by ⅝ inch.	8 pods	85	25	2	Trace	-	-	-	5	78	.4	420	.11	.15	.8	17

[4] Measure and weight apply to entire vegetable or fruit including parts not usually aten.

[5] Based on yellow varieties; white varieties contain only a trace of cryptoxanthin and carotenes, the pigments in corn that have biological activity.

TABLE 36—*Continued*

Food, Approximate Measure, and Weight (in Grams)			Food Energy	Protein	Fat (Total Lipid)	Fatty acids			Carbohydrate	Calcium	Iron	Vitamin A Value	Thiamine	Riboflavin	Niacin	Ascorbic Acid
						Saturated (Total)	Unsaturated									
							Oleic	Linoleic								
VEGETABLES AND VEGETABLE PRODUCTS—Continued																
		Grams	(Calories)	(Gm.)	(Gm.)	(Gm.)	(Gm.)	(Gm.)	(Gm.)	(Mg.)	(Mg.)	(I.U.)	(Mg.)	(Mg.)	(Mg.)	(Mg.)
Onions:																
Mature:																
Raw, onion 2½-inch diameter.	1 onion	110	40	2	Trace	----	----	----	10	30	0.6	40	0.04	0.04	0.2	11
Cooked	1 cup	210	60	3	Trace	----	----	----	14	50	.8	80	.06	.06	.4	14
Young green, small, without tops.	6 onions	50	20	1	Trace	----	----	----	5	20	.3	Trace	.02	.02	.2	12
Parsley, raw, chopped	1 tablespoon	3.5	1	Trace	Trace	----	----	----	Trace	7	.2	300	Trace	.01	Trace	6
Parsnips, cooked	1 cup	155	100	2	1	----	----	----	23	70	.9	50	.11	.13	.2	16
Peas, green:																
Cooked	1 cup	160	115	9	1	----	----	----	19	37	2.9	860	.44	.17	3.7	33
Canned, solids and liquid.	1 cup	249	165	9	1	----	----	----	31	50	4.2	1,120	.23	.13	2.2	22
Canned, strained (baby food).	1 ounce	28	15	1	Trace	----	----	----	3	3	.4	140	.02	.02	.4	3
Peppers, hot, red, without seeds, dried (ground chili powder, added seasonings).	1 tablespoon	15	50	2	2	----	----	----	8	40	2.3	9,750	.03	.17	1.3	2
Peppers, sweet:																
Raw, medium, about 6 per pound:																
Green pod without stem and seeds.	1 pod	62	15	1	Trace	----	----	----	3	6	.4	260	.05	.05	.3	79
Red pod without stem and seeds.	1 pod	60	20	1	Trace	----	----	----	4	8	.4	2,670	.05	.05	.3	122
Canned, pimientos, medium.	1 pod	38	10	Trace	Trace	----	----	----	2	3	.6	870	.01	.02	.1	36

Baked, peeled after baking.	1 potato	99	90	3	Trace				21	9	.7	Trace	.10	.04	1.7	20
Boiled:																
Peeled after boiling	1 potato	136	105	3	Trace				23	10	.8	Trace	.13	.05	2.0	22
Peeled before boiling	1 potato	122	30	2	Trace				18	7	.6	Trace	.11	.04	1.4	20
French-fried, piece 2 by ½ by ½ inch:																
Cooked in deep fat	10 pieces	57	155	2	7	2	2	4	20	9	.7	Trace	.07	.04	1.8	12
Frozen, heated	10 pieces	57	125	2	5	1	1	2	19	5	1.0	Trace	.08	.01	1.5	12
Mashed:																
Milk added	1 cup	195	125	4	1				25	47	.8	50	.16	.10	2.0	19
Milk and butter added.	1 cup	195	185	4	8	4	3	Trace	24	47	.8	330	.16	.10	1.9	18
Potato chips, medium, 2-inch diameter.	10 chips	20	115	1	8	2	2	4	10	8	.4	Trace	.04	.01	1.0	3
Pumpkin, canned	1 cup	228	75	2	1				18	57	.9	14,590	.07	.12	1.3	12
Radishes, raw, small, without tops.	4 radishes	40	5	Trace	Trace				1	12	.4	Trace	.01	.01	.1	10
Sauerkraut, canned, solids and liquid.	1 cup	235	45	2	Trace				9	85	1.2	120	.07	.09	.4	33
Spinach:																
Cooked	1 cup	180	40	5	1				6	167	4.0	14,580	.13	.25	1.0	50
Canned, drained solids	1 cup	180	45	5	1				6	212	4.7	14,400	.03	.21	.6	24
Canned, strained or chopped (baby food).	1 ounce	28	10	1	Trace				2	18	.2	1,420	.01	.04	.1	2
Sprouts, raw:																
Mung bean	1 cup	90	30	3	Trace				6	17	1.2	20	.12	.12	.7	17
Soybean	1 cup	107	40	6	2				4	46	.7	90	.17	.16	.8	4
Squash:																
Cooked:																
Summer, diced	1 cup	210	30	2	Trace				7	52	.8	820	.10	.16	1.6	21
Winter, baked, mashed.	1 cup	205	130	4	1				32	57	1.6	8,610	.10	.27	1.4	27
Canned, winter, strained and chopped (baby food).	1 ounce	28	10	Trace	Trace				2	7	.1	510	.01	.01	.1	1

TABLE 36—*Continued*

Food, Approximate Measure, and Weight (in Grams)			Food Energy	Protein	Fat (Total Lipid)	Fatty acids			Carbohydrate	Calcium	Iron	Vitamin A Value	Thiamine	Riboflavin	Niacin	Ascorbic Acid
						Saturated (Total)	Unsaturated									
							Oleic	Linoleic								
VEGETABLES AND VEGETABLE PRODUCTS—Continued																
Sweetpotatoes:																
Cooked, medium, 5 by 2 inches, weight raw about 6 ounces:		*Grams*	(Calories)	(Gm.)	(Gm.)	(Gm.)	(Gm.)	(Gm.)	(Gm.)	(Mg.)	(Mg.)	(I.U.)	(Mg.)	(Mg.)	(Mg.)	(Mg.)
Baked, peeled after baking.	1 sweetpotato.	110	155	2	1				36	44	1.0	8,910	0.10	0.07	0.7	24
Boiled, peeled after boiling.	1 sweetpotato.	147	170	2	1				39	47	1.0	11,610	.13	.09	.9	25
Candied, 3½ by 2¼ inches.	1 sweetpotato.	175	295	2	6	2	3	1	60	65	1.6	11,030	.10	.08	.8	17
Canned, vacuum or solid pack.	1 cup	218	235	4	Trace				54	54	1.7	17,000	.10	.10	1.4	30
Tomatoes:																
Raw, medium, 2 by 2½ inches, about 3 per pound.	1 tomato	150	35	2	Trace				7	20	.8	1,350	.10	.06	1.0	[6]34
Canned	1 cup	242	50	2	Trace				10	15	1.2	2,180	.13	.07	1.7	40
Tomato juice, canned	1 cup	242	45	2	Trace				10	17	2.2	1,940	.13	.07	1.8	39
Tomato catsup	1 tablespoon	17	15	Trace	Trace				4	4	.1	240	.02	.01	.3	3
Turnips, cooked, diced	1 cup	155	35	1	Trace				8	54	.6	Trace	.06	.08	.5	33
Turnip greens:																
Cooked:																
In small amount of water, short time.	1 cup	145	30	3	Trace				5	267	1.6	9,140	.21	.36	.8	100
In large amount of water, long time.	1 cup	145	25	3	Trace				5	252	1.4	8,260	.14	.33	.8	68
Canned, solids and liquid	1 cup	232	40	3	1				7	232	3.7	10,900	.04	.21	1.4	44
FRUITS AND FRUIT PRODUCTS																
Apples, raw, medium, 2½-inch diameter, about 3	1 apple	150	70	Trace	Trace				18	8	.4	50	.04	.02	.1	3

canned.																
Applesauce, canned:																
Sweetened	1 cup	254	230	1	Trace				60	10	1.3	100	.05	.03	.1	3
Unsweetened or artificially sweetened.	1 cup	239	100	Trace	Trace				2[illegible]	10	1.2	100	.04	.02	.1	2
Applesauce and apricots, canned, strained or junior (baby food).	1 ounce	28	25	Trace	Trace				[illegible]	1	.1	170	Trace	Trace	Trace	1
Apricots:																
Raw, about 12 per pound.[4]	3 apricots	114	55	1	Trace				1[illegible]	18	.5	2,890	.03	.04	.7	10
Canned in heavy sirup:																
Halves and sirup	1 cup	259	220	2	Trace				5[illegible]	28	.8	4,510	.05	.06	.9	10
Halves (medium) and sirup.	4 halves; 2 table-spoons sirup.	122	105	1	Trace				2[illegible]	13	.4	2,120	.02	.03	.4	5
Dried:																
Uncooked, 40 halves, small.	1 cup	150	390	8	1				10[illegible]	100	8.2	16,350	.02	.23	4.9	19
Cooked, unsweetened, fruit and liquid.	1 cup	285	240	5	1				6[illegible]	63	5.1	8,550	.01	.13	2.8	8
Apricot nectar, canned	1 cup	250	140	1	Trace				3[illegible]	22	.5	2,380	.02	.02	.5	7
Avocados, raw:																
California varieties, mainly Fuerte:																
10-ounce avocado, about 3⅓ by 4¼ inches, peeled, pitted.	½ avocado	108	135	2	18	4	8	2	[illegible]	11	.6	310	.12	.21	1.7	15
½-inch cubes	1 cup	152	250	3	26	5	12	3	[illegible]	15	.9	440	.16	.30	2.4	21
Florida varieties:																
13-ounce avocado, about 4 by 3 inches, peeled, pitted.	½ avocado	123	150	2	14	3	6	2	11	12	.7	360	.13	.24	2.0	17
½-inch cubes	1 cup	152	195	2	17	3	8	2	1[illegible]	15	.9	440	.16	.30	2.4	21
Bananas, raw, 6 by 1½ inches, about 3 per pound.[4]	1 banana	150	85	1	Trace				2[illegible]	8	.7	190	.05	.06	.7	10
Blackberries, raw	1 cup	144	85	2	1				1[illegible]	46	1.3	290	.05	.06	.5	30
Blueberries, raw	1 cup	140	85	1	1				21	21	1.4	140	.04	.08	.6	20
Cantaloups, raw; medium, 5-inch diameter, about 1⅔ pounds.[4]	½ melon	385	60	1	Trace				14	27	.8	[7]6,540	.08	.06	1.2	63

[4] Measure and weight apply to entire vegetable or fruit including parts not usually eaten.

[6] Year-round average. Samples marketed from November through May average around 15 milligrams per 150-gram tomato; from June through October, around 39 milligrams.

[7] Value based on varieties with orange-colored flesh, for green-fleshed varieties value is about 540 I.U. per ½ melon.

TABLE 36—*Continued*

Food, Approximate Measure, and Weight (in Grams)			Food Energy	Protein	Fat (Total Lipid)	Fatty acids			Carbohydrate	Calcium	Iron	Vitamin A Value	Thiamine	Riboflavin	Niacin	Ascorbic Acid
						Saturated (Total)	Unsaturated									
							Oleic	Linoleic								
FRUITS AND FRUIT PRODUCTS—Con.																
		Grams	(Calories)	(Gm.)	(Gm.)	(Gm.)	(Gm.)	(Gm.)	(Gm.)	(Mg.)	(Mg.)	(I.U.)	(Mg.)	(Mg.)	(Mg.)	(Mg.)
Cherries:																
Raw, sweet, with stems [4]	1 cup	130	80	2	Trace				20	26	0.5	130	0.06	0.07	0.5	12
Canned, red, sour, pitted, heavy sirup.	1 cup	260	230	2	1				59	36	.8	1,680	.07	.06	.4	13
Cranberry juice cocktail, canned.	1 cup	250	160	Trace	Trace				41	12	.8	Trace	.02	.02	.1	(8)
Cranberry sauce, sweetened, canned, strained.	1 cup	277	405	Trace	1				104	17	.6	40	.03	.03	.1	5
Dates, domestic, natural and dry, pitted, cut.	1 cup	178	490	4	1				130	105	5.3	90	.16	.17	3.9	0
Figs:																
Raw, small, 1½-inch diameter, about 12 per pound.	3 figs	114	90	1	Trace				23	40	.7	90	.07	.06	.5	2
Dried, large, 2 by 1 inch	1 fig	21	60	1	Trace				15	26	.6	20	.02	.02	.1	0
Fruit cocktail, canned in heavy sirup, solids and liquid.	1 cup	256	195	1	1				50	23	1.0	360	.04	.03	1.1	5
Grapefruit:																
Raw, medium, 4¼-inch diameter, size 64:																
White [4]	½ grapefruit	285	55	1	Trace				14	22	.6	10	.05	.02	.2	52
Pink or red [4]	½ grapefruit	285	60	1	Trace				15	23	.6	640	.05	.02	.3	52
Raw sections, white	1 cup	194	75	1	Trace				20	31	.8	20	.07	.03	.3	72
Canned, white:																
Sirup pack, solids and liquid.	1 cup	249	175	1	Trace				44	32	.7	20	.07	.04	.5	75
Water pack, solids and liquid.	1 cup	240	70	1	Trace				18	31	.7	20	.07	.04	.5	72
Grapefruit juice:																
Fresh	1 cup	246	95	1	Trace				23	22	.5	(9)	.09	.04	.4	92
Canned, white:																
Unsweetened	1 cup	247	100	1	Trace				24	20	1.0	20	.07	.04	.4	84

Frozen, concentrate, unsweetened:																
Undiluted, can, 6 fluid ounces.	1 can	207	300	4	1	------	------	------	72	70	.8	60	.29	.12	1.4	286
Diluted with 3 parts water, by volume.	1 cup	247	100	1	Trace	------	------	------	24	25	.2	20	.10	.04	.5	96
Frozen, concentrate, sweetened:																
Undiluted, can, 6 fluid ounces.	1 can	211	350	3	1	------	------	------	85	59	.6	50	.24	.11	1.2	245
Diluted with 3 parts water, by volume.	1 cup	249	115	1	Trace	------	------	------	28	20	.2	20	.08	.03	.4	82
Dehydrated:																
Crystals, can, net weight 4 ounces.	1 can	114	430	5	1	------	------	------	103	99	1.1	90	.41	.18	2.0	399
Prepared with water (1 pound yields about 1 gallon).	1 cup	247	100	1	Trace	------	------	------	24	22	.2	20	.10	.05	.5	92
Grapes, raw:																
American type (slip skin), such as Concord, Delaware, Niagara, Catawba, and Scuppernong.[4]	1 cup	153	65	1	1	------	------	------	15	15	.4	100	.05	.03	.2	3
European type (adherent skin), such as Malaga, Muscat, Thompson Seedless, Emperor, and Flame Tokay.[4]	1 cup	160	95	1	Trace	------	------	------	25	17	.6	140	.07	.04	.4	6
Grape juice, bottled or canned.	1 cup	254	165	1	Trace	------	------	------	42	28	.8	------	.10	.05	.6	Trace
Lemons, raw, medium, 2⅕-inch diameter, size 150.[4]	1 lemon	106	20	1	Trace	------	------	------	6	18	.4	10	.03	.01	.1	38
Lemon juice:																
Fresh	1 cup	246	60	1	Trace	------	------	------	20	17	.5	40	.08	.03	.2	113
	1 tablespoon	15	5	Trace	Trace	------	------	------	1	1	Trace	Trace	Trace	Trace	Trace	7
Canned, unsweetened	1 cup	245	55	1	Trace	------	------	------	19	17	.5	40	.07	.03	.2	102
Lemonade concentrate, frozen, sweetened:																
Undiluted, can, 6 fluid ounces.	1 can	220	430	Trace	Trace	------	------	------	112	9	.4	40	.05	.06	.7	66
Diluted with 4⅓ parts water, by volume.	1 cup	248	110	Trace	Trace	------	------	------	28	2	.1	10	.01	.01	.2	17

[4] Measure and weight apply to entire vegetable or fruit including parts not usually eaten.

[8] About 5 milligrams per 8 fluid ounces is from cranberries. Ascorbic acid is usually added to approximately 100 milligrams per 8 fluid ounces.

[9] For white-fleshed varieties value is about 20 I.U. per cup; for red-fleshed varieties, 1,080 I.U. per cup.

TABLE 36—*Continued*

Food, Approximate Measure, and Weight (in Grams)			Food Energy	Protein	Fat (Total Lipid)	Fatty acids: Saturated (Total)	Fatty acids: Unsaturated: Oleic	Fatty acids: Unsaturated: Linoleic	Carbohydrate	Calcium	Iron	Vitamin A Value	Thiamine	Riboflavin	Niacin	Ascorbic Acid
FRUITS AND FRUIT PRODUCTS—Con.		*Grams*	(Calories)	(Gm.)	(Gm.)	(Gm.)	(Gm.)	(Gm.)	(Gm.)	(Mg.)	(Mg.)	(I.U.)	(Mg.)	(Mg.)	(Mg.)	(Mg.)
Lime juice:																
Fresh	1 cup	246	65	1	Trace				22	22	0.5	30	0.05	0.03	0.3	80
Canned	1 cup	246	65	1	Trace				22	22	.5	30	.05	.03	.3	52
Limeade concentrate, frozen, sweetened:																
Undiluted, can, 6 fluid ounces.	1 can	218	410	Trace	Trace				108	11	.2	Trace	.02	.02	.2	26
Diluted with 4⅓ parts water, by volume.	1 cup	248	105	Trace	Trace				27	2	Trace	Trace	Trace	Trace	Trace	6
Oranges, raw:																
California, Navel (winter), 2⅘-inch diameter, size 88.[4]	1 orange	180	60	2	Trace				16	49	.5	240	.12	.05	.5	75
Florida, all varieties, 3-inch diameter.[4]	1 orange	210	75	1	Trace				19	67	.3	310	.16	.06	.6	70
Orange juice:																
Fresh:																
California, Valencia (summer).	1 cup	249	115	2	1				26	27	.7	500	.22	.06	.9	122
Florida varieties:																
Early and midseason.	1 cup	247	100	1	Trace				23	25	.5	490	.22	.06	.9	127
Late season, Valencia.	1 cup	248	110	1	Trace				26	25	.5	500	.22	.06	.9	92
Canned, unsweetened	1 cup	249	120	2	Trace				28	25	1.0	500	.17	.05	.6	100
Frozen concentrate:																
Undiluted, can, 6 fluid ounces.	1 can	210	330	5	Trace				80	69	.8	1,490	.63	.10	2.4	332
Diluted with 3 parts water, by volume.	1 cup	248	110	2	Trace				27	22	.2	500	.21	.03	.8	112
Dehydrated:																
Crystals, can, net weight 4 ounces.	1 can	113	430	6	2				100	95	1.9	1,900	.76	.24	3.3	406

Prepared with water, 1 pound yields about 1 gallon.	1 cup	248	115	1	Trace	----	----	----	27	25	.5	500	.20	.06	.9	108
Orange and grapefruit juice:																
Frozen concentrate:																
Undiluted, can, 6 fluid ounces.	1 can	209	325	4	1	----	----	----	78	61	.8	790	.47	.06	2.3	301
Diluted with 3 parts water, by volume.	1 cup	248	110	1	Trace	----	----	----	26	20	.2	270	.16	.02	.8	102
Papayas, raw, ½-inch cubes.	1 cup	182	70	1	Trace	----	----	----	18	36	.5	3,190	.07	.08	.5	102
Peaches:																
Raw:																
Whole, medium, 2-inch diameter, about 4 per pound.[4]	1 peach	114	35	1	Trace	----	----	----	10	9	.5	[10]1,320	.02	.05	1.0	7
Sliced	1 cup	168	65	1	Trace	----	----	----	16	15	.8	[10]2,230	.03	.08	1.6	12
Canned, yellow-fleshed, solids and liquid:																
Sirup pack, heavy:																
Halves or slices	1 cup	257	200	1	Trace	----	----	----	52	10	.8	1,100	.02	.06	1.4	7
Halves (medium) and sirup.	2 halves and 2 tablespoons sirup.	117	90	Trace	Trace	----	----	----	24	5	.4	500	.01	.03	.7	3
Water pack	1 cup	245	75	1	Trace	----	----	----	20	10	.7	1,100	.02	.06	1.4	7
Strained or chopped (baby food).	1 ounce	28	25	Trace	Trace	----	----	----	6	2	.1	140	Trace	.01	.2	1
Dried:																
Uncooked	1 cup	160	420	5	1	----	----	----	109	77	9.6	6,240	.02	.31	8.5	28
Cooked, unsweetened, 10–12 halves and 6 tablespoons liquid.	1 cup	270	220	3	1	----	----	----	58	41	5.1	3,290	.01	.15	4.2	6
Frozen:																
Carton, 12 ounces, not thawed.	1 carton	340	300	1	Trace	----	----	----	77	14	1.7	2,210	.03	.14	2.4	[11]135
Can, 16 ounces, not thawed.	1 can	454	400	2	Trace	----	----	----	103	18	2.3	2,950	.05	.18	3.2	[11]181
Peach nectar, canned	1 cup	250	120	Trace	Trace	----	----	----	31	10	.5	1,080	.02	.05	1.0	1
Pears:																
Raw, 3 by 2½-inch diameter.[4]	1 pear	182	100	1	1	----	----	----	25	13	.5	30	.04	.07	.2	7

[4] Measure and weight apply to entire vegetable or fruit including parts not usually eaten.

[10] Based on yellow-fleshed varieties; for white-fleshed varieties value is about 50 I.U per 114-gram peach and 80 I.U. per cup of sliced peaches.

[11] Average weighted in accordance with commercial freezing practices. For products without added ascorbic acid, value is about 37 milligrams per 12-ounce carton and 50 milligrams per 16-ounce can; for those with added ascorbic acid, 139 milligrams per 12 ounces and 186 milligrams per 16 ounces.

TABLE 36—*Continued*

Food, Approximate Measure, and Weight (in Grams)			Food Energy	Protein	Fat (Total Lipid)	Fatty acids			Carbohydrate	Calcium	Iron	Vitamin A Value	Thiamine	Riboflavin	Niacin	Ascorbic Acid
						Saturated (Total)	Unsaturated									
							Oleic	Linoleic								
FRUITS AND FRUIT PRODUCTS—Con.																
Pears—Continued																
Canned, solids and liquid:			(Calories)	(Gm.)	(Gm.)	(Gm.)	(Gm.)	(Gm.)	(Gm.)	(Mg.)	(Mg.)	(I.U.)	(Mg.)	(Mg.)	(Mg.)	(Mg.)
Sirup pack, heavy:		*Grams*														
Halves or slices	1 cup	255	195	1	1				50	13	0.5	Trace	0.03	0.05	0.3	4
Halves (medium) and sirup.	2 halves and 2 tablespoons sirup.	117	90	Trace	Trace				23	6	.2	Trace	.01	.02	.2	2
Water pack	1 cup	243	80	Trace	Trace				20	12	.5	Trace	.02	.05	.3	4
Strained or chopped (baby food).	1 ounce	28	20	Trace	Trace				5	2	.1	10	Trace	.01	.1	1
Pear nectar, canned	1 cup	250	130	1	Trace				33	8	.2	Trace	.01	.05	Trace	1
Persimmons, Japanese or kaki, raw, seedless, 2½-inch diameter.[4]	1 persimmon	125	75	1	Trace				20	6	.4	2,740	.03	.02	.1	11
Pineapple:																
Raw, diced	1 cup	140	75	1	Trace				19	24	.7	100	.12	.04	.3	24
Canned, heavy sirup pack, solids and liquid:																
Crushed	1 cup	260	195	1	Trace				50	29	.8	120	.20	.06	.5	17
Sliced, slices and juice.	2 small or 1 large and 2 tablespoons juice.	122	90	Trace	Trace				24	13	.4	50	.09	.03	.2	8
Pineapple juice, canned	1 cup	249	135	1	Trace				34	37	.7	120	.12	.04	.5	22
Plums, all except prunes:																
Raw, 2-inch diameter, about 2 ounces.[4]	1 plum	60	25	Trace	Trace				7	7	.3	140	.02	.02	.3	3
Canned, sirup pack (Italian prunes):																
Plums (with pits) and juice.[4]	1 cup	256	205	1	Trace				53	22	2.2	2,970	.05	.05	.9	4

pits) and juice.	and 2 table- spoons juice.															
Prunes, dried, "softenized", medium:																
Uncooked [4]	4 prunes	32	70	1	Trace				18	14	1.1	440	.02	.04	.4	1
Cooked, unsweetened, 17–18 prunes and ⅓ cup liquid.[4]	1 cup	270	295	2	1				78	60	4.5	1,860	.08	.18	1.7	2
Prunes with tapioca, canned, strained or junior (baby food).	1 ounce	28	25	Trace	Trace				6	2	.3	110	.01	.02	.1	1
Prune juice, canned	1 cup	256	200	1	Trace				49	36	10.5		.02	.03	1.1	4
Raisins, dried	1 cup	160	460	4	Trace				124	99	5.6	30	.18	.13	.9	2
Raspberries, red:																
Raw	1 cup	123	70	1	1				17	27	1.1	160	.04	.11	1.1	31
Frozen, 10-ounce carton, not thawed.	1 carton	284	275	2	1				70	37	1.7	200	.06	.17	1.7	59
Rhubarb, cooked, sugar added.	1 cup	272	385	1	Trace				98	212	1.6	220	.06	.15	.7	17
Strawberries:																
Raw, capped	1 cup	149	55	1	1				13	31	1.5	90	.04	.10	1.0	88
Frozen, 10-ounce carton, not thawed.	1 carton	284	310	1	1				79	40	2.0	90	.06	.17	1.5	150
Frozen, 16-ounce can, not thawed.	1 can	454	495	2	1				126	64	3.2	150	.09	.27	2.4	240
Tangerines, raw, medium, 2½-inch diameter, about 4 per pound.[4]	1 tangerine	114	40	1	Trace				10	34	.3	350	.05	.02	.1	26
Tangerine juice:																
Canned, unsweetened	1 cup	248	105	1	Trace				25	45	.5	1,040	.14	.04	.3	56
Frozen concentrate:																
Undiluted, can, 6 fluid ounces.	1 can	210	340	4	1				80	130	1.5	3,070	.43	.12	.9	202
Diluted with 3 parts water, by volume.	1 cup	248	115	1	Trace				27	45	.5	1,020	.14	.04	.3	67
Watermelon, raw, wedge, 4 by 8 inches (1/16 of 10 by 16-inch melon, about 2 pounds with rind).[4]	1 wedge	925	115	2	1				27	30	2.1	2,510	.13	.13	.7	30

[4] Measure and weight apply to entire vegetable or fruit including parts not usually eaten.

TABLE 36—*Continued*

Food, Approximate Measure, and Weight (in Grams)			Food Energy	Protein	Fat (Total Lipid)	Fatty acids: Saturated (Total)	Fatty acids: Unsaturated: Oleic	Fatty acids: Unsaturated: Linoleic	Carbohydrate	Calcium	Iron	Vitamin A Value	Thiamine	Riboflavin	Niacin	Ascorbic Acid
GRAIN PRODUCTS		*Grams*	(Calories)	(Gm.)	(Gm.)	(Gm.)	(Gm.)	(Gm.)	(Gm.)	(Mg.)	(Mg.)	(I.U.)	(Mg.)	(Mg.)	(Mg.)	(Mg.)
Barley, pearled, light, uncooked.	1 cup	203	710	17	2	Trace	1	1	160	32	4.1	0	0.25	0.17	6.3	0
Biscuits, baking powder with enriched flour, 2½-inch diameter.	1 biscuit	38	140	3	6	2	3	1	17	46	.6	Trace	.08	.08	.7	Trace
Bran flakes (40 percent bran) added thiamine.	1 ounce	28	85	3	1	------	------	------	23	20	1.2	0	.11	.05	1.7	0
Breads:																
Boston brown bread, slice, 3 by ¾ inch.	1 slice	48	100	3	1	------	------	------	22	43	.9	0	.05	.03	.6	0
Cracked-wheat bread:																
Loaf, 1-pound, 20 slices.	1 loaf	454	1,190	39	10	2	5	2	236	399	5.0	Trace	.53	.42	5.8	Trace
Slice	1 slice	23	60	2	1	------	------	------	12	20	.3	Trace	.03	.02	.3	Trace
French or vienna bread:																
Enriched, 1-pound loaf.	1 loaf	454	1,315	41	14	3	8	2	251	195	10.0	Trace	1.26	.98	11.3	Trace
Unenriched, 1-pound loaf.	1 loaf	454	1,315	41	14	3	8	2	251	195	3.2	Trace	.39	.39	3.6	Trace
Italian bread:																
Enriched, 1-pound loaf.	1 loaf	454	1,250	41	4	Trace	1	2	256	77	10.0	0	1.31	.93	11.7	0
Unenriched, 1-pound loaf.	1 loaf	454	1,250	41	4	Trace	1	2	256	77	3.2	0	.39	.27	3.6	0
Raisin bread:																
Loaf, 1-pound, 20 slices.	1 loaf	454	1,190	30	13	3	8	2	243	322	5.9	Trace	.24	.42	3.0	Trace
Slice	1 slice	23	60	2	1	------	------	------	12	16	.3	Trace	.01	.02	.2	Trace
Rye bread:																
American, light (1/3 rye, 2/3 wheat):																
Loaf, 1-pound, 20 slices.	1 loaf	454	1,100	41	5	------	------	------	236	340	7.3	0	.81	.33	6.4	0

[illegible], loaf, 1 pound.	1 loaf	454	1,115	41	5				241	381	10.9	0	1.05	.63	5.4	0
White bread, enriched:																
1 to 2 percent nonfat dry milk:																
Loaf, 1-pound, 20 slices.	1 loaf	454	1,225	39	15	3	8	2	229	318	10.9	Trace	1.13	.77	10.4	Trace
Slice	1 slice	23	60	2	1	Trace	Trace	Trace	12	16	.6	Trace	.06	.04	.5	Trace
3 to 4 percent nonfat dry milk: [12]																
Loaf, 1-pound	1 loaf	454	1,225	39	15	3	8	2	229	381	11.3	Trace	1.13	.95	10.8	Trace
Slice, 20 per loaf	1 slice	23	60	2	1	Trace	Trace	Trace	12	19	.6	Trace	.06	.05	.6	Trace
Slice, toasted	1 slice	20	60	2	1	Trace	Trace	Trace	12	19	.6	Trace	.05	.05	.6	Trace
Slice, 26 per loaf	1 slice	17	45	1	1	Trace	Trace	Trace	9	14	.4	Trace	.04	.04	.4	Trace
5 to 6 percent nonfat dry milk:																
Loaf, 1-pound, 20 slices.	1 loaf	454	1,245	41	17	4	10	2	228	435	11.3	Trace	1.22	.91	11.0	Trace
Slice	1 slice	23	65	2	1	Trace	Trace	Trace	12	22	.6	Trace	.06	.05	.6	Trace
White bread, unenriched:																
1 to 2 percent nonfat dry milk:																
Loaf, 1-pound, 20 slices.	1 loaf	454	1,225	39	15	3	8	2	229	318	3.2	Trace	.40	.36	5.6	Trace
Slice	1 slice	23	60	2	1	Trace	Trace	Trace	12	16	.2	Trace	.02	.02	.3	Trace
3 to 4 percent nonfat dry milk: [12]																
Loaf, 1-pound	1 loaf	454	1,225	39	15	3	8		229	381	3.2	Trace	.31	.39	5.0	Trace
Slice, 20 per loaf	1 slice	23	60	2	1	Trace	Trace	Trace	12	19	.2	Trace	.02	.02	.3	Trace
Slice, toasted	1 slice	20	60	2	1	Trace	Trace	Trace	12	19	.2	Trace	.01	.02	.3	Trace
Slice, 26 per loaf	1 slice	17	45	1	1	Trace	Trace	Trace	9	14	.1	Trace	.01	.01	.2	Trace
5 to 6 percent nonfat dry milk:																
Loaf, 1 pound, 20 slices.	1 loaf	454	1,245	41	17	4	10	2	228	435	3.2	Trace	.32	.59	4.1	Trace
Slice	1 slice	23	65	2	1	Trace	Trace	Trace	12	22	.2	Trace	.02	.03	.2	Trace
Whole-wheat bread, made with 2 percent nonfat dry milk:																
Loaf, 1-pound, 20 slices	1 loaf	454	1,105	48	14	3	6	3	216	449	10.4	Trace	1.17	.56	12.9	Trace
Slice	1 slice	23	55	2	1	Trace	Trace	Trace	11	23	.5	Trace	.06	.03	.7	Trace
Slice, toasted	1 slice	19	55	2	1	Trace	Trace	Trace	11	22	.5	Trace	.05	.03	.6	Trace
Breadcrumbs, dry, grated	1 cup	88	345	11	4	1	2	1	65	107	3.2	Trace	.19	.26	3.1	Trace
Cakes: [13]																
Angelfood cake; sector, 2-inch (1/12 of 8-inch-diameter cake).	1 sector	40	110	3	Trace				24	4	.1	0	Trace	.06	.1	0

[12] When the amount of nonfat dry milk in commercial white bread is unknown, values for bread with 3 to 4 percent nonfat dry milk are suggested.

[13] Unenriched cake flour and vegetable cooking fat used unless otherwise specified.

TABLE 36—*Continued*

Food, Approximate Measure, and Weight (in Grams)	Measure	Weight	Food Energy	Protein	Fat (Total Lipid)	Fatty acids: Saturated (Total)	Fatty acids: Unsaturated: Oleic	Fatty acids: Unsaturated: Linoleic	Carbohydrate	Calcium	Iron	Vitamin A Value	Thiamine	Riboflavin	Niacin	Ascorbic Acid
GRAIN PRODUCTS—Continued																
Cakes [13]—Continued		*Grams*	(Calories)	(Gm.)	(Gm.)	(Gm.)	(Gm.)	(Gm.)	(Gm.)	(Mg.)	(Mg.)	(I.U.)	(Mg.)	(Mg.)	(Mg.)	(Mg.)
Chocolate cake, chocolate icing; sector, 2-inch (1/16 of 10-inch-diameter layer cake).	1 sector	120	445	5	20	8	10	1	67	84	1.2	[14] 190	0.03	0.12	0.3	Trace
Fruitcake, dark (made with enriched flour); piece, 2 by 2 by ½ inch.	1 piece	30	115	1	5	1	3	1	18	22	.8	[14] 40	.04	.04	.2	Trace
Gingerbread (made with enriched flour); piece, 2 by 2 by 2 inches.	1 piece	55	175	2	6	1	4	Trace	29	37	1.3	50	.06	.06	.5	0
Plain cake and cupcakes, without icing:																
Piece, 3 by 2 by 1½ inches.	1 piece	55	200	2	8	2	5	1	31	35	.2	[14] 90	.01	.05	.1	Trace
Cupcake, 2¾-inch diameter.	1 cupcake	40	145	2	6	1	3	Trace	22	26	.2	[14] 70	.01	.03	.1	Trace
Plain cake and cupcakes, with chocolate icing:																
Sector, 2-inch (1/16 of 10-inch-layer cake).	1 sector	100	370	4	14	5	7	1	59	63	.6	[14] 180	.02	.09	.2	Trace
Cupcake, 2¾-inch diameter.	1 cupcake	50	185	2	7	2	4	Trace	30	32	.3	[14] 90	.01	.04	.1	Trace
Poundcake, old-fashioned (equal weights flour, sugar, fat, eggs); slice, 2¾ by 3 by ⅝ inch.	1 slice	30	140	2	9	2	5	1	14	6	.2	[14] 80	.01	.03	.1	0
Sponge cake; sector, 2-inch (1/12 of 8-inch-diameter cake).	1 sector	40	120	3	2	1	1	Trace	22	12	.5	180	.02	.06	.1	Trace
Cookies:																
Plain and assorted,	1 cooky	25	120	1	5	------	------	------	18	9	.2	20	.01	.01	.1	Trace

Corn, rice and wheat flakes, mixed, added nutrients.	1 ounce	28	110	2	Trace				24	11	.5	0	.11		.9	0
Corn flakes, added nutrients:																
Plain	1 ounce	28	110	2	Trace				24	5	.4	0	.12	.02	.6	0
Sugar-covered	1 ounce	28	110	1	Trace				26	3	.3	0	.12	.01	.5	0
Corn grits, degermed, cooked:																
Enriched	1 cup	242	120	3	Trace				27	2	[15] .7	[16] 150	[15] .10	[15] .07	[15] 1.0	0
Unenriched	1 cup	242	120	3	Trace				27	2	.2	[16] 150	.05	.02	.5	0
Cornmeal, white or yellow, dry:																
Whole ground, unbolted	1 cup	118	420	11	5	1	2	2	87	24	2.8	[16] 600	.45	.13	2.4	0
Degermed, enriched	1 cup	145	525	11	2	Trace	1	[illegible]	114	9	[15] 4.2	[16] 640	[15] .64	[15] .38	[15] 5.1	0
Corn muffins, made with enriched degermed cornmeal and enriched flour; muffin, 2¾-inch diameter.	1 muffin	48	150	3	5	2	2	Trace	23	50	.8	[17] 80	.09	.11	.8	Trace
Corn, puffed, pre-sweetened, added nutrients.	1 ounce	28	110	1	Trace				26	3	.5	0	.12	.05	.6	0
Corn, shredded, added nutrients.	1 ounce	28	110	2	Trace				25	1	.7	0	.12	.05	.6	0
Crackers:																
Graham, plain	4 small or 2 medium.	14	55	1	1				10	6	.2	0	.01	.03	.2	0
Saltines, 2 inches square.	2 crackers	8	35	1	1				6	2	.1	0	Trace	Trace	.1	0
Soda:																
Cracker, 2½ inches square.	2 crackers	11	50	1	1	Trace	1	Trace	8	2	.2	0	Trace	Trace	.1	0
Oyster crackers	10 crackers	10	45	1	1	Trace	1	Trace	7	2	.2	0	Trace	Trace	.1	0
Cracker meal	1 tablespoon	10	45	1	1	Trace	1	Trace	7	2	.1	0	.01	Trace	.1	0
Doughnuts, cake type	1 doughnut	32	125	1	6	1	4	Trace	16	13	[18] .4	30	[18] .05	[18] .05	[18] .4	Trace
Farina, regular, enriched, cooked.	1 cup	238	100	3	Trace				21	10	[15] .7	0	[15] .11	[15] .07	[15] 1.0	0

[13] Unenriched cake flour and vegetable cooking fat used unless otherwise specified.

[14] If the fat used in the recipe is butter or fortified margarine, the vitamin A value for chocolate cake with chocolate icing will be 490 I.U. per 2-inch sector, item 360; 100 I.U. for fruitcake, item 361; for plain cake without icing, 300 I.U. per piece, item 363; 220 I.U. per cupcake, item 364; for plain cake with icing, 440 I.U. per 2-inch sector, item 365; 220 I.U. per cupcake, item 365; and 300 I.U. for poundcake, item 367.

[15] Iron, thiamine, riboflavin, and niacin are based on the minimum levels of enrichment specified in standards of identity promulgated under the Federal Food, Drug, and Cosmetic Act.

[16] Vitamin A value based on yellow product. White product contains only a trace.

[17] Based on recipe using white cornmeal; if yellow cornmeal is used, the vitamin A value is 140 I.U. per muffin.

[18] Based on product made with enriched flour. With unenriched flour, approximate values per doughnut are: Iron, 0.2 milligram; thiamine, 0.01 milligram; riboflavin, 0.03 milligram; niacin, 0.2 milligram.

TABLE 36—*Continued*

Food, Approximate Measure, and Weight (in Grams)			Food Energy	Protein	Fat (Total Lipid)	Fatty acids: Saturated (Total)	Fatty acids: Unsaturated: Oleic	Fatty acids: Unsaturated: Linoleic	Carbohydrate	Calcium	Iron	Vitamin A Value	Thiamine	Riboflavin	Niacin	Ascorbic Acid
GRAIN PRODUCTS—Continued																
Macaroni, cooked:																
Enriched:		*Grams*	(Calories)	(Gm.)	(Gm.)	(Gm.)	(Gm.)	(Gm.)	(Gm.)	(Mg.)	(Mg.)	(I.U.)	(Mg.)	(Mg.)	(Mg.)	(Mg.)
Cooked, firm stage (8 to 10 minutes; undergoes additional cooking in a food mixture).	1 cup	130	190	6	1	------	------	------	39	14	[15] 1.4	0	[15] 0.23	[15] 0.14	[15] 1.9	0
Cooked until tender	1 cup	140	155	5	1	------	------	------	32	11	[15] 1.3	0	[15] .19	[15] .11	[15] 1.5	0
Unenriched:																
Cooked, firm stage (8 to 10 minutes; undergoes additional cooking in a food mixture).	1 cup	130	190	6	1	------	------	------	39	14	.6	0	.02	.02	.5	0
Cooked until tender	1 cup	140	155	5	1	------	------	------	32	11	.6	0	.02	.02	.4	0
Macaroni (enriched) and cheese, baked.	1 cup	220	470	18	24	11	10	1	44	398	2.0	950	.22	.44	2.0	Trace
Muffins, with enriched white flour; muffin, 2¾-inch diameter.	1 muffin	48	140	4	5	1	3	Trace	20	50	.8	50	.08	.11	.7	Trace
Noodles (egg noodles), cooked:																
Enriched	1 cup	160	200	7	2	1	1	Trace	37	16	[15] 1.4	110	[15] .23	[15] .14	[15] 1.8	0
Unenriched	1 cup	160	200	7	2	1	1	Trace	37	16	1.0	110	.04	.03	.7	0
Oats (with or without corn) puffed, added nutrients.	1 ounce	28	115	3	2	Trace	1	1	21	50	1.3	0	.28	.05	.5	0
Oatmeal or rolled oats, regular or quick-cooking, cooked.	1 cup	236	130	5	2	Trace	1	1	23	21	1.4	0	.19	.05	.3	0
Pancakes (griddlecakes), 4-inch diameter:																
Wheat, enriched flour	1 cake	27	60	2	2	Trace	1	Trace	9	27	.4	30	.05	.06	.3	Trace

with egg and milk).																
Piecrust, plain, baked:																
Enriched flour:																
Lower crust, 9-inch shell.	1 crust	135	675	8	45	10	29	3	59	19	2.3	0	.27	.19	2.4	0
Double crust, 9-inch pie.	1 double crust	270	1,350	16	90	21	58	7	118	38	4.6	0	.55	.39	4.9	0
Unenriched flour:																
Lower crust, 9-inch shell.	1 crust	135	675	8	45	10	29	3	59	19	.7	0	.04	.04	.6	0
Double crust, 9-inch pie.	1 double crust	270	1,350	16	90	21	58	7	118	38	1.4	0	.08	.07	1.3	0
Pies (piecrust made with unenriched flour); sector, 4-inch, ⅐ of 9-inch-diameter pie:																
Apple	1 sector	135	345	3	15	4	9	1	51	11	.4	40	.03	.02	.5	1
Cherry	1 sector	135	355	4	15	4	10	1	52	19	.4	590	.03	.03	.6	1
Custard	1 sector	130	280	8	14	5	8	1	30	125	.8	300	.07	.21	.4	0
Lemon meringue	1 sector	120	305	4	12	4	7	1	45	17	.6	200	.04	.10	.2	4
Mince	1 sector	135	365	3	16	4	10	1	56	38	1.4	Trace	.09	.05	.5	1
Pumpkin	1 sector	130	275	5	15	5	7	1	32	66	.6	3,210	.04	.13	.6	Trace
Pizza (cheese); 5½-inch sector; ⅛ of 14-inch-diameter pie.	1 sector	75	185	7	6	2	3	Trace	27	107	.7	290	.04	.12	.7	4
Popcorn, popped, with added oil and salt.	1 cup	14	65	1	3	2	Trace	Trace	8	1	.3	------	------	.01	.2	0
Pretzels, small stick	5 sticks	5	20	Trace	Trace	------	------	------	4	1	0	0	Trace	Trace	Trace	0
Rice, white (fully milled or polished), enriched, cooked:																
Common commercial varieties, all types.	1 cup	168	185	3	Trace	------	------	------	41	17	[19] 1.5	0	[19] .19	[19] .01	[19] 1.6	0
Long grain, parboiled	1 cup	176	185	4	Trace	------	------	------	41	33	[19] 1.4	0	[19] .19	[19] .02	[19] 2.0	0
Rice, puffed, added nutrients (without salt).	1 cup	14	55	1	Trace	------	------	------	13	3	.3	0	.06	.01	.6	0

[15] Iron, thiamine, riboflavin, and niacin are based on the minimum levels of enrichment specified in standards of identity promulgated under the Federal Food, Drug, and Cosmetic Act.

[19] Iron, thiamine, and niacin are based on the minimum levels of enrichment specified in standards of identity promulgated under the Federal Food, Drug, and Cosmetic Act. Riboflavin is based on unenriched rice. When the minimum level of enrichment for riboflavin specified in the standards of identity becomes effective the value will be 0.12 milligram per cup of parboiled rice and of white rice.

TABLE 36—*Continued*

Food, Approximate Measure, and Weight (in Grams)			Food Energy	Protein	Fat (Total Lipid)	Fatty acids: Saturated (Total)	Fatty acids: Unsaturated: Oleic	Fatty acids: Unsaturated: Linoleic	Carbohydrate	Calcium	Iron	Vitamin A Value	Thiamine	Riboflavin	Niacin	Ascorbic Acid
GRAIN PRODUCTS—Continued		*Grams*	(Calories)	(Gm.)	(Gm.)	(Gm.)	(Gm.)	(Gm.)	(Gm.)	(Mg.)	(Mg.)	(I.U.)	(Mg.)	(Mg.)	(Mg.)	(Mg.)
Rice flakes, added nutrients.	1 cup	30	115	2	Trace	----	----	----	26	9	0.5	0	0.10	0.02	1.6	0
Rolls:																
Plain, pan; 12 per 16 ounces:																
Enriched	1 roll	38	115	3	2	Trace	1	Trace	20	28	.7	Trace	.11	.07	.8	Trace
Unenriched	1 roll	38	115	3	2	Trace	1	Trace	20	28	.3	Trace	.02	.03	.3	Trace
Hard, round; 12 per 22 ounces.	1 roll	52	160	5	2	Trace	1	Trace	31	24	.4	Trace	.03	.05	.4	Trace
Sweet, pan; 12 per 18 ounces.	1 roll	43	135	4	4	1	2	Trace	21	37	.3	30	.03	.06	.4	Trace
Rye wafers, whole-grain, 1⅞ by 3½ inches.	2 wafers	13	45	2	Trace	----	----	----	10	7	.5	0	.04	.03	.2	0
Spaghetti:																
Cooked, tender stage (14 to 20 minutes):																
Enriched	1 cup	140	155	5	1	----	----	----	32	11	[15] 1.3	0	[15] .19	[15] .11	[15] 1.5	0
Unenriched	1 cup	140	155	5	1	----	----	----	32	11	.6	0	.02	.02	.4	0
Spaghetti with meat balls in tomato sauce (home recipe).	1 cup	250	335	19	12	4	6	1	39	125	3.8	1,600	.26	.30	4.0	22
Spaghetti in tomato sauce with cheese (home recipe).	1 cup	250	260	9	9	2	5	1	37	80	2.2	1,080	.24	.18	2.4	14
Waffles, with enriched flour, ½ by 4½ by 5½ inches.	1 waffle	75	210	7	7	2	4	1	28	85	1.3	250	.13	.19	1.0	Trace
Wheat, puffed:																
With added nutrients (without salt).	1 ounce	28	105	4	Trace	----	----	----	22	8	1.2	0	.15	.07	2.2	0
[illegible]	1 [illegible]	28	105	2	1				25	7	.9	0	.14	.05	1.8	0

Wheat, rolled; cooked....	1 cup....	236	175	5	1	----	----	----	40	19	1.7	0	.17	.06	2.1	0
Wheat, shredded, plain (long, round, or bite-size).	1 ounce....	28	100	3	1	----	----	----	23	12	1.0	0	.06	.03	1.2	0
Wheat and malted barley flakes, with added nutrients.	1 ounce....	28	110	2	Trace	----	----	----	24	14	.7	0	.13	.03	1.1	0
Wheat flakes, with added nutrients.	1 ounce....	28	100	3	Trace	----	----	----	23	12	1.2	0	.18	.04	1.4	0
Wheat flours:																
Whole-wheat, from hard wheats, stirred.	1 cup....	120	400	16	2	Trace	1	1	85	49	4.0	0	.66	.14	5.2	0
All-purpose or family flour:																
Enriched, sifted....	1 cup....	110	400	12	1	Trace	Trace	Trace	84	18	[15] 3.2	0	[15] .48	[15] .29	[15] 3.8	0
Unenriched, sifted....	1 cup....	110	400	12	1	Trace	Trace	Trace	84	18	.9	0	.07	.05	1.0	0
Self-rising, enriched....	1 cup....	110	385	10	1	Trace	Trace	Trace	82	292	[15] 3.2	0	[15] .49	[15] .29	[15] 3.9	0
Cake or pastry flour, sifted.	1 cup....	100	365	8	1	Trace	Trace	Trace	79	17	.5	0	.03	.03	.7	0
Wheat germ, crude, commercially milled.	1 cup....	68	245	18	7	1	2	4	32	49	6.4	0	1.36	.46	2.9	0
FATS, OILS																
Butter, 4 sticks per pound:																
Sticks, 2....	1 cup....	227	1,625	1	184	101	61	6	1	45	0	[20] 7,500	----	----	----	0
Stick, ⅛....	1 tablespoon..	14	100	Trace	11	6	4	Trace	Trace	3	0	[20] 460	----	----	----	0
Pat or square (64 per pound).	1 pat....	7	50	Trace	6	3	2	Trace	Trace	1	0	[20] 230	----	----	----	0
Fats, cooking:																
Lard....	1 cup....	220	1,985	0	220	84	101	22	0	0	0	0	0	0	0	0
Lard....	1 tablespoon..	14	125	0	14	5	6	1	0	0	0	0	0	0	0	0
Vegetable fats....	1 cup....	200	1,770	0	200	46	130	14	0	0	0	----	0	0	0	0
Vegetable fats....	1 tablespoon..	12.5	110	0	12	3	8	1	0	0	0	----	0	0	0	0
Margarine, 4 sticks per pound:																
Sticks, 2....	1 cup....	227	1,635	1	184	37	105	33	1	45	0	[21] 7,500	----	----	----	0
Stick, ⅛....	1 tablespoon..	14	100	Trace	11	2	6	2	Trace	3	0	[21] 460	----	----	----	0
Pat or square (64 per pound).	1 pat....	7	50	Trace	6	1	3	1	Trace	1	0	[21] 230	----	----	----	0
Oils, salad or cooking:																
Corn....	1 tablespoon..	14	125	0	14	1	4	7	0	0	0	----	0	0	0	0
Cottonseed....	1 tablespoon..	14	125	0	14	4	3	7	0	0	0	----	0	0	0	0
Olive....	1 tablespoon..	14	125	0	14	2	11	1	0	0	0	----	0	0	0	0
Soybean....	1 tablespoon..	14	125	0	14	2	3	7	0	0	0	----	0	0	0	0

[15] Iron, thiamine, riboflavin, and niacin are based on the minimum levels of enrichment specified in standards of identity promulgated under the Federal Food, Drug, and Cosmetic Act.

[20] Year-round average.

[21] Based on the average vitamin A content of fortified margarine. Federal specifications for fortified margarine require a minimum of 15,000 I.U. of vitamin A per pound.

TABLE 36—*Continued*

Food, Approximate Measure, and Weight (in Grams)			Food Energy	Protein	Fat (Total Lipid)	Fatty acids: Saturated (Total)	Fatty acids: Unsaturated: Oleic	Fatty acids: Unsaturated: Linoleic	Carbohydrate	Calcium	Iron	Vitamin A Value	Thiamine	Riboflavin	Niacin	Ascorbic Acid
FATS, OILS—Continued																
		Grams	(Calories)	(Gm.)	(Gm.)	(Gm.)	(Gm.)	(Gm.)	(Gm.)	(Mg.)	(Mg.)	(I.U.)	(Mg.)	(Mg.)	(Mg.)	(Mg.)
Salad dressings:																
Blue cheese	1 tablespoon	16	80	1	8	2	2	4	1	13	Trace	30	Trace	0.02	Trace	Trace
Commercial, mayonnaise type.	1 tablespoon	15	65	Trace	6	1	1	3	2	2	Trace	30	Trace	Trace	Trace	------
French	1 tablespoon	15	60	Trace	6	1	1	3	3	2	.1	------	------	------	------	------
Home cooked, boiled	1 tablespoon	17	30	1	2	1	1	Trace	3	15	.1	80	.01	.03	Trace	Trace
Mayonnaise	1 tablespoon	15	110	Trace	12	2	3	6	Trace	3	.1	40	Trace	.01	Trace	------
Thousand island	1 tablespoon	15	75	Trace	8	1	2	4	2	2	.1	50	Trace	Trace	Trace	Trace
SUGARS, SWEETS																
Candy:																
Caramels	1 ounce	28	115	1	3	2	1	Trace	22	42	.4	Trace	.01	.05	Trace	Trace
Chocolate, milk, plain	1 ounce	28	150	2	9	5	3	Trace	16	65	.3	80	.02	.09	.1	Trace
Fudge, plain	1 ounce	28	115	1	3	2	1	Trace	21	22	.3	Trace	.01	.03	.1	Trace
Hard candy	1 ounce	28	110	0	Trace	------	------	------	28	6	.5	0	0	0	0	0
Marshmallows	1 ounce	28	90	1	Trace	------	------	------	23	5	.5	0	0	Trace	Trace	0
Chocolate sirup, thin type	1 tablespoon	20	50	Trace	Trace	Trace	Trace	Trace	13	3	.3	------	Trace	.01	.1	0
Honey, strained or extracted.	1 tablespoon	21	65	Trace	0	------	------	------	17	1	.1	0	Trace	.01	.1	Trace
Jams and preserves	1 tablespoon	20	55	Trace	Trace	------	------	------	14	4	.2	Trace	Trace	.01	Trace	Trace
Jellies	1 tablespoon	20	55	Trace	Trace	------	------	------	14	4	.3	Trace	Trace	.01	Trace	1
Molasses, cane:																
Light (first extraction)	1 tablespoon	20	50	------	------	------	------	------	13	33	.9	------	.01	.01	Trace	------
Blackstrap (third extraction).	1 tablespoon	20	45	------	------	------	------	------	11	137	3.2	------	.02	.04	.4	------
Sirup, table blends (chiefly corn, light and dark).	1 tablespoon	20	60	0	0	------	------	------	15	9	.8	0	0	0	0	0
Sugars (cane or beet):																
Granulated	1 cup	200	770	0	0	------	------	------	199	0	.2	0	0	0	0	0
	1 tablespoon	12	45	0	0	------	------	------	12	0	Trace	0	0	0	0	0
Lump, 1⅛ by ¾ by ⅜	1 lump	6	25	0	0	------	------	------	6	0	Trace	0	0	0	0	0
Powdered, stirred before measuring.	1 cup	128	495	0	0	------	------	------	127	0	.1	0	0	0	0	0
	1 tablespoon	8	30	0	0	------	------	------	8	0	Trace	0	0	0	0	0

… firm packed	1 cup	220	820	0	0	----	----	----	212	187	7.5	0	.02	.07	.4	0
	1 tablespoon	14	50	0	0	----	----	----	13	12	.5	0	Trace	Trace	Trace	0
MISCELLANEOUS ITEMS																
Beer (average 3.6 percent alcohol by weight).	1 cup	240	100	1	0	----	----	----	9	12	Trace	----	.01	.07	1.6	----
Beverages, carbonated:																
Cola type	1 cup	240	95	0	0	----	----	----	24	----	----	0	0	0	0	0
Ginger ale	1 cup	230	70	0	0	----	----	----	18	----	----	0	0	0	0	0
Bouillon cube, ⅝ inch	1 cube	4	5	1	Trace	----	----	----	Trace	----	----	----	----	----	----	----
Chili powder. *See* Vegetables, peppers.																
Chili sauce (mainly tomatoes).	1 tablespoon	17	20	Trace	Trace	----	----	----	4	3	.1	240	.02	.01	.3	3
Chocolate:																
Bitter or baking	1 ounce	28	145	3	15	8	6	Trace	8	22	1.9	20	.01	.07	.4	0
Sweet	1 ounce	28	150	1	10	6	4	Trace	16	27	.4	Trace	.01	.04	.1	Trace
Cider. *See* Fruits, apple juice.																
Gelatin, dry:																
Plain	1 tablespoon	10	35	9	Trace	----	----	----	----	----	----	----	----	----	----	----
Dessert powder, 3-ounce package.	½ cup	85	315	8	0	----	----	----	75	----	----	----	----	----	----	----
Gelatin dessert, ready-to-eat:																
Plain	1 cup	239	140	4	0	----	----	----	34	----	----	----	----	----	----	----
With fruit	1 cup	241	160	3	Trace	----	----	----	40	----	----	----	----	----	----	----
Olives, pickled:																
Green	4 medium or 3 extra large or 2 giant.	16	15	Trace	2	Trace	2	Trace	Trace	8	.2	40	----	----	----	----
Ripe: Mission	3 small or 2 large.	10	15	Trace	2	Trace	2	Trace	Trace	9	.1	10	Trace	Trace	----	----
Pickles, cucumber:																
Dill, large, 4 by 1¾ inches.	1 pickle	135	15	1	Trace	----	----	----	3	35	1.4	140	Trace	.03	Trace	8
Sweet, 2¾ by ¾ inches	1 pickle	20	30	Trace	Trace	----	----	----	7	2	.2	20	Trace	Trace	Trace	1
Popcorn. *See* Grain products.																
Sherbet, orange	1 cup	193	260	2	2	----	----	----	59	31	Trace	110	.02	.06	Trace	4
Soups, canned; ready-to-serve (prepared with equal volume of water):																
Bean with pork	1 cup	250	170	8	6	1	2	2	22	62	2.2	650	.14	.07	1.0	2
Beef noodle	1 cup	250	70	4	3	1	1	1	7	8	1.0	50	.05	.06	1.1	Trace
Beef bouillon, broth, consomme.	1 cup	240	30	5	0	0	0	0	3	Trace	.5	Trace	Trace	.02	1.2	----

TABLE 36—*Continued*

Food, Approximate Measure, and Weight (in Grams)			Food Energy	Protein	Fat (Total Lipid)	Fatty acids: Saturated (Total)	Fatty acids: Unsaturated: Oleic	Fatty acids: Unsaturated: Linoleic	Carbohydrate	Calcium	Iron	Vitamin A Value	Thiamine	Riboflavin	Niacin	Ascorbic Acid
MISCELLANEOUS ITEMS—Continued			(Calories)	(Gm.)	(Gm.)	(Gm.)	(Gm.)	(Gm.)	(Gm.)	(Mg.)	(Mg.)	(I.U.)	(Mg.)	(Mg.)	(Mg.)	(Mg.)
Soups, canned; ready-to-serve—Con.		*Grams*		*Grams*	*Grams*	*Grams*										
Chicken noodle	1 cup	250	65	4	2	Trace	1	1	8	10	0.5	50	0.02	0.02	0.8	Trace
Clam chowder	1 cup	255	85	2	3	----	----	----	13	36	1.0	920	.03	.03	1.0	----
Cream soup (mushroom)	1 cup	240	135	2	10	1	3	5	10	41	.5	70	.02	.12	.7	Trace
Minestrone	1 cup	245	105	5	3	----	----	----	14	37	1.0	2,350	.07	.05	1.0	----
Pea, green	1 cup	245	130	6	2	1	1	Trace	23	44	1.0	340	.05	.05	1.0	7
Tomato	1 cup	245	90	2	2	Trace	1	1	16	15	.7	1,000	.06	.05	1.1	12
Vegetable with beef broth.	1 cup	250	80	3	2	----	----	----	14	20	.8	3,250	.05	.02	1.2	----
Starch (cornstarch)	1 cup	128	465	Trace	Trace	----	----	----	112	0	0	0	0	0	0	0
	1 tablespoon	8	30	Trace	Trace	----	----	----	7	0	0	0	0	0	0	0
Tapioca, quick-cooking granulated, dry, stirred before measuring.	1 cup	152	535	1	Trace	----	----	----	131	15	.6	0	0	0	0	0
	1 tablespoon	10	35	Trace	Trace	----	----	----	9	1	Trace	0	0	0	0	0
Vinegar	1 tablespoon	15	2	0	----	----	----	----	1	1	.1	----	----	----	----	----
White sauce, medium	1 cup	265	430	10	33	18	11	1	23	305	.5	1,220	.12	.44	.6	Trace
Yeast:																
Baker's:																
Compressed	1 ounce	28	25	3	Trace	----	----	----	3	4	1.4	Trace	.20	.47	3.2	Trace
Dry active	1 ounce	28	80	10	Trace	----	----	----	11	12	4.6	Trace	.66	1.53	10.4	Trace
Brewer's, dry, debittered.	1 tablespoon	8	25	3	Trace	----	----	----	3	17	1.4	Trace	1.25	.34	3.0	Trace
Yoghurt. *See* Milk, cream, cheese; related products.																

APPENDIX 2

Data Used for Calculating Energy Values of Foods or Food Groups by the Atwater System

TABLE 37

Food or Food Group	Protein			Fat			Carbohydrate		
	Coefficient of digestibility (Pct.)	Heat of combustion less 1.25* (Cal./gm.)	Factor to be applied to ingested nutrients (Cal./gm.)	Coefficient of digestibility (Pct.)	Heat of combustion (Cal./gm.)	Factor to be applied to ingested nutrients (Cal./gm.)	Coefficient of digestibility (Pct.)	Heat of combustion (Cal./gm.)	Factor to be applied to ingested nutrients (Cal./gm.)
Eggs, Meat products, Milk products:									
Eggs	97	4.50	4.36	95	9.50	9.02	98	3.75	3.68
Gelatin	97	4.02	3.90	95	9.50	9.02	...	...	...
Glycogen	...	...	...	...	...	...	98	4.19	4.11
Meat, fish	97	4.40	4.27	95	9.50	9.02	...	...	†
Milk, milk products	97	4.40	4.27	95	9.25	8.79	98	3.95	3.87
Fats, separated:									
Butter	97	4.40	4.27	95	9.25	8.79	98	3.95	3.87
Other animal fats	...	...	...	95	9.50	9.02	...	...	...
Margarine, vegetable	97	4.40	4.27	95	9.30	8.84	98	3.95	3.87
Other vegetable fats and oils	...	...	...	95	9.30	8.84	...	...	...
Fruits:									
All (except lemons, limes)	85	3.95	3.36	90	9.30	8.37	90	4.00	3.60
All fruit juice (except lemon, lime) unsweetened	85	3.95	3.36	90	9.30	8.37	98‡	4.00	3.92‡
Lemons, limes	85	3.95	3.36	90	9.30	8.37	90‡	2.75	2.48‡
Lemon juice, lime juice, unsweetened	85	3.95	3.36	90	9.30	8.37	98	2.75	2.70
Grain products:									
Barley, pearled	78	4.55	3.55	90	9.30	8.37	94	4.20	3.95
Buckwheat flour, dark	74	4.55	3.37	90	9.30	8.37	90	4.20	3.78
Buckwheat flour, light	78	4.55	3.55	90	9.30	8.37	94	4.20	3.95
Cornmeal, whole-ground	60	4.55	2.73	90	9.30	8.37	96	4.20	4.03
Cornmeal, degermed	76	4.55	3.46	90	9.30	8.37	99	4.20	4.16
Dextrin	...	...	...	...	...	...	98	4.11	4.03
Macaroni, spaghetti	86	4.55	3.91	90	9.30	8.37	98	4.20	4.12
Oatmeal, rolled oats	76	4.55	3.46	90	9.30	8.37	98	4.20	4.12
Rice, brown	75	4.55	3.41	90	9.30	8.37	98	4.20	4.12
Rice, white or polished	84	4.55	3.82	90	9.30	8.37	99	4.20	4.16

* The correction, 1.25 calories, has been subtracted from the heat of combustion. This gives values applicable to grams of digested protein and is identical with Atwater's factors per gram of available protein.

† Carbohydrate factor, 3.87 for brain, heart, kidney, liver; 4.11 for tongue and shellfish.

‡ Unpublished revision made since 1955.

TABLE 37—*Continued*

Food or Food Group	Protein: Coefficient of digestibility (Pct.)	Protein: Heat of combustion less 1.25* (Cal./gm.)	Protein: Factor to be applied to ingested nutrients (Cal./gm.)	Fat: Coefficient of digestibility (Pct.)	Fat: Heat of combustion (Cal./gm.)	Fat: Factor to be applied to ingested nutrients (Cal./gm.)	Carbohydrate: Coefficient of digestibility (Pct.)	Carbohydrate: Heat of combustion (Cal./gm.)	Carbohydrate: Factor to be applied to ingested nutrients (Cal./gm.)
Rye flour, dark	65	4.55	2.96	90	9.30	8.37	90	4.20	3.78
Rye flour, whole-grain	67	4.55	3.05	90	9.30	8.37	92	4.20	3.86
Rye flour, medium	71	4.55	3.23	90	9.30	8.37	95	4.20	3.99
Rye flour, light	75	4.55	3.41	90	9.30	8.37	97	4.20	4.07
Sorghum (kaoliang), whole or nearly whole meal	20	4.55	.91	90	9.30	8.37	96	4.20	4.03
Wheat, 97–100 per cent extraction	79	4.55	3.59	90	9.30	8.37	90	4.20	3.78
Wheat, 85–93 per cent extraction	83	4.55	3.78	90	9.30	8.37	94	4.20	3.95
Wheat, 70–74 per cent extraction	89	4.55	4.05	90	9.30	8.37	98	4.20	4.12
Wheat, flaked, puffed, rolled, shredded, whole meal	79	4.55	3.59	90	9.30	8.37	90	4.20	3.78
Wheat bran (100 per cent)	40	4.55	1.82	90	9.30	8.37	56	4.20	2.35
Other cereals, refined	85	4.55	3.87	90	9.30	8.37	98	4.20	4.12
Wild rice	78	4.55	3.55	90	9.30	8.37	94	4.20	3.95
Legumes, Nuts:									
Mature dry beans, cowpeas, peas, other legumes; nuts	78	4.45	3.47	90	9.30	8.37	97	4.20	4.07
Immature Lima beans, cowpeas, peas, other legumes	78	4.45	3.47	90	9.30	8.37	97	4.20	4.07
Soybeans, dry; soy flour, flakes, grits	78	4.45	3.47	90	9.30	8.37	97	4.20	4.07
Sugars:									
Cane or beet sugar (sucrose)	.....	.....	.....	.....	.....	.....	98	3.95	3.87
Glucose	.....	.....	.....	.....	.....	.....	98	3.75	3.68
Vegetables:									
Mushrooms	70	3.75	2.62	90	9.30	8.37	85	4.10	3.48
Potatoes and starchy roots	74	3.75	2.78	90	9.30	8.37	96	4.20	4.03
Other underground crops§	74	3.75	2.78	90	9.30	8.37	96	4.00	3.84
Other vegetables	65	3.75	2.44	90	9.30	8.37	85	4.20	3.57
Miscellaneous foods:									
Alcohol‖	.....	.....	.....	.....	.....	.....	.....	.....	.....
Chocolate, cocoa	42	4.35	1.83	90	9.30	8.37	32	4.16	1.33
Vinegar	.....	.....	.....	.....	.....	.....	98	2.45	2.40
Yeast	80	3.75	3.00	90	9.30	8.37	80	4.20	3.35

§ Vegetables such as beets, carrots, onions, parsnips, radishes.

‖ Coefficient of digestibility, 98 per cent; heat of combustion, 7.07 calories per gram; factor to apply to ingested alcohol, 6.93 calories per gram.

APPENDIX 3

Beverages—Alcoholic and Carbonated Non-alcoholic

Alcoholic beverages.—Food energy was calculated for alcoholic beverages as the total potential calories from any nutrients present (protein, fat, carbohydrate) plus those from alcohol. The factor 6.93 was applied to the alcoholic content by weight.

Dessert wines as classified in Table 38 include those containing more than 15 per cent alcohol (by volume), such as apple, muscatel, sherries, port, and tokay. Apertif wines and vermouths will also fall in this classification. Table wines to which the data in this table apply include those containing less than 15 per cent alcohol (by volume), such as barbera, burgundy, cabernet, chablis, champagnes, chianti, claret, Rhine wines, rosé, and sauternes. Cherry, peach, berry, and varietal wines usually fall in this class, although some may be high enough in alcohol content to be classified with dessert wines.

Within each group there is a rather wide range in total carbohydrate content. The carbohydrate is less in dry wines than in sweet wines.

TABLE 38

COMPOSITION OF BEVERAGES—ALCOHOLIC AND CARBONATED NON-ALCOHOLIC PER 100 GRAMS*

	Food Energy	Protein	Carbo-hydrate	Calcium	Phosphorus	Iron	Thiamine	Riboflavin	Niacin
Beverages, alcoholic and carbonated non-alcoholic:									
Alcoholic:									
Beer, alcohol 4.5% by volume (3.6% by weight)	42	.3	3.8	5	30	Trace	Trace	.03	.6
Gin, rum, vodka, whisky:									
80-proof (33.4% alcohol by weight)	231		Trace						
86-proof (36.0% alcohol by weight)	249		Trace						
90-proof (37.9% alcohol by weight)	263		Trace						
94-proof (39.7% alcohol by weight)	275		Trace						
100-proof (42.5% alcohol by weight)	295		Trace						
Wines:									
Dessert, alcohol 18.8% by volume (15.3% by weight)	137	.1	7.7	8			.01	.02	.2
Table, alcohol 12.2% by volume (9.9% by weight)	85	.1	4.2	9	10	.4	Trace	.01	.1
Carbonated, non-alcoholic:									
Carbonated waters:									
Sweetened (quinine sodas)	31		8						
Unsweetened (club sodas)									
Cola type	39		10						
Cream sodas	43		11						
Fruit-flavored sodas (citrus, cherry, grape, strawberry, Tom Collins mixer, other) (10%–13% sugar)	46		12						
Ginger ale, pale dry and golden	31		8						
Root beer	41		10.5						
Special dietary drinks with artificial sweetener (less than 1 calorie per ounce)									

* From *Composition of Foods—Raw, Processed, Prepared* (U.S. Department of Agriculture, Agriculture Handbook, No. 8 [December, 1963]).

APPENDIX 4

Cholesterol Content of Foods*

TABLE 39

Item	Amount of Cholesterol in:		Refuse from Item as Purchased (Percent)
	100 grams edible portion‡ (Mg.)	Edible portion of 1 pound as purchased (Mg.)	
Beef, raw:			
With bone†	70	270	15
Without bone†	70	320	0
Brains, raw	>2,000	>9,000	0
Butter	250	1,135	0
Cavier or fish roe	>300	>1,300	0
Cheese:			
Cheddar	100	455	0
Cottage, creamed	15	70	0
Cream	120	545	0
Other (25% to 30% fat)	85	385	0
Cheese spread	65	295	0
Chicken, flesh only, raw	60	....	0
Crab:			
In shell†	125	270	52
Meat only†	125	565	0
Egg, whole	550	2,200	12
Egg white	0	0	0
Egg yolk:			
Fresh	1,500	6,800	0
Frozen	1,280	5,800	0
Dried	2,950	13,380	0
Fish:			
Steak†	70	265	16
Fillet†	70	320	0
Heart, raw	150	680	0
Ice cream	45	205	0
Kidney, raw	375	1,700	0
Lamb, raw:			
With bone†	70	265	16
Without bone†	70	320	0
Lard and other animal fat	95	430	0
Liver, raw	300	1,360	0
Lobster:			
Whole†	200	235	74
Meat only†	200	900	0
Margarine:			
All vegetable fat	0	0	0
Two-thirds animal fat, one-third vegetable fat	65	295	0
Milk:			
Fluid, whole	11	50	0
Dried, whole	85	385	0
Fluid, skim	3	15	0

* From *Composition of Foods—Raw, Processed, Prepared*, Department of Agriculture, Agriculture Handbook, No. 8 [December, 1963]).

† Designate items that have the same chemical composition for the edible portion but differ in the amount of refuse.

‡ Data apply to 100 grams of edible portion of the item, although it may be purchased with the refuse indicated and described or implied in the first column.

TABLE 39—*Continued*

Item	Amount of Cholesterol in:		Refuse from Item as Purchased (Percent)
	100 grams edible portion‡ (Mg.)	Edible portion of 1 pound as purchased (Mg.)	
Mutton:			
With bone†	65	250	16
Without bone†	65	295	0
Oysters:			
In shell†	>200	> 90	90
Meat only†	>200	>900	0
Pork:			
With bone†	70	260	18
Without bone†	70	320	0
Shrimp:			
In shell†	125	390	31
Flesh only†	125	565	0
Sweetbreads (thymus)	250	1,135	0
Veal:			
With bone†	90	320	21
Without bone†	90	410	0

APPENDIX 5

Amino Acid Content of Foods

The following table is taken from a compilation prepared by M. L. Orr and B. K. Watt, as Home Economics Research Report No. 4 (1957), Household Economics Research Division, Institute of Home Economics, Agricultural Research Service, U.S. Department of Agriculture. The original report contains data on 18 amino acids in 202 food items. Only the average amounts of 8 "essential" amino acids, plus arginine and histidine, have been included in the following table. This table is useful when an average protein content may be assumed. When specific nitrogen or protein content of a food is known, reference may be made to the original publication.

TABLE 40

Amino Acid Content of Foods, 100 Gm., Edible Portion

Protein Content, and Nitrogen Conversion Factor	Tryptophan (Gm.)	Threonine (Gm.)	Isoleucine (Gm.)	Leucine (Gm.)	Lysine (Gm.)	Methionine (Gm.)	Cystine (Gm.)	Phenylalanine (Gm.)	Tyrosine (Gm.)	Valine (Gm.)	Arginine (Gm.)	Histidine (Gm.)
Milk; Milk Products												
Milk (Protein, N×6.38):												
cow:												
fluid, whole and non-fat (3.5% protein)	0.049	0.161	0.223	0.344	0.272	0.086	0.031	0.170	0.178	0.240	0.128	0.092
canned:												
evaporated, unsweetened (7.0% protein)	0.099	0.323	0.447	0.688	0.545	0.171	0.063	0.340	0.357	0.481	0.256	0.185
condensed, sweetened (8.1% protein)	0.114	0.374	0.518	0.796	0.631	0.198	0.072	0.393	0.413	0.557	0.296	0.214
dried:												
whole (25.8% protein)	0.364	1.191	1.648	2.535	2.009	0.632	0.231	1.251	1.316	1.774	0.944	0.680
non-fat (35.6% protein)	0.502	1.641	2.271	3.493	2.768	0.870	0.318	1.724	1.814	2.444	1.300	0.937
goat (3.3% protein)	0.039	0.217	0.087	0.278	0.312	0.065	......	0.121	......	0.139	0.174	0.068
human (1.4% protein)	0.023	0.062	0.075	0.124	0.090	0.028	0.027	0.060	0.071	0.086	0.055	0.030
Indian buffalo (4.2% protein)	0.059	0.212	0.204	0.420	0.331	0.112	0.058	0.177	......	0.255	0.136	0.086
Milk products:												
buttermilk (3.5% protein, N×6.38)	0.038	0.165	0.219	0.348	0.291	0.082	0.032	0.186	0.137	0.262	0.168	0.099
casein (100.0% protein, N×6.29)	1.335	4.277	6.550	10.048	8.013	3.084	0.382	5.389	5.819	7.393	4.070	3.021
cheese (protein, N×6.38):												
blue mold (21.5% protein)	0.293	0.799	1.449	2.096	1.577	0.559	0.121	1.153	1.028	1.543	0.785	0.701
Camembert (17.5% protein)	0.239	0.650	1.179	1.706	1.284	0.455	0.099	0.938	0.837	1.256	0.639	0.571
Cheddar (25.0% protein)	0.341	0.929	1.685	2.437	1.834	0.650	0.141	1.340	1.195	1.794	0.913	0.815
Cheddar processed (23.2% protein)	0.316	0.862	1.563	2.262	1.702	0.604	0.131	1.244	1.109	1.665	0.847	0.756
cheese foods, Cheddar (20.5% protein)	0.280	0.761	1.382	1.998	1.504	0.533	0.116	1.099	0.980	1.472	0.749	0.668
cottage (17.0% protein)	0.179	0.794	0.989	1.826	1.428	0.469	0.147	0.917	0.917	0.978	0.802	0.549

TABLE 40—*Continued*

Protein Content, and Nitrogen Conversion Factor	Tryptophan (Gm.)	Threonine (Gm.)	Isoleucine (Gm.)	Leucine (Gm.)	Lysine (Gm.)	Methionine (Gm.)	Cystine (Gm.)	Phenylalanine (Gm.)	Tyrosine (Gm.)	Valine (Gm.)	Arginine (Gm.)	Histidine (Gm.)
MILK PRODUCTS—*Continued*												
cream cheese (9.0% protein)	0.080	0.408	0.519	0.923	0.721	0.229	0.085	0.547	0.408	0.538	0.313	0.278
Limburger (21.2% protein)	0.289	0.788	1.429	2.067	1.555	0.552	0.120	1.136	1.014	1.522	0.774	0.691
Parmesan (36.0% protein)	0.491	1.337	2.426	3.510	2.641	0.937	0.203	1.930	1.721	2.584	1.315	1.174
Swiss (27.5% protein)	0.375	1.021	1.853	2.681	2.017	0.715	0.155	1.474	1.315	1.974	1.004	0.896
Swiss processed (26.4% protein)	0.360	0.981	1.779	2.574	1.937	0.687	0.149	1.415	1.262	1.895	0.964	0.861
lactalbumin (100.0% protein, N×6.49)	2.203	5.239	6.209	12.342	9.060	2.250	3.405	4.360	3.806	5.686	3.498	1.911
whey (Protein, N×6.49)												
fluid (0.9% protein)	0.010	0.048	0.052	0.074	0.055	0.013	0.018	0.023	0.009	0.045	0.017	0.011
dried (12.7% protein)	0.147	0.677	0.734	1.043	0.769	0.188	0.250	0.323	0.131	0.640	0.235	0.159
EGGS, CHICKEN (Protein, N×6.25)												
Fresh or stored:												
whole (12.8% protein)	0.211	0.637	0.850	1.126	0.819	0.401	0.299	0.739	0.551	0.950	0.840	0.307
whites (10.8% protein)	0.164	0.477	0.698	0.950	0.648	0.420	0.263	0.689	0.449	0.842	0.634	0.233
yolks (16.3% protein)	0.235	0.827	0.996	1.372	1.074	0.417	0.274	0.717	0.756	1.121	1.132	0.368
Dried:												
whole (46.8% protein)	0.771	2.329	3.108	4.118	2.995	1.468	1.093	2.703	2.014	3.474	3.070	1.123
whites (85.9% protein)	1.306	3.793	5.553	7.559	5.154	3.340	2.089	5.484	3.573	6.693	5.044	1.855
yolks (31.2% protein)	0.449	1.582	1.907	2.626	2.057	0.799	0.524	1.373	1.448	2.147	2.167	0.704
MEAT; POULTRY; FISH AND SHELLFISH; THEIR PRODUCTS												
Meat (Protein, N×6.25):												
beef carcass or side:												
thin (18.8% protein)	0.220	0.830	0.984	1.540	1.642	0.466	0.238	0.773	0.638	1.044	1.212	0.653
medium fat (17.5% protein)	0.204	0.773	0.916	1.434	1.529	0.434	0.221	0.720	0.594	0.972	1.128	0.608
fat (16.3% protein)	0.190	0.720	0.853	1.335	1.424	0.404	0.206	0.670	0.553	0.905	1.051	0.566
very fat (13.7% protein)	0.160	0.605	0.717	1.122	1.197	0.340	0.173	0.563	0.465	0.761	0.883	0.476
medium fat, trimmed to retail basis (18.2% protein)	0.213	0.804	0.952	1.491	1.590	0.451	0.230	0.748	0.617	1.010	1.174	0.632

TABLE 40—*Continued*

Protein Content, and Nitrogen Conversion Factor	Tryptophan (Gm.)	Threonine (Gm.)	Isoleucine (Gm.)	Leucine (Gm.)	Lysine (Gm.)	Methionine (Gm.)	Cystine (Gm.)	Phenylalanine (Gm.)	Tyrosine (Gm.)	Valine (Gm.)	Arginine (Gm.)	Histidine (Gm.)
MEAT; POULTRY; FISH—*Continued*												
beef cuts, medium fat:												
chuck (18.6% protein)	0.217	0.821	0.973	1.524	1.625	0.461	0.235	0.765	0.631	1.033	1.199	0.646
flank (19.9% protein)	0.232	0.879	1.041	1.630	1.738	0.494	0.252	0.818	0.675	1.105	1.283	0.691
hamburger (16.0% protein)	0.187	0.707	0.837	1.311	1.398	0.397	0.202	0.658	0.543	0.888	1.032	0.556
porterhouse (16.4% protein)	0.192	0.724	0.858	1.343	1.433	0.407	0.207	0.674	0.556	0.911	1.057	0.569
rib roast (17.4% protein)	0.203	0.768	0.910	1.425	1.520	0.432	0.220	0.715	0.590	0.966	1.122	0.604
round (19.5% protein)	0.228	0.861	1.020	1.597	1.704	0.484	0.246	0.802	0.661	1.083	1.257	0.677
rump (16.2% protein)	0.189	0.715	0.848	1.327	1.415	0.402	0.205	0.666	0.550	0.899	1.045	0.562
sirloin (17.3% protein)	0.202	0.764	0.905	1.417	1.511	0.429	0.219	0.711	0.587	0.960	1.116	0.601
beef, canned (25.0% protein)	0.292	1.104	1.308	2.048	2.184	0.620	0.316	1.028	0.848	1.388	1.612	0.868
beef, dried or chipped (34.3% protein)	0.401	1.515	1.795	2.810	2.996	0.851	0.434	1.410	1.163	1.904	2.212	1.191
lamb carcass or side:												
thin (17.1% protein)	0.222	0.782	0.886	1.324	1.384	0.410	0.224	0.695	0.594	0.843	1.114	0.476
medium fat (15.7% protein)	0.203	0.718	0.814	1.216	1.271	0.377	0.206	0.638	0.545	0.774	1.022	0.437
fat (13.0% protein)	0.168	0.595	0.674	1.007	1.052	0.312	0.171	0.528	0.451	0.641	0.847	0.362
lamb cuts, medium fat:												
leg (18.0% protein)	0.233	0.824	0.933	1.394	1.457	0.432	0.236	0.732	0.625	0.887	1.172	0.501
rib (14.9% protein)	0.193	0.682	0.772	1.154	1.206	0.358	0.195	0.606	0.517	0.734	0.970	0.415
shoulder (15.6% protein)	0.202	0.714	0.809	1.208	1.263	0.374	0.205	0.634	0.542	0.769	1.016	0.434
pork, packer's carcass or side:												
thin (14.1% protein)	0.183	0.654	0.724	1.038	1.157	0.352	0.165	0.555	0.503	0.733	0.864	0.487
medium fat (11.9% protein)	0.154	0.552	0.611	0.876	0.977	0.297	0.139	0.468	0.425	0.619	0.729	0.411
fat (9.8% protein)	0.127	0.455	0.503	0.721	0.804	0.245	0.114	0.386	0.350	0.510	0.601	0.339
pork cuts, medium fat, fresh:												
ham (15.2% protein)	0.197	0.705	0.781	1.119	1.248	0.379	0.178	0.598	0.542	0.790	0.931	0.525
loin (16.4% protein)	0.213	0.761	0.842	1.207	1.346	0.409	0.192	0.646	0.585	0.853	1.005	0.567
miscellaneous lean cuts (14.5% protein)	0.188	0.673	0.745	1.067	1.190	0.362	0.169	0.571	0.517	0.754	0.889	0.501

TABLE 40—*Continued*

Protein Content, and Nitrogen Conversion Factor	Tryptophan (Gm.)	Threonine (Gm.)	Isoleucine (Gm.)	Leucine (Gm.)	Lysine (Gm.)	Methionine (Gm.)	Cystine (Gm.)	Phenylalanine (Gm.)	Tyrosine (Gm.)	Valine (Gm.)	Arginine (Gm.)	Histidine (Gm.)
MEAT; POULTRY; FISH—*Continued*												
pork, cured:												
bacon, medium fat (9.1% protein)	0.095	0.306	0.399	0.728	0.587	0.141	0.105	0.434	0.234	0.434	0.622	0.246
fat back or salt pork (3.9% protein)	0.006	0.141	0.110	0.367	0.317	0.055	0.043	0.157	0.052	0.168	0.379	0.035
ham (16.9% protein)	0.162	0.692	0.841	1.306	1.420	0.411	0.273	0.646	0.652	0.879	1.068	0.544
luncheon meat:												
boiled ham (22.8% protein)	0.219	0.934	1.135	1.762	1.915	0.554	0.368	0.872	0.879	1.186	1.441	0.733
canned, spiced (14.9% protein)	0.143	0.610	0.741	1.151	1.252	0.362	0.241	0.570	0.575	0.775	0.942	0.479
rabbit, domesticated, flesh only (21.0% protein)	......	1.021	1.082	1.636	1.818	0.541	......	0.793	......	1.021	1.176	0.474
veal, carcass or side:												
thin (19.7% protein)	0.258	0.854	1.040	1.444	1.645	0.451	0.233	0.801	0.709	1.018	1.283	0.634
medium fat (19.1% protein)	0.251	0.828	1.008	1.400	1.595	0.437	0.226	0.776	0.688	0.987	1.244	0.614
fat (18.5% protein)	0.243	0.802	0.977	1.356	1.545	0.423	0.219	0.752	0.666	0.956	1.205	0.595
veal cuts, medium fat:												
round (19.5% protein)	0.256	0.846	1.030	1.429	1.629	0.446	0.231	0.792	0.702	1.008	1.270	0.627
shoulder (19.4% protein)	0.255	0.841	1.024	1.422	1.620	0.444	0.230	0.788	0.698	1.003	1.263	0.624
stew meat (18.3% protein)	0.240	0.793	0.966	1.341	1.528	0.419	0.217	0.744	0.659	0.946	1.192	0.589
Poultry (*Protein*, $N \times 6.25$):												
chicken, flesh only:												
broilers or fryers (20.6% protein)	0.250	0.877	1.088	1.490	1.810	0.537	0.277	0.811	0.725	1.012	1.302	0.593
hens (21.3% protein)	0.259	0.907	1.125	1.540	1.871	0.556	0.286	0.838	0.750	1.046	1.346	0.613
ducks, domesticated, flesh only (21.4% protein)	......	0.935	1.109	1.657	1.842	0.531	......	0.842	......	1.027	1.301	0.486
turkey, flesh only (24.0% protein)	......	1.014	1.260	1.836	2.173	0.664	0.330	0.960	......	1.187	1.513	0.649

TABLE 40—*Continued*

Protein Content, and Nitrogen Conversion Factor	Tryptophan (Gm.)	Threonine (Gm.)	Isoleucine (Gm.)	Leucine (Gm.)	Lysine (Gm.)	Methionine (Gm.)	Cystine (Gm.)	Phenylalanine (Gm.)	Tyrosine (Gm.)	Valine (Gm.)	Arginine (Gm.)	Histidine (Gm.)
MEAT; POULTRY; FISH—*Continued*												
Fish and shellfish (Protein, N×6.25):												
bluefish (20.5% protein)	0.203	0.889	1.040	1.548	1.797	0.597	0.276	0.761	0.554	1.092	1.155	......
cod:												
fresh (16.5% protein)	0.164	0.715	0.837	1.246	1.447	0.480	0.222	0.612	0.446	0.879	0.929	......
dried (81.8% protein)	0.811	3.547	4.149	6.178	7.172	2.382	1.099	3.036	2.212	4.358	4.607	......
croaker (17.8% protein)	0.177	0.772	0.903	1.344	1.561	0.518	0.239	0.661	0.481	0.948	1.002	......
eel (18.6% protein)	0.185	0.806	0.943	1.405	1.631	0.542	0.250	0.690	0.503	0.991	1.048	......
flounder (14.9% protein)	0.148	0.646	0.756	1.125	1.306	0.434	0.200	0.553	0.403	0.794	0.839	......
haddock (18.2% protein)	0.181	0.789	0.923	1.374	1.596	0.530	0.245	0.676	0.492	0.970	1.025	......
halibut (18.6% protein)	0.185	0.806	0.943	1.405	1.631	0.542	0.250	0.690	0.503	0.991	1.048	......
herring:												
Atlantic (18.3% protein)	0.182	0.793	0.928	1.382	1.605	0.533	0.246	0.679	0.495	0.975	1.031	......
lake (18.5% protein)	0.184	0.802	0.938	1.397	1.622	0.539	0.249	0.687	0.500	0.986	1.042	......
Pacific (16.6% protein)	0.165	0.720	0.842	1.254	1.455	0.483	0.223	0.616	0.449	0.884	0.935	......
mackerel:												
raw, common Atlantic (18.7% protein)	0.186	0.811	0.948	1.412	1.640	0.545	0.251	0.694	0.506	0.996	1.053	......
canned, solids and liquid:												
Atlantic (19.3% protein)	0.191	0.837	0.979	1.458	1.692	0.562	0.259	0.716	0.522	1.028	1.087	......
Pacific (21.1% protein)	0.209	0.915	1.070	1.593	1.850	0.614	0.284	0.783	0.571	1.124	1.188	......
salmon:												
raw, Pacific (Chinook or King) (17.4% protein)	0.173	0.754	0.883	1.314	1.526	0.507	0.234	0.646	0.470	0.927	0.980	......
canned, solids and liquid (sockeye or red) (20.2% protein)	0.200	0.876	1.025	1.526	1.771	0.588	0.271	0.750	0.546	1.076	1.138	......
sardines, canned, solids and liquid:												
Atlantic type (21.1% protein)	0.209	0.915	1.070	1.593	1.850	0.614	0.284	0.783	0.571	1.124	1.188	......
Pacific type (17.7% protein)	0.176	0.767	0.898	1.337	1.552	0.515	0.238	0.657	0.479	0.943	0.997	......
shrimp, canned, solids and liquid (18.7% protein)	0.186	0.811	0.948	1.412	1.640	0.545	0.251	0.694	0.506	0.996	1.053	......

TABLE 40—*Continued*

Protein Content, and Nitrogen Conversion Factor	Tryptophan (Gm.)	Threonine (Gm.)	Isoleucine (Gm.)	Leucine (Gm.)	Lysine (Gm.)	Methionine (Gm.)	Cystine (Gm.)	Phenylalanine (Gm.)	Tyrosine (Gm.)	Valine (Gm.)	Arginine (Gm.)	Histidine (Gm.)
MEAT; POULTRY; FISH—*Continued*												
Products from meat, poultry, and fish (Protein, N×6.25):												
brains (10.4% protein)	0.138	0.494	0.504	0.845	0.760	0.220	0.145	0.506	0.433	0.536	0.614	0.278
chitterlings (8.6% protein)	0.094	0.398	0.308	0.457	0.670	0.193	0.109	0.359	0.228	0.462	1.406	0.169
fish flour (76.0% protein)	0.754	4.378	4.232	6.189	7.381	2.019	....	2.845	....	3.916	5.204	1.289
gelatin (85.6% protein, N×5.55)	0.006	1.912	1.357	2.930	4.226	0.787	0.077	2.036	0.401	2.421	7.866	0.771
gizzard, chicken (23.1% protein)	0.207	1.072	1.094	1.689	1.567	0.554	0.218	0.968	0.680	1.116	1.741	0.480
heart:												
beef or pork (16.9% protein)	0.219	0.776	0.857	1.509	1.387	0.403	0.168	0.765	0.627	0.973	1.068	0.433
chicken (20.5% protein)	0.266	0.941	1.040	1.830	1.683	0.489	0.203	0.928	0.761	1.181	1.296	0.525
kidney:												
beef (15.0% protein)	0.221	0.665	0.730	1.301	1.087	0.307	0.182	0.706	0.557	0.876	0.934	0.377
pork (16.3% protein)	0.240	0.722	0.793	1.414	1.181	0.334	0.198	0.767	0.605	0.952	1.015	0.409
sheep (16.6% protein)	0.244	0.736	0.807	1.440	1.203	0.340	0.202	0.781	0.616	0.969	1.033	0.417
liver:												
beef or pork (19.7% protein)	0.296	0.936	1.031	1.819	1.475	0.463	0.243	0.993	0.738	1.239	1.201	0.523
calf (19.0% protein)	0.286	0.903	0.994	1.754	1.423	0.447	0.234	0.958	0.711	1.195	1.158	0.505
chicken (22.1% protein)	0.332	1.050	1.156	2.040	1.655	0.520	0.272	1.114	0.827	1.390	1.347	0.587
sheep or lamb (21.0% protein)	0.316	0.998	1.099	1.939	1.572	0.494	0.259	1.058	0.786	1.320	1.280	0.558
pancreas:												
beef (13.5% protein)	0.175	0.626	0.683	1.054	0.996	0.244	....	0.562	0.590	0.724	0.771	0.266
pork (14.5% protein)	0.188	0.673	0.733	1.132	1.070	0.262	....	0.603	0.633	0.777	0.828	0.285
pork or beef, canned (14.3% protein)	0.151	0.618	0.730	1.190	1.345	0.327	0.261	0.579	0.570	0.810	1.050	0.460
potted meat (16.1% protein)	0.149	0.662	0.641	1.203	1.061	0.361	....	0.641	....	0.943	1.002	0.322

TABLE 40—*Continued*

Protein Content, and Nitrogen Conversion Factor	Tryptophan (Gm.)	Threonine (Gm.)	Isoleucine (Gm.)	Leucine (Gm.)	Lysine (Gm.)	Methionine (Gm.)	Cystine (Gm.)	Phenylalanine (Gm.)	Tyrosine (Gm.)	Valine (Gm.)	Arginine (Gm.)	Histidine (Gm.)
MEAT; POULTRY; FISH—*Continued*												
sausage:												
Bologna (14.8% protein)	0.126	0.606	0.718	1.061	1.191	0.313	0.185	0.540	0.481	0.744	1.028	0.398
Braunschweiger (15.4% protein)	0.172	0.668	0.754	1.291	1.200	0.320	0.187	0.700	0.471	0.956	0.954	0.458
frankfurters (14.2% protein)	0.120	0.582	0.688	1.018	1.143	0.300	0.177	0.518	0.461	0.713	0.986	0.382
head cheese (15.0% protein)	0.079	0.418	0.509	0.946	0.907	0.250	0.209	0.569	0.569	0.617	1.075	0.278
liverwurst (16.7% protein)	0.187	0.724	0.818	1.400	1.301	0.347	0.203	0.759	0.510	1.037	1.034	0.497
pork, links or bulk, raw (10.8% protein)	0.092	0.442	0.524	0.774	0.869	0.228	0.135	0.394	0.351	0.543	0.750	0.290
pork, bulk, canned (15.4% protein)	0.131	0.631	0.747	1.104	1.239	0.325	0.192	0.562	0.500	0.774	1.069	0.414
salami (23.9% protein)	0.203	0.979	1.159	1.713	1.923	0.505	0.298	0.872	0.776	1.201	1.660	0.642
Vienna sausage, canned (15.8% protein)	0.134	0.647	0.766	1.133	1.272	0.334	0.197	0.576	0.513	0.794	1.097	0.425
tongue:												
beef (16.4% protein)	0.197	0.708	0.792	1.286	1.364	0.357	0.207	0.661	0.548	0.840	1.065	0.412
pork (16.8% protein)	0.202	0.726	0.812	1.317	1.398	0.366	0.212	0.677	0.562	0.860	1.091	0.422
veal and pork loaf, canned (17.2% protein)	0.198	0.627	0.859	1.236	1.258	0.418	0.209	0.619	0.468	0.958	0.916	0.388
LEGUMES (DRY SEED); COMMON NUTS; OTHER NUTS AND DRY SEEDS; THEIR PRODUCTS:												
Legume seeds and their products:												
beans (*Phaseolus vulgaris*) (N×6.25):												
pinto and red Mexican (23.0% protein)	0.213	0.997	1.306	1.976	1.708	0.232	0.228	1.270	0.887	1.395	1.384	0.655
red kidney:												
raw (23.1% protein)	0.214	1.002	1.312	1.985	1.715	0.233	0.229	1.275	0.891	1.401	1.390	0.658
canned, solids and liquid (5.7% protein)	0.053	0.247	0.324	0.490	0.423	0.057	0.057	0.315	0.220	0.346	0.343	0.162

TABLE 40—*Continued*

Protein Content, and Nitrogen Conversion Factor	Trypto-phan (Gm.)	Threo-nine (Gm.)	Iso-leucine (Gm.)	Leucine (Gm.)	Lysine (Gm.)	Methi-onine (Gm.)	Cystine (Gm.)	Phenyl-alanine (Gm.)	Tyro-sine (Gm.)	Valine (Gm.)	Argi-nine (Gm.)	Histi-dine (Gm.)
LEGUMES; SEEDS; NUTS—*Continued*												
other common beans including navy, peabean, white marrow:												
raw (21.4% protein)	0.199	0.928	1.216	1.839	1.589	0.216	0.212	1.181	0.825	1.298	1.287	0.609
baked with pork, canned (5.8% protein)	0.057	0.274	0.291	0.486	0.354	0.059	0.018	0.333	0.165	0.312	0.251	0.186
black gram, raw (23.6% protein, N×6.25)	0.242	0.801	1.390	2.062	1.510	0.332	0.287	1.242	0.551	1.450	1.552	0.559
broadbeans, raw (25.4% protein, N×6.25)	0.236	0.829	1.593	2.211	1.426	0.106	0.179	1.057	0.687	1.276	1.780	0.748
chickpeas (20.8% protein, N±6.25)	0.170	0.739	1.195	1.538	1.434	0.276	0.296	1.012	0.692	1.025	1.551	0.559
cowpeas (22.9% protein, N×6.25	0.220	0.901	1.110	1.715	1.491	0.352	0.297	1.198	0.678	1.293	1.473	0.692
dolichos, twinflower (21.6% protein, N×6.25)	0.221	0.836	1.448	1.707	1.700	0.294	0.480	1.486	0.560	1.286	1.230	0.650
lentils, whole (25.0% protein, N×6.25)	0.216	0.896	1.316	1.760	1.528	0.180	0.204	1.104	0.664	1.360	1.908	0.548
lima beans (20.7% protein, N×6 25	0.195	0.980	1.199	1.722	1.378	0.331	0.311	1.222	0.543	1.298	1.315	0.669
lupine (32.3% protein, N×6.25)	......	1.101	1.618	1.964	1.447	0.114	......	1.271	......	1.328	2.718	0.811
moth beans (24.4% protein, N×6.25)	0.164	......	1.093	1.484	1.202	0.191	0.109	1.003	1.245	0.695	......	0.722
mung beans (24.4% protein, 6.25)	0.180	0.765	1.351	2.202	1.667	0.265	0.152	1.167	0.390	1.444	1.370	0.543
peanuts (26.9% protein, N×5.46)	0.340	0.828	1.266	1.872	1.099	0.271	0.463	1.557	1.104	1.532	3.296	0.749
peanut flour (51.2% protein, N×5.46)	0.647	1.575	2.410	3.563	2.091	0.516	0.881	2.963	2.100	2.916	6.273	1.425
peanut butter (26.1% protein, N×5.46)	0.330	0.803	1.228	1.816	1.066	0.263	0.449	1.510	1.071	1.487	3.198	0.727

TABLE 40—*Continued*

Protein Content, and Nitrogen Conversion Factor	Tryptophan (Gm.)	Threonine (Gm.)	Isoleucine (Gm.)	Leucine (Gm.)	Lysine (Gm.)	Methionine (Gm.)	Cystine (Gm.)	Phenylalanine (Gm.)	Tyrosine (Gm.)	Valine (Gm.)	Arginine (Gm.)	Histidine (Gm.)
LEGUMES; SEEDS; NUTS—*Continued*												
peas (*Pisum sativum*) (N×6.25):												
entire seeds (23.8% protein)	0.251	0.918	1.340	1.969	1.744	0.286	0.308	1.200	0.960	1.333	2.102	0.651
split (24.5% protein)	0.259	0.945	1.380	2.027	1.795	0.294	0.318	1.235	0.988	1.372	2.164	0.670
pigeonpeas, without seed coat (21.9% protein, N×6.25)	0.119	0.834	1.346	1.717	1.580	0.256	0.308	1.875	0.725	1.153	1.489	0.617
soybeans, whole (34.9% protein, N×5.71)	0.526	1.504	2.054	2.946	2.414	0.513	0.678	1.889	1.216	2.005	2.763	0.911
soybean flour, flakes, and grits (protein, N×5.71):												
low fat (44.7% protein)	0.673	1.926	2.630	3.773	3.092	0.658	0.869	2.419	1.558	2.568	3.538	1.166
medium fat (42.5% protein)	0.640	1.831	2.501	3.588	2.940	0.625	0.826	2.300	1.481	2.441	3.364	1.109
full fat (35.9% protein)	0.541	1.547	2.112	3.030	2.483	0.528	0.698	1.943	1.251	2.062	2.842	0.937
soybean curd (7.0% protein, N×5.71)	......	......	......	......	......	0.081	0.091	......	......	......	......	......
soybean milk (3.4% protein, N×5.71)	0.051	0.176	0.175	0.305	0.269	0.054	0.071	0.195	0.193	0.186	0.302	0.121
vetch (28.8% protein, N×6.25)	0.203	0.899	2.198	2.290	1.898	0.346	0.336	1.014	0.369	1.442	2.249	0.659
Common nuts and their products:												
almonds (18.6 protein, N×5.18)	0.176	0.610	0.873	1.454	0.582	0.259	0.377	1.146	0.618	1.124	2.729	0.517
Brazil nuts (14.4% protein, N×5.46)	0.187	0.422	0.593	1.129	0.443	0.941	0.504	0.617	0.483	0.823	2.247	0.367
cashews (18.5% protein, N×5.30)	0.471	0.737	1.222	1.522	0.792	0.353	0.527	0.946	0.712	1.592	2.098	0.415
coconut (3.4% protein, N×5.30)	0.033	0.129	0.180	0.269	0.152	0.071	0.062	0.174	0.101	0.212	0.486	0.069
coconut meal (20.3% protein, N×5.30)	0.199	0.770	1.076	1.605	0.908	0.421	0.372	1.038	0.605	1.268	2.899	0.414
filberts (12.7% protein, N×5.30)	0.211	0.415	0.853	0.939	0.417	0.139	0.165	0.537	0.434	0.934	2.171	0.288
peanuts. *See* Legumes.												
pecans (9.4% protein, N×5.30)	0.138	0.389	0.553	0.773	0.435	0.153	0.216	0.564	0.316	0.525	1.185	0.273
walnuts (English or Persian) (15.0% protein, N×5.30)	0.175	0.589	0.767	1.228	0.441	0.306	0.320	0.767	0.583	0.974	2.287	0.405

TABLE 40—*Continued*

Protein Content, and Nitrogen Conversion Factor	Tryptophan (Gm.)	Threonine (Gm.)	Isoleucine (Gm.)	Leucine (Gm.)	Lysine (Gm.)	Methionine (Gm.)	Cystine (Gm.)	Phenylalanine (Gm.)	Tyrosine (Gm.)	Valine (Gm.)	Arginine (Gm.)	Histidine (Gm.)
LEGUMES; SEEDS; NUTS—*Continued*												
Other nuts and seeds and their products												
(*Protein N×5:30*):												
acorns (10.4% protein)	0.126	0.434	0.561	0.808	0.636	0.139	0.184	0.473	......	0.718	0.722	0.251
amaranth (14.6% protein)	0.149	0.332	0.382	1.209	1.074	0.372	0.521	1.141	......	0.849	1.747	0.441
balsam pear seed meal (41.9% protein)	......	......	......	......	1.265	......	0.142	2.609	0.617	......	5.914	0.917
breadnut tree, Ramon (9.6% protein)	0.261	0.373	0.543	1.041	0.418	0.056	......	0.453	......	0.927	0.884	0.147
Chinese tallow tree-nut flour (57.6% protein)	0.837	2.174	3.510	4.347	1.587	0.924	0.696	2.847	2.011	4.510	10.031	1.587
chocolate tree, Nicaragua (38.5% protein)	0.588	1.496	2.092	3.952	2.223	0.276	......	2.630	......	2.404	4.220	0.683
cottonseed flour and meal (42.3% protein)	0.591	1.764	1.884	2.945	2.139	0.686	0.814	2.610	1.365	2.458	5.603	1.325
earpod tree, Guanacaste (34.1% protein)	0.444	1.165	2.213	4.581	1.930	0.360	......	1.325	......	1.570	2.857	1.004
lead tree (24.1% protein)	0.191	0.328	1.651	1.787	1.164	0.055	......	0.855	......	0.864	2.410	0.564
pumpkin seed (30.9% protein)	0.560	0.333	1.737	2.437	1.411	0.577	......	1.749	......	1.679	4.810	0.711
safflower seed meal (42.1% protein)	0.675	1.462	1.914	2.740	1.525	0.731	......	2.605	......	2.446	4.623	0.985
sesame:												
seed (19.3% protein)	0.331	0.707	0.951	1.679	0.583	0.637	0.495	1.457	0.951	0.885	1.992	0.441
meal (33.4% protein)	0.573	1.223	1.645	2.905	1.008	1.103	0.857	2.521	1.645	1.531	3.447	0.763
sunflower:												
kernel (23.0% protein)	0.343	0.911	1.276	1.736	0.868	0.443	0.464	1.220	0.647	1.354	2.370	0.586
meal (39.5% protein)	0.589	1.565	2.191	2.981	1.491	0.750	0.797	2.094	1.110	2.325	4.069	1.006

TABLE 40—*Continued*

Protein Content, and Nitrogen Conversion Factor	Tryptophan (Gm.)	Threonine (Gm.)	Isoleucine (Gm.)	Leucine (Gm.)	Lysine (Gm.)	Methionine (Gm.)	Cystine (Gm.)	Phenylalanine (Gm.)	Tyrosine (Gm.)	Valine (Gm.)	Arginine (Gm.)	Histidine (Gm.)
GRAINS AND THEIR PRODUCTS												
Barley (12.8% protein, N×5.83)	0.160	0.433	0.545	0.889	0.433	0.184	0.257	0.661	0.466	0.643	0.659	0.239
Bread, white (4% non-fat dry milk, flour basis) (8.5% protein, N×5.70)	0.091	0.282	0.429	0.668	0.225	0.142	0.200	0.465	0.243	0.435	0.340	0.192
Buckwheat flour:												
dark (11.7% protein, N×6.25)	0.165	0.461	0.440	0.683	0.687	0.206	0.228	0.442	0.240	0.607	0.930	0.256
light (6.4% protein, N×6.25)	0.090	0.252	0.241	0.374	0.376	0.113	0.125	0.242	0.131	0.332	0.509	0.140
Cañihua (14.7% protein, N×6.25)	0.118	0.706	1.000	0.851	0.882	0.263	0.162	0.529	0.294	0.677	1.162	0.367
Cereal combinations:												
corn and soy grits (18.0% protein, N×6.25)	0.161	0.792	0.841	1.656	0.772	0.271	0.311	0.832	0.562	1.054	0.982	0.472
infant food, precooked, mixed cereals with non-fat dry milk and yeast (19.4% protein, N×6.25)	0.118	......	......	......	0.273	0.310	0.137	0.543	0.447	......	0.447	0.233
oat-corn-rye mixture, puffed (14.5% protein, N×5.83)	0.172	0.545	0.841	1.368	0.343	0.388	0.234	0.933	0.622	0.900	0.776	0.326
Corn, field (10.0% protein, N×6.25)	0.061	0.398	0.462	1.296	0.288	0.186	0.130	0.454	0.611	0.510	0.352	0.206
Corn flour (7.8% protein, N×6.25)	0.047	0.311	0.361	1.011	0.225	0.145	0.101	0.354	0.477	0.398	0.275	0.161
Corn grits (8.7% protein, N×6.25)	0.053	0.347	0.402	1.128	0.251	0.161	0.113	0.395	0.532	0.444	0.306	0.180
Cornmeal:												
whole ground (9.2% protein, N×6.25)	0.056	0.367	0.425	1.192	0.265	0.171	0.119	0.418	0.562	0.470	0.324	0.190
de-germed (7.9% protein, N×6.25)	0.048	0.315	0.365	1.024	0.228	0.147	0.102	0.359	0.483	0.403	0.278	0.163
Corn products:												
flakes (8.1% protein, N×6.25)	0.052	0.275	0.306	1.047	0.154	0.135	0.152	0.354	0.283	0.386	0.231	0.226
germ (14.5% protein, N×6.25)	0.144	0.622	0.578	1.030	0.791	0.232	0.130	0.483	0.343	0.789	1.134	0.464
gluten (10.0% protein, N×6.25)	0.059	0.344	0.443	1.563	0.179	0.282	0.141	0.558	0.582	0.512	0.322	0.200
hominy (8.7% protein, N×6.25)	0.084	0.316	0.349	0.810	0.358	0.099	......	0.333	0.331	0.398	0.444	0.203
masa (2.8% protein, N×6.25)	0.010	......	......	......	0.103	0.108	0.030	......	......	......	......	......
pozol (5.9% protein, N×6.25)	0.042	0.336	0.304	0.591	0.234	0.087	......	0.254	......	0.267	0.197	0.122
tortilla (5.8% protein, N×6.25)	0.031	0.235	0.345	0.939	0.145	0.111	......	0.252	......	0.304	0.223	0.128
zein (16.1% protein, N×6.25)	0.010	0.495	0.822	3.184	......	0.281	0.162	1.664	0.981	0.654	0.286	0.216
Job's tears (13.8% protein, N×5.83)	0.066	0.620	1.065	3.506	0.362	0.459	0.265	0.703	......	......	0.518	0.317

TABLE 40—*Continued*

Protein Content, and Nitrogen Conversion Factor	Tryptophan (Gm.)	Threonine (Gm.)	Isoleucine (Gm.)	Leucine (Gm.)	Lysine (Gm.)	Methionine (Gm.)	Cystine (Gm.)	Phenylalanine (Gm.)	Tyrosine (Gm.)	Valine (Gm.)	Arginine (Gm.)	Histidine (Gm.)
GRAINS AND PRODUCTS—*Continued*												
Millets:												
foxtail millet (9.7% protein, N×5.83)	0.103	0.323	0.790	1.737	0.218	0.291	....	0.697	....	0.717	0.374	0.218
little millet (7.2% protein, N×5.83)	0.047	0.262	0.517	0.841	0.138	0.178	....	0.370	....	0.471	0.363	0.147
pearl millet (11.4% protein, N×5.83)	0.248	0.456	0.635	1.746	0.383	0.270	0.152	0.506	....	0.682	0.524	0.240
ragimillet (6.2% protein, N×5.83)	0.085	0.270	0.398	0.620	0.202	0.270	0.187	0.263	....	0.473	0.100	0.079
Oatmeal and rolled oats (14.2% protein, N×5.83)	0.183	0.470	0.733	1.065	0.521	0.209	0.309	0.758	0.524	0.845	0.935	0.261
Quinoa (11.0% protein, N×6.25)	0.120	0.523	0.722	0.781	0.729	0.273	0.107	0.394	0.253	0.447	0.820	0.297
Rice:												
brown (7.5% protein, N×5.95)	0.081	0.294	0.352	0.646	0.296	0.135	0.102	0.377	0.343	0.524	0.432	0.126
white and converted (7.6% protein, N×5.95)	0.082	0.298	0.356	0.655	0.300	0.137	0.103	0.382	0.347	0.531	0.438	0.128
Rice products:												
flakes or puffed (5.9% protein, N×5.95)	0.046	....	....	....	0.056	....	0.044	0.286	0.124	....	0.137	0.137
germ (14.2% protein, N×5.95)	0.270	2.177	0.630	0.838	1.707	0.420	0.169	0.750	0.929	0.938	1.559	0.430
Rye (12.1% protein, N×5.83)	0.137	0.443	0.515	0.813	0.494	0.191	0.221	0.571	0.390	0.631	0.591	0.276
Rye flour:												
light (9.4% protein, N×5.83)	0.106	0.343	0.400	0.632	0.384	0.143	0.187	0.443	0.303	0.490	0.459	0.214
medium (11.4% protein, N×5.83)	0.129	0.422	0.485	0.766	0.465	0.180	0.227	0.538	0.368	0.594	0.557	0.260
Sorghum (11.0% protein, N×6.25)	0.123	0.394	0.598	1.767	0.299	0.190	0.183	0.547	0.303	0.628	0.417	0.211
Teosinte (22.0% protein, N×6.25)	0.049	....	....	....	0.343	0.496	....	....	....	....	....	....
Wheat, whole grain:												
hard red spring (14.0% protein, N×5.83)	0.173	0.403	0.607	0.939	0.384	0.214	0.307	0.691	0.523	0.648	0.670	0.286
hard red winter (12.3% protein, N 5.83)	0.152	0.354	0.534	0.825	0.338	0.188	0.270	0.608	0.460	0.570	0.589	0.251
soft red winter (10.2% protein, N×5.83)	0.126	0.294	0.443	0.684	0.280	0.156	0.224	0.504	0.382	0.472	0.488	0.208
white (9.4% protein, N×5.83)	0.116	0.271	0.408	0.630	0.258	0.143	0.206	0.464	0.351	0.435	0.450	0.192
durum (12.7% protein, N×5.83)	0.157	0.366	0.551	0.852	0.348	0.194	0.279	0.627	0.475	0.588	0.608	0.259

TABLE 40—*Continued*

Protein Content, and Nitrogen Conversion Factor	Trypto-phan (Gm.)	Threo-nine (Gm.)	Iso-leucine (Gm.)	Leucine (Gm.)	Lysine (Gm.)	Methi-onine (Gm.)	Cystine (Gm.)	Phenyl-alanine (Gm.)	Tyro-sine (Gm.)	Valine (Gm.)	Argi-nine (Gm.)	Histi-dine (Gm.)
GRAINS AND PRODUCTS—*Continued*												
Wheat flour:												
whole grain (13.3% protein, N×5.83)	0.164	0.383	0.577	0.892	0.365	0.203	0.292	0.657	0.497	0.616	0.636	0.271
intermediate extraction (12.0% protein, N×5.70)	......	0.392	0.619	0.924	0.356	0.198	0.320	0.732	0.335	0.583	0.549	0.286
white (10.5% protein, N×5.70)	0.129	0.302	0.483	0.809	0.239	0.138	0.210	0.577	0.359	0.453	0.466	0.210
Wheat products:												
bran (12.0% protein, N×6.31)	0.196	0.342	0.485	0.717	0.491	0.145	0.270	0.434	0.259	0.552	0.742	0.280
burghul (12.4% protein, N×5.83)	0.070	......	......	......	0.430	0.300	0.319	......	......	......	......	......
farina (10.9% protein, N×5.70)	0.124	......	......	......	0.199	0.143	0.184	0.579	0.447	......	0.424	0.268
flakes (10.8% protein, N×5.70)	0.121	0.356	0.496	0.891	0.360	0.127	0.191	0.478	0.311	0.572	0.559	0.231
germ (25.2% protein, N×5.80)	0.265	1.343	1.177	1.708	1.534	0.404	0.287	0.908	0.882	1.364	1.825	0.687
gluten, commercial (80.0% protein, N×5.70)	0.856	2.119	3.677	5.993	1.530	1.389	1.726	4.351	2.596	3.789	3.481	1.825
gluten flour (41.4% protein, N×5.70)	0.443	1.097	1.903	3.101	0.792	0.719	0.893	2.252	1.344	1.961	1.801	0.944
macaroni or spaghetti (12.8% protein, N×5.70)	0.150	0.499	0.642	0.849	0.413	0.193	0.243	0.669	0.422	0.728	0.582	0.303
noodles, containing egg solids (12.6% protein, N×5.70)	0.133	0.533	0.621	0.834	0.411	0.212	0.245	0.610	0.312	0.745	0.621	0.301
Shredded Wheat (10.1% protein, N×5.83)	0.085	0.405	0.449	0.684	0.331	0.139	0.204	0.481	0.236	0.577	0.523	0.236
whole wheat with added germ (12.8% protein, N×5.83)	0.136	......	......	......	0.466	......	0.246	0.755	0.481	......	0.742	0.371
FRUITS (Protein, N×6.25)												
Abiu (1.7% protein)	0.028	......	......	......	0.085	0.013	......	......	......	......	......	......
Avocados (1.3% protein)	0.014	......	......	......	0.074	0.012	......	......	......	......	......	......
Bananas ripe												
common (1.2% protein)	0.018	......	......	......	0.055	0.011	......	......	0.031	......	......	......
dwarf (1.2% protein)	0.012	......	......	......	0.049	0.004	......	......	......	......	......	......
Dates (2.2% protein)	0.061	0.061	0.074	0.077	0.065	0.027	......	0.063	......	0.094	0.049	0.049

TABLE 40—*Continued*

Protein Content, and Nitrogen Conversion Factor	Tryptophan (Gm.)	Threonine (Gm.)	Isoleucine (Gm.)	Leucine (Gm.)	Lysine (Gm.)	Methionine (Gm.)	Cystine (Gm.)	Phenylalanine (Gm.)	Tyrosine (Gm.)	Valine (Gm.)	Arginine (Gm.)	Histidine (Gm.)
FRUITS—*Continued*												
Grapefruit (0.5% protein)	0.001	......	......	......	0.026	0.000	......	......	......	......	......	......
Guavas, common (1.0% protein)	0.010	......	......	......	0.030	0.010	......	......	......	......	......	......
Limes (0.8% protein)	0.003	......	......	......	0.015	0.002	......	......	......	......	......	......
Mamey (0.5% protein)	0.006	......	......	......	0.040	0.007	......	......	......	......	......	......
Mangos (0.7% protein)	0.014	......	......	......	0.093	0.008	......	......	......	......	......	......
Muskmelons (0.6% protein)	0.001	......	......	......	0.015	0.002	......	......	......	......	......	......
Oranges, sweet (0.9% protein)	0.003	......	......	......	0.024	0.003	......	......	......	......	......	......
Orange juice (0.8% protein)	0.003	......	......	......	0.021	0.002	......	......	......	......	......	......
Oranges, mandarin including tangerines (0.8% protein)	0.005	......	......	......	0.028	0.004	......	......	......	......	......	......
Papayas (0.6% protein)	0.012	......	......	......	0.038	0.002	......	......	......	......	......	......
Pineapple (0.4% protein)	0.005	......	......	......	0.009	0.001	......	......	......	......	......	......
Plantain or baking banana (1.1% protein)	0.010	0.027	0.056	0.059	0.050	0.005	0.016	0.049	......	0.065	0.045	......
Soursop (1.0% protein)	0.011	......	......	......	0.060	0.007	......	......	......	......	......	......
Sugarapple (1.8% protein)	0.009	......	......	......	0.071	0.008	......	......	......	......	......	......
VEGETABLES												
Immature seeds (Protein, N×6.25):												
corn, sweet, white or yellow:												
raw (3.7% protein)	0.023	0.151	0.137	0.407	0.137	0.072	0.062	0.207	0.124	0.231	0.174	0.095
canned, solids and liquid (2.0% protein)	0.012	0.082	0.074	0.220	0.074	0.039	0.033	0.112	0.067	0.125	0.094	0.052
cowpeas (9.4% protein)	0.099	0.353	0.465	0.653	0.617	0.131	......	0.523	......	0.513	0.615	0.310
lima beans:												
raw (7.5% protein)	0.097	0.338	0.460	0.605	0.474	0.080	0.083	0.389	0.259	0.485	0.454	0.247
canned, solids and liquid (3.8% protein)	0.049	0.171	0.233	0.306	0.240	0.041	0.042	0.197	0.131	0.246	0.230	0.125
peas:												
raw (6.7% protein)	0.056	0.245	0.308	0.418	0.315	0.054	0.073	0.257	0.163	0.274	0.595	0.109
canned, solids and liquid (3.4% protein)	0.028	0.125	0.156	0.212	0.160	0.027	0.037	0.131	0.083	0.139	0.302	0.055

TABLE 40—*Continued*

Protein Content, and Nitrogen Conversion Factor	Tryptophan (Gm.)	Threonine (Gm.)	Isoleucine (Gm.)	Leucine (Gm.)	Lysine (Gm.)	Methionine (Gm.)	Cystine (Gm.)	Phenylalanine (Gm.)	Tyrosine (Gm.)	Valine (Gm.)	Arginine (Gm.)	Histidine (Gm.)
VEGETABLES—*Continued*												
Leafy vegetables, raw (*Protein, N×6.25*):												
amaranth (3.5% protein)	0.038	0.056	0.164	0.206	0.141	0.025	0.024	0.096	0.105	0.136	0.134	0.069
beet greens (2.0% protein)	0.024	0.076	0.084	0.129	0.108	0.034	......	0.116	......	0.101	0.083	0.026
Brussels sprouts (4.4% protein)	0.044	0.153	0.186	0.194	0.197	0.046	......	0.148	......	0.193	0.279	0.106
cabbage (1.4% protein)	0.011	0.039	0.040	0.057	0.066	0.013	0.028	0.030	0.030	0.043	0.105	0.025
chard (1.4% protein)	0.014	0.058	0.060	0.076	0.055	0.004	......	0.046	......	0.055	0.035	0.018
chicory (1.6% protein)	0.024	......	......	......	0.052	0.016	0.006	......	0.040	......	......	0.024
collards (3.9% protein)	0.055	0.114	0.121	0.218	0.202	0.046	0.059	0.124	0.151	0.195	0.258	0.087
kale (3.9% protein)	0.042	0.139	0.133	0.252	0.121	0.035	0.036	0.158	......	0.184	0.202	0.062
lettuce (1.2% protein)	0.012	......	......	......	0.070	0.004	......	......	......	......	......	......
mustard greens (2.3% protein)	0.037	0.060	0.075	0.062	0.111	0.024	0.035	0.074	0.121	0.108	0.167	0.041
parsley, curly garden (2.5% protein)	0.050	......	......	......	0.160	0.012	......	......	......	......	......	......
spinach (2.3% protein)	0.037	0.102	0.107	0.176	0.142	0.039	0.046	0.099	0.073	0.126	0.116	0.049
turnip greens (2.9% protein)	0.045	0.125	0.107	0.207	0.129	0.052	0.045	0.146	0.105	0.149	0.167	0.051
watercress (1.7% protein)	0.028	0.084	0.076	0.131	0.091	0.010	......	0.062	0.036	0.084	0.053	0.034
Starchy roots and tubers (*Protein, N×6.25*):												
Apio arracacia (1.2% protein)	0.008	......	......	......	0.042	0.003	......	......	......	......	......	......
cassava:												
flour (1.6% protein)	0.021	0.044	0.045	0.066	0.066	0.010	0.018	0.045	0.030	0.049	0.159	0.025
root (1.1% protein)	0.014	0.030	0.031	0.045	0.045	0.007	0.012	0.031	0.021	0.033	0.110	0.017
potatoes:												
raw (2.0% protein)	0.021	0.079	0.088	0.100	0.107	0.025	0.019	0.088	0.036	0.107	0.099	0.029
canned, solids and liquid (1.7% protein)	0.018	0.067	0.075	0.085	0.091	0.021	0.016	0.075	0.030	0.091	0.084	0.024
flour (7.1% protein)	0.076	0.279	0.311	0.353	0.378	0.089	0.068	0.314	0.127	0.379	0.350	0.102

TABLE 40—*Continued*

Protein Content, and Nitrogen Conversion Factor	Tryptophan (Gm.)	Threonine (Gm.)	Isoleucine (Gm.)	Leucine (Gm.)	Lysine (Gm.)	Methionine (Gm.)	Cystine (Gm.)	Phenylalanine (Gm.)	Tyrosine (Gm.)	Valine (Gm.)	Arginine (Gm.)	Histidine (Gm.)
VEGETABLES—*Continued*												
sweet potatoes (*Ipomaea batatas*):												
raw (1.8% protein)	0.031	0.085	0.087	0.103	0.085	0.033	0.029	0.100	0.081	0.135	0.094	0.036
dehydrated (5.0% protein)	0.087	0.235	0.241	0.286	0.236	0.093	0.080	0.278	0.225	0.374	0.261	0.099
taro (1.9% protein)	0.035	0.089	0.099	0.169	0.110	0.021	......	0.099	......	0.114	0.118	0.032
yam (*Dioscorea* spp.) (2.1% protein)	0.035	......	......	......	0.110	0.034	......	......	......	......	......	......
Yautia malanga (1.7% protein)	0.023	......	......	......	0.067	0.016	......	......	......	......	......	......
Other vegetables (Protein, N×6.25):												
asparagus:												
raw (2.2% protein)	0.027	0.066	0.080	0.096	0.103	0.032	......	0.069	......	0.106	0.123	0.036
canned, solids and liquid (1.9% protein)	0.023	0.057	0.069	0.083	0.089	0.027	......	0.060	......	0.092	0.106	0.031
beans, snap:												
raw (2.4% protein)	0.033	0.091	0.109	0.139	0.126	0.035	0.024	0.057	0.050	0.115	0.101	0.045
canned, solids and liquid (1.0% protein)	0.014	0.038	0.045	0.058	0.052	0.014	0.010	0.024	0.021	0.048	0.042	0.019
beets:												
raw (1.6% protein)	0.014	0.034	0.051	0.055	0.086	0.006	......	0.027	......	0.049	0.028	0.022
canned, solids and liquid (0.9% protein)	0.008	0.019	0.029	0.031	0.048	0.003	......	0.015	......	0.028	0.016	0.012
broccoli (3.3% protein)	0.037	0.122	0.126	0.163	0.147	0.050	......	0.119	......	0.170	0.192	0.063
carrots:												
raw (1.2% protein)	0.010	0.043	0.046	0.065	0.052	0.010	0.029	0.042	0.020	0.056	0.041	0.017
canned, solids and liquid (0.5% protein)	0.004	0.018	0.019	0.027	0.022	0.004	0.012	0.018	0.008	0.023	0.017	0.007
cauliflower (2.4% protein)	0.033	0.102	0.104	0.162	0.134	0.047	......	0.075	0.034	0.144	0.110	0.048
celery (1.3% protein)	0.012	......	......	......	0.021	0.015	0.006	......	0.016	......	......	......
chayote (0.6% protein)	0.008	......	......	......	0.038	0.001	......	......	......	......	......	......
cowpeas, yardlong, immature pod (3.4% protein)	0.034	......	......	......	0.203	0.021	......	......	......	......	......	......
cucumbers (0.7% protein)	0.005	0.019	0.022	0.030	0.031	0.007	......	0.016	......	0.024	0.053	0.001
cushaw (1.5% protein)	0.014	......	......	......	0.044	0.008	......	......	......	......	......	......
eggplant (1.1% protein)	0.010	0.038	0.056	0.068	0.030	0.006	......	0.048	......	0.065	0.037	0.019
mallow (3.7% protein)	0.144	0.155	......	0.259	0.155	0.030	......	0.166	......	0.181	0.189	0.063

TABLE 40—*Continued*

Protein Content, and Nitrogen Conversion Factor	Tryptophan (Gm.)	Threonine (Gm.)	Isoleucine (Gm.)	Leucine (Gm.)	Lysine (Gm.)	Methionine (Gm.)	Cystine (Gm.)	Phenylalanine (Gm.)	Tyrosine (Gm.)	Valine (Gm.)	Arginine (Gm.)	Histidine (Gm.)
VEGETABLES—*Continued*												
mushrooms:												
(*Agaricus campestris*)*	0.006	......	0.532	0.281	......	0.167	......	......	......	0.378	0.235	......
(*Lactarius* spp.)†	0.006	0.156	0.201	0.139	0.088	0.021	......	0.018	......	0.116	0.021	0.027
okra (1.8% protein)	0.018	0.066	0.069	0.101	0.076	0.022	0.017	0.065	0.079	0.091	0.093	0.030
onions, mature (1.4% protein)	0.021	0.022	0.021	0.037	0.064	0.013	......	0.039	0.046	0.031	0.180	0.014
peppers (1.2% protein)	0.009	0.050	0.046	0.046	0.051	0.016	......	0.055	......	0.033	0.024	0.014
prickly pears (1.1% protein)	0.009	0.053	0.044	0.057	0.044	0.008	......	0.059	......	0.041	0.032	0.016
pumpkin (1.2% protein)	0.016	0.028	0.044	0.063	0.058	0.011	......	0.032	0.016	0.045	0.043	0.019
radishes (1.2% protein)	0.005	0.059	......	......	0.034	0.002	......	......	......	0.030	......	......
seepweed (2.6% protein)	0.027	0.089	0.113	0.152	0.089	0.013	......	0.116	......	0.091	0.062	0.036
soybean sprouts (6.2% protein)	......	0.159	0.225	0.265	0.211	0.045	......	0.186	......	0.225	0.225	0.133
squash, summer (0.6% protein)	0.005	0.014	0.019	0.027	0.023	0.008	......	0.016	......	0.022	0.027	0.009
tomatoes and cherry tomatoes (1.0% protein)	0.009	0.033	0.029	0.041	0.042	0.007	......	0.028	0.014	0.028	0.029	0.015
turnips (1.1% protein)	......	......	0.020	......	0.057	0.012	......	0.020	0.029	......	......	......
waxgourd, Chinese (0.4% protein)	0.002	......	......	......	0.009	0.003	......	......	......	......	......	......
MISCELLANEOUS FOOD ITEMS												
Vegetable patty or steak (principally wheat protein) (15% protein, N×5.70)	0.142	0.411	0.884	1.079	0.321	0.253	......	0.811	......	0.705	0.597	0.321
Yeast:												
baker's, compressed‡ (N×6.25)	0.122	0.655	0.655	1.151	0.914	0.248	0.120	0.607	0.580	0.840	0.536	0.353
brewer's, dried§ (N×6.25)	0.710	2.353	2.398	3.226	3.300	0.836	0.548	1.902	1.902	2.723	2.250	1.251
primary, dried:												
(*Saccharomyces cerevisiae*)§ (N×6.25)	0.636	2.353	2.708	3.300	3.337	0.851	0.444	1.813	2.472	2.553	1.931	1.103
(*Torulopsis utilis*)§ (N×6.25)	0.636	2.331	3.323	3.707	3.648	0.710	0.422	2.361	2.464	2.901	3.337	1.251

* Total nitrogen is 0.58%. This is equivalent to 2.4% protein on the basis that two-thirds of the nitrogen is protein nitrogen. If total nitrogen is used for the calculation, the protein content is 3.6%.

† Total nitrogen is 0.69%. This is equivalent to 2.9% protein on the basis that two-thirds of the nitrogen is protein nitrogen. If total nitrogen is used for the calculation, the protein content is 4.3%.

‡ Total nitrogen is 2.1%. This is equivalent to 10.6% protein on the basis that four-fifths of the nitrogen is protein nitrogen. If total nitrogen is used for the calculation, the protein content is 13.1%.

§ Total nitrogen is 7.4%. This is equivalent to 36.9% protein on the basis that four-fifths of the nitrogen is protein nitrogen. If total nitrogen is used for the calculation, the protein content is 46.1%.

APPENDIX 6

Sodium and Potassium Content of Foods, 100 Grams Edible Portion[1]

TABLE 41

Food and description	Sodium (Mg.)	Potassium (Mg.)
Almonds:		
Dried	4	773
Roasted and salted	198	773
Apples:		
Raw, pared	1	110
Frozen, sliced, sweetened	14	68
Apple Brown Betty	153	100
Apple butter	2	252
Apple juice, canned or bottled	1	101
Applesauce, canned, sweetened	2	65
Apricots:		
Raw	1	281
Canned, syrup pack, light	1	239
Dried, sulfured, cooked, fruit, and liquid	8	318
Apricot nectar, canned (approx. 40% fruit)	Trace	151
Asparagus:		
Cooked spears, boiled, drained	1	183
Canned spears, green:		
Regular pack, solids and liquid	236[2]	166
Special dietary pack (low-sodium), solids and liquids	3	166
Frozen:		
Cuts and tips, cooked, boiled, drained	1	220
Spears, cooked, boiled, drained	1	238
Avocados, raw, all commercial varieties	4	604
Bacon, cured, cooked, broiled or fried, drained	1,021	236
Bacon, Canadian, cooked, broiled or fried, drained	2,555	432
Baking powders:		
Home use:		
Straight phosphate	8,220	170
Special low-sodium preparations	6	10,948
Bananas, raw, common	1	370
Barbecue sauce	815	174
Bass, black sea, raw	68	256
Beans, common, mature seeds, dry:		
White:		
Cooked	7	416
Canned, solids and liquid, with pork and tomato sauce	463	210
Red, cooked	3	340
Beans, Lima:		
Immature seeds:		
Cooked, boiled, drained	1	422
Canned:		
Regular pack, solids and liquid	236[2]	222
Special dietary pack (low-sodium), solids and liquid	4	222
Frozen, thin-seeded types, commonly called baby Limas, cooked, boiled, drained	129	394
Mature seeds, dry, cooked	2	612

1. Numbers in parentheses denote values imputed—usually from another form of the food or from a similar food. Dashes denote lack of reliable data for a constituent believed to be present in measurable amount. Values are selected from *Composition of Foods—Raw, Processed, Prepared* (U.S. Department of Agriculture, Agriculture Handbook No. 8 [December, 1963]).

2. Estimated average based on addition of salt in the amount of 0.6 percent of the finished product.

TABLE 41—*Continued*

Food and description	Sodium (Mg.)	Potassium (Mg.)
Beans, mung, sprouted seeds, cooked, boiled, drained	4	156
Beans, snap:		
Green:		
Cooked, boiled, drained	4	151
Canned:		
Regular pack, solids and liquid	236[2]	95
Special dietary pack (low sodium), solids and liquid	2	95
Frozen, cut, cooked, boiled, drained	1	152
Yellow or wax:		
Cooked, boiled, drained	3	151
Canned:		
Regular pack, solids and liquid	236[2]	95
Special dietary pack (low-sodium), solids and liquid	2	95
Frozen, cut, cooked, boiled, drained	1	164
Beans and frankfurters, canned	539	262
Beef:		
Retail cuts, trimmed to retail level:		
Round	60	370
Rump	60	370
Hamburger, regular ground, cooked	47	450
Beef and vegetable stew, canned	411	174
Beef, corned, boneless:		
Cooked, medium-fat	1,740	150
Canned corned-beef hash (with potato)	540	200
Beef, dried, cooked, creamed	716	153
Beef potpie, commercial, frozen, unheated	366	93
Beets, common, red:		
Canned:		
Regular pack, solids and liquid	236[2]	167
Special dietary pack (low-sodium), solids and liquid	46	167
Beet greens, common, cooked, boiled, drained	76	332
Beverages, alcoholic:		
Beer, alcohol 4.5% by volume (3.6% by weight)	7	25
Gin, rum, vodka, whisky:		
80-proof (33.4% alcohol by weight)	1	2
86-proof (36.0% alcohol by weight)	1	2
90-proof (37.9% alcohol by weight)	1	2
94-proof (39.7% alcohol by weight)	1	2
100-proof (42.5% alcohol by weight)	1	2
Wines:		
Dessert, alcohol 18.8% by volume (15.3% by weight)	4	75
Table, alcohol 12.2% by volume (9.9% by weight)	5	92
Biscuits, baking powder, made with enriched flour	626	117
Biscuit dough, commercial, frozen	910	86
Biscuit mix, with enriched flour, and biscuits baked from mix:		
Mix, dry form	1,300	80
Biscuits, made with milk	973	116
Blackberries, including dewberries, boysenberries, and youngberries, raw	1	170
Blackberries, canned, solids and liquid:		
Water pack, with or without artificial sweetener	1	115
Syrup pack, heavy	1	109
Blueberries:		
Raw	1	81
Frozen, not thawed, sweetened	1	66
Bluefish, cooked:		
Baked or broiled	104	....
Fried	146	....

TABLE 41—*Continued*

Food and description	Sodium (Mg.)	Potassium (Mg.)
Boston brown bread	251	292
Bouillon cubes or powder	24,000	100
Boysenberries, frozen, not thawed, sweetened	1	105
Bran, added sugar and malt extract	1,060	1,070
Bran flakes (40% bran), added thiamine	925	....
Bran flakes with raisins, added thiamine	800	....
Brazil nuts	1	715
Breads:		
Cracked-wheat	529	134
French or Vienna, enriched	580	90
Italian, enriched	585	74
Raisin	365	233
Rye, American (⅓ rye, ⅔ clear flour)	557	145
White, enriched, made with 3%–4% non-fat dry milk	507	105
Whole-wheat, made with 2% non-fat dry milk	527	273
Bread crumbs, dry, grated	736	152
Bread stuffing mix and stuffings prepared from mix:		
Mix, dry form	1,331	172
Broccoli:		
Cooked spears, boiled, drained	10	267
Frozen, spears, cooked, boiled, drained	12	220
Brussels sprouts, frozen, cooked, boiled, drained	14	295
Buffalo fish, raw	52	293
Bulgur (parboiled wheat):		
Canned, made from hard red winter wheat:		
Unseasoned[3]	599	87
Seasoned[4]	460	112
Butter[5]	987	23
Buttermilk, fluid, cultured (made from skim milk)	130	140
Cabbage:		
Common varieties (Danish, domestic, and pointed types):		
Raw	20	233
Cooked, boiled until tender, drained, shredded, cooked in small amount of water	14	163
Red, raw	26	268
Cabbage, Chinese (also called celery cabbage or petsai)	23	253
Cakes:		
Baked from home recipes:		
Angelfood	283	88
Fruitcake, made with enriched flour, dark	158	496
Gingerbread, made with enriched flour	237	454
Plain cake or cupcake, without icing	300	79
Pound, modified	178	78
Frozen, commercial, devil's food, with chocolate icing	420	119
Candy:		
Caramels, plain or chocolate	226	192
Chocolate, sweet	33	269
Chocolate-coated, chocolate fudge	228	193
Gum drops, starch jelly pieces	35	5
Hard	32	4
Marshmallows	39	6
Peanut bars	10	448
Carp, raw	50	286

3. Processed, partially debranned, whole-kernel wheat with salt added.

4. Processed, partially debranned, whole-kernel wheat with chicken fat, chicken stock base, dehydrated onion flakes, salt, monosodium glutamate, and herbs.

5. Values apply to salted butter. Unsalted butter contains less than 10 mg. of either sodium or potassium per 100 grams. Value for vitamin A is the year-round average.

TABLE 41—*Continued*

Food and description	Sodium (Mg.)	Potassium (Mg.)
Carrots:		
Raw	47	341
Canned:		
Regular pack, solids and liquid	236[2]	120
Special dietary pack (low-sodium), solids and liquid	39	120
Cashew nuts	15[6]	464
Catfish, freshwater, raw	60	330
Cauliflower:		
Cooked, boiled, drained	9	206
Frozen, cooked, boiled, drained	10	207
Caviar, sturgeon, granular	2,200	180
Celery, all, including green and yellow varieties:		
Raw	126	341
Cooked, boiled, drained	88	239
Chard, Swiss, cooked, boiled, drained	86	321
Cheese straws	721	63
Cheeses:		
Natural cheeses:		
Cheddar (domestic type, commonly called American)	700	82
Cottage (large or small curd):		
Creamed	229	85
Uncreamed	290	72
Cream	250	74
Parmesan	734	149
Swiss (domestic)	710	104
Pasteurized process cheese, American	1,367[7]	80
Pasteurized process cheese spread, American	1,625[7]	240
Cherries:		
Raw, sweet	2	191
Canned:		
Sour, red, solids and liquid, water pack	2	130
Sweet, solids and liquid, syrup pack, light	1	128
Frozen, not thawed, sweetened	2	130
Chicken:		
All classes:		
Light meat without skin, cooked, roasted	64	411
Dark meat without skin, cooked, roasted	86	321
Chicken potpie, commercial, frozen, unheated	411	153
Chicory, Witloof (also called French or Belgian endive), bleached head (forced), raw	7	182
Chili con carne, canned, with beans	531	233
Chocolate, bitter or baking	4	830
Chocolate syrup, fudge type	89	284
Chop suey, with meat, canned	551	138
Chow mein, chicken (without noodles), canned	290	167
Citron, candied	290	120
Clams, raw:		
Soft, meat only	36	235
Hard or round, meat only	205	311
Clams, canned, including hard, soft, razor, and unspecified:		
Solids and liquid	....	140

6. Applies to unsalted nuts. For salted nuts, value is approximately 200 mg. per 100 grams.

7. Values for phosphorus and sodium are based on use of 1.5 per cent anhydrous disodium phosphate as the emulsifying agent. If emulsifying agent does not contain either phosphorus or sodium, the content of these two nutrients in milligrams per 100 grams is as follows:

	P	Na
American process cheese	444	650
Swiss process cheese	540	681
American cheese food	427	.....
American cheese spread	548	1,139

TABLE 41—*Continued*

Food and description	Sodium (Mg.)	Potassium (Mg.)
Cocoa and chocolate-flavored beverage powders:		
Cocoa powder with non-fat dry milk	525	800
Mix for hot chocolate	382	605
Cocoa, dry powder:		
High-fat or breakfast:		
Plain	6	1,522
Processed with alkali	717	651
Coconut cream (liquid expressed from grated coconut meat)	4	324
Coconut meat, fresh	23	256
Cod:		
Cooked, broiled	110	407
Dehydrated, lightly salted	8,100	160
Coffee, instant, water-soluble solids:		
Dry powder	72	3,256
Beverage	1	36
Coleslaw, made with French dressing (commercial)	268	205
Collards, cooked, boiled, drained, leaves, including stems, cooked in small amount of water	25	234
Cookies:		
Assorted, packaged, commercial	365	67
Butter, thin, rich	418	60
Gingersnaps	571	462
Molasses	386	138
Oatmeal with raisins	162	370
Sandwich type	483	38
Vanilla wafer	252	72
Cookie dough, plain, chilled in roll, baked	548	48
Corn, sweet:		
Cooked, boiled, drained, white and yellow, kernels, cut off cob before cooking	Trace	165
Canned:		
Regular pack, cream style, white and yellow, solids and liquid	236[2]	(97)
Special dietary pack (low-sodium), cream style, white and yellow, solids and liquid	2	(97)
Frozen, kernels cut off cob, cooked, boiled, drained	1	184
Corn fritters	477	133
Corn grits, degermed, enriched, dry form	1	80
Corn products used mainly as ready-to-eat breakfast cereals:		
Corn flakes, added nutrients	1,005	120
Corn, puffed, added nutrients	1,060	....
Corn, rice, and wheat flakes, mixed, added nutrients	950	....
Cornbread, baked from home recipes, southern style, made with degermed cornmeal, enriched	591	157
Cornbread mix and cornbread baked from mix, cornbread, made with egg, milk	744	127
Cornmeal, white or yellow, degermed, enriched, dry form	1	120
Cornstarch	Trace	Trace
Cowpeas, including blackeye peas:		
Immature seeds, canned, solids and liquid	236[2]	352
Young pods, with seeds, cooked, boiled, drained	3	196
Crab, canned	1,000	110
Crackers:		
Butter	1,092	113
Graham, plain	670	384
Saltines	(1,100)	(120)
Sandwich type, peanut-cheese	992	226
Soda	1,100	120

TABLE 41—*Continued*

Food and description	Sodium (Mg.)	Potassium (Mg.)
Cranberries, raw	2	82
Cranberry juice cocktail, bottled (approx. 33% cranberry juice)	1	10
Cranberry sauce, sweetened, canned, strained	1	30
Cream, fluid, light, coffee, or table, 20% fat	43	122
Cream substitutes, dried, containing:		
Cream, skim milk (calcium reduced), and lactose	575	....
Cream puffs with custard filling	83	121
Cress, garden, raw	14	606
Croaker, Atlantic, cooked, baked	120	323
Cucumbers, raw, pared	6	160
Custard, baked	79	146
Dates, domestic, natural and dry	1	648
Doughnuts, cake type	501	90
Duck, domesticated, raw, flesh only	74	285
Eggs, chicken:		
Raw:		
Whole, fresh and frozen	122	129
Whites, fresh and frozen	146	139
Yolks, fresh	52	98
Eggplant, cooked, boiled, drained	1	150
Endive (curly endive and escarole), raw	14	294
Farina:		
Enriched:		
Regular:		
Dry form	2	83
Cooked	144	9
Quick-cooking, cooked	165	10
Instant-cooking, cooked	188	13
Unenriched, regular, dry form	2	83
Figs, canned, solids and liquid, syrup pack, light	2	152
Flatfishes (flounders, soles, and sand dabs), raw	78	342
Fruit cocktail, canned, solids and liquid, water pack, with or without artificial sweetener	5	168
Garlic, cloves, raw	19	529
Ginger root, fresh	6	264
Gizzard, chicken, all classes, cooked, simmered	57	211
Goose, domesticated, flesh only, cooked, roasted	124	605
Gooseberries, canned, solids and liquid, syrup pack, heavy	1	98
Grapefruit:		
Raw, pulp, pink, red, white, all varieties	1	135
Canned, juice, sweetened	1	162
Grapefruit juice and orange juice blended, canned, sweetened	1	184
Grapes, raw, American type (slip skin) such as Concord, Delaware, Niagara, Catawba, and Scuppernong	3	158
Grapejuice, canned or bottled	2	116
Guavas, whole, raw, common	4	289
Haddock, cooked, fried	177	348
Hake, including Pacific hake, squirrel hake, and silver hake or whiting; raw	74	363
Halibut, Atlantic and Pacific, cooked, broiled	134	525
Ham croquette	342	83
Heart, beef, lean, cooked, braised	104	232
Herring:		
Raw, Pacific	74	420
Smoked, hard	6,231	157

TABLE 41—*Continued*

Food and description	Sodium (Mg.)	Potassium (Mg.)
Honey, strained or extracted	5	51
Horse-radish, prepared	96	290
Ice cream and frozen custard:		
Regular, approximately 10% fat	63[8]	181
Ice cream cones	232	244
Ice milk	68[8]	195
Jams and preserves	12	88
Kale, cooked, boiled, drained, leaves including stems	43	221
Kingfish; southern, gulf, and northern (whiting); raw	83	250
Lake herring (cisco), raw	47	319
Lamb, retail cuts	70	290
Lemon juice, canned or bottled, unsweetened	1	141
Lettuce, raw, crisphead varieties such as Iceberg, New York, and Great Lakes strains	9	175
Lime juice, canned or bottled, unsweetened	1	104
Liver, beef, cooked, fried	184	380
Lobster, northern, canned or cooked	210	180
Loganberries, canned, solids and liquid, syrup pack, light	1	111
Macadamia nuts	....	264
Macaroni, unenriched, dry form	2	197
Macaroni and cheese, canned	304	58
Margarine[9]	987	23
Marmalade, citrus	14	33
Milk, cow:		
Fluid (pasteurized and raw):		
Whole, 3.7% fat	50	144
Skim	52	145
Canned, evaporated (unsweetened)	118	303
Dry, skim (non fat solids), regular	532	1,745
Malted:		
Dry powder	440	720
Beverage	91	200
Chocolate drink, fluid, commercial:		
Made with skim milk	46	142
Made with whole (3.5% fat) milk	47	146
Molasses, cane:		
First extraction or light	15	917
Third extraction or blackstrap	96	2,927
Muffin mixes, corn, and muffins baked from mixes:		
Muffins, made with egg, milk	479	110
Muffins, made with egg, water	346	104
Mushrooms:		
Raw	15	414
Canned, solids and liquid	400	197
Muskmelons, raw, cantaloupes, other netted varieties	12	251
Mussels, Atlantic and Pacific, raw, meat only	289	315
Mustard greens, cooked, boiled, drained	18	220
Mustard, prepared:		
Brown	1,307	130
Yellow	1,252	130
Nectarines, raw	6	294
New Zealand spinach, cooked, boiled, drained	92	463
Noodles, egg noodles, enriched, cooked	2	44

8. Value for product without added salt.

9. Values apply to salted margarine. Unsalted margarine contains less than 10 mg. per 100 grams of either sodium or potassium. Vitamin A value based on the minimum required to meet federal specifications for margarine with vitamin A added, namely 15,000 I.U. of vitamin A per pound.

TABLE 41—*Continued*

Food and description	Sodium (Mg.)	Potassium (Mg.)
Oat products used mainly as hot breakfast cereals:		
Oatmeal or rolled oats:		
Dry form	2	352
Cooked	218	61
Oat products used mainly as ready-to-eat breakfast cereals:		
Oats (with or without corn), puffed, added nutrients	1,267	....
Ocean perch, Atlantic (redfish):		
Raw	79	269
Cooked, fried	153	284
Ocean perch, Pacific, raw	63	390
Oils, salad or cooking	0	0
Okra:		
Raw	3	249
Cooked, boiled, drained	2	174
Olives, pickled; canned or bottled:		
Green	2,400	55
Ripe, Ascolano (extra large, mammoth, giant jumbo)	813	34
Ripe, salt-cured, oil-coated, Greek style	3,288	....
Onions, mature (dry), raw	10	157
Onions, young green (bunching varieties), raw:		
Bulb and entire top	5	231
Oranges, raw, peeled fruit, all commercial varieties	1	200
Orange juice:		
Raw, all commercial varieties	1	200
Canned, unsweetened	1	199
Frozen concentrate, unsweetened, diluted with 3 parts water, by volume	1	186
Oysters:		
Raw, meat only, Eastern	73	121
Cooked, fried	206	203
Frozen, solids and liquid	380	210
Oyster stew, commercial frozen, prepared with equal volume of milk	366	176
Pancake and waffle mixes and pancakes baked from mixes:		
Plain and buttermilk, made with egg, milk	564	154
Parsnips, cooked, boiled, drained	8	379
Peaches:		
Raw	1	202
Canned, solids and liquid, water pack, with or without artificial sweetener	2	137
Frozen, sliced, sweetened, not thawed	2	124
Peanuts:		
Roasted, with skins	5	701
Roasted and salted	418	674
Peanut butters made with small amounts of added fat, salt	607	670
Pears:		
Raw, including skin	2	130
Canned, solids and liquid, syrup pack, light	1	85
Peas, green, immature:		
Cooked, boiled, drained	1	196
Canned, Alaska (Early or June peas):		
Regular pack, solids and liquid	236[2]	96
Special dietary pack (low-sodium), solids and liquid	3	96
Frozen, cooked, boiled, and drained	115	135
Peas, mature seeds, dry, whole, raw	35	1,005

TABLE 41—*Continued*

Food and description	Sodium (Mg.)	Potassium (Mg.)
Peas and carrots, frozen, cooked, boiled, drained	84	157
Pecans	Trace	603
Peppers, hot, chili, mature, red, raw, pods excluding seeds	25	564
Peppers, sweet, garden varieties, immature, green, raw	13	213
Perch, yellow, raw	68	230
Pickles, cucumber, dill	1,428	200
Pies:		
Baked, piecrust made with unenriched flour:		
Apple	301	80
Cherry	304	105
Mince	448	178
Pumpkin	214	160
Piecrust or plain pastry, made with, enriched flour, baked	611	50
Pike, walleye, raw	51	319
Pineapple:		
Raw	1	146
Frozen chunks, sweetened, not thawed	2	100
Pizza, with cheese, from home recipe, baked:		
With cheese topping	702	130
With sausage topping	729	168
Plate dinners, frozen, commercial, unheated:		
Beef pot roast, whole oven-browned potatoes, peas, and corn	259	244
Chicken, fried; mashed potatoes; mixed vegetables (carrots, peas, corn, beans)	344	112
Meat loaf with tomato sauce, mashed potatoes, and peas	393	115
Turkey, sliced; mashed potatoes; peas	400	176
Plums:		
Raw, Damson	2	299
Canned, solids and liquid, purple (Italian prunes), syrup pack, light	1	145
Popcorn, popped:		
Plain	(3)	....
Oil and salt added	1,940	....
Pork, fresh:		
Retail cuts, trimmed to retail level:		
Loin	65	390
Pork, cured, light-cure, commercial, ham, medium-fat class, separable lean, cooked, roasted	930	326
Pork, cured, canned:		
Ham, contents of can	(1,100)	(340)
Potatoes:		
Cooked, boiled in skin	3[10]	407
Dehydrated mashed:		
Flakes without milk:		
Dry form	89	(1,600)
Prepared, water, milk, table fat added	231	286
Pretzels	1,680[11]	130
Prunes:		
Dried, "softenized," cooked (fruit and liquid), with added sugar	3	262
Pudding mixes and puddings made from mixes:		
With starch base:		
Pudding made with milk, cooked	129	136
Pudding made with milk, without cooking	124	129

10. Applies to product without added salt. If salt is added, an estimated average value for sodium is 236 mg. per 100 grams.

11. Sodium content is variable. For example, very thin pretzel sticks contain about twice the average amount listed.

TABLE 41—*Continued*

Food and description	Sodium (Mg.)	Potassium (Mg.)
Pumpkin, canned	2	240
Radishes, raw, common	18	322
Raisins, natural (unbleached):		
Cooked, fruit and liquid, added sugar	13	355
Raspberries:		
Canned, solids and liquid, water pack, with or without artificial sweetener, red	1	114
Frozen, red, sweetened, not thawed	1	100
Rennin products:		
Tablet (salts, starch, rennin enzyme)	22,300	....
Dessert mixes and desserts prepared from mixes:		
Chocolate, dessert made with milk	52	125
Other flavors (vanilla, caramel, fruit flavorings):		
Mix, dry form	6	....
Dessert made with milk	46	128
Rhubarb, cooked, added sugar	2	203
Rice:		
Brown:		
Raw	9	214
Cooked	282	70
White (fully milled or polished):		
Enriched:		
Common commercial varieties, all types:		
Raw	5	92
Cooked	374	28
Rice products used mainly as ready-to-eat breakfast cereals:		
Rice flakes, added nutrients	987	180
Rice puffed; added nutrients, without salt	2	100
Rice, puffed or open-popped, presweetened, honey and added nutrients	706	....
Rockfish, including black, canary, yellowtail, rasphead, and bocaccio, cooked, oven-steamed	68	446
Roe, cooked, baked or broiled, cod and shad[12]	73	132
Rolls and buns:		
Commercial:		
Ready-to-serve:		
Danish pastry	366	112
Hard rolls, enriched	625	97
Plain (pan rolls), enriched	506	95
Sweet rolls	389	124
Rusk	246	161
Rutabagas, cooked, boiled, drained	4	167
Rye, flour, medium	(1)	203
Rye wafers, whole-grain	882	600
Salad dressings, commercial:[13]		
Blue and Roquefort cheese:		
Regular	1,094	37
Special dietary (low-calorie):		
Low-fat (approx. 5 cal. per tsp.)	1,108	34
French:		
Regular	1,370	79
Special dietary (low-calorie):		
Low-fat (approx. 5 cal. per tsp.)	787	79
Mayonnaise	597	34
Thousand island:		
Regular	700	113

12. Prepared with butter or margarine, lemon juice or vinegar.

13. Values apply to products containing salt. For those without salt, sodium content is low, ranging from less than 10 mg. to 50 mg. per 100 grams; the amount usually is indicated on the label.

TABLE 41—*Continued*

Food and description	Sodium (Mg.)	Potassium (Mg.)
Salad dressings, commercial:[12]—*Continued:*		
Thousand island—*Continued:*		
Special dietary (low-calorie, approx. 10 cal. per tsp.)	700	113
Salmon:		
Coho (silver):		
Raw	48[15]	421
Canned, solids and liquid	351[14]	339
Salt pork, raw	1,212	42
Salt sticks, regular type	1,674	92
Sandwich spread (with chopped pickle):		
Regular	626	92
Special dietary (low-calorie, approx. 5 cal. per tsp.)	626	92
Sardines, Atlantic, canned in oil, drained solids	823	590
Sardines, Pacific, in tomato sauce, solids and liquid	400	320
Sauerkraut, canned, solids and liquid	747[16]	140
Sausage, cold cuts, and luncheon meats:		
Bologna, all samples	1,300	230
Frankfurters, raw, all samples	1,100	220
Luncheon meat, pork, cured ham or shoulder, chopped, spiced or unspiced, canned	1,234	222
Pork sausage, links or bulk, cooked	958	269
Scallops, bay and sea, cooked, steamed	265	476
Soups, commercial, canned:		
Beef broth, bouillon, and consomme, prepared with equal volume of water	326	54
Chicken noodle, prepared with equal volume of water	408	23
Tomato:		
Prepared with equal volume of water	396	94
Prepared with equal volume of milk	422	167
Vegetable beef, prepared with equal volume of water	427	66
Soy sauce	7,325	366
Spaghetti, enriched, cooked, tender stage	1	61
Spaghetti, in tomato sauce with cheese, canned	382	121
Spinach:		
Cooked, boiled, drained	50	324
Canned:		
Regular pack, drained solids	236[2]	250
Special dietary pack (low-sodium), solids and liquid	34	250
Frozen, chopped, cooked, boiled, drained	52	333
Squash, summer, all varieties, cooked, boiled, drained	1	141
Squash, frozen:		
Summer, yellow crookneck, cooked, boiled, drained	3	167
Winter, heated	1	207
Strawberries:		
Raw	1	164
Frozen, sweetened, not thawed, sliced	1	112
Sturgeon, cooked, steamed	108	235
Succotash (corn and Lima beans), frozen:		
Cooked, boiled, drained	38	246
Sugars, beet or cane, brown	30	344
Sweet potatoes:		
Cooked, all, baked in skin	12	300
Canned, liquid pack, solids and liquid, regular pack in syrup	48	(120)
Dehydrated flakes, prepared with water	45	140

14. For product canned without added salt, value is approximately the same as for raw salmon.

15. Sample dipped in brine contained 215 mg. sodium per 100 grams.

16. Values for sauerkraut and sauerkraut juice are based on salt content of 1.9 and 2.0 per cent, respectively, in the finished products. The amounts in some samples may vary significantly from this estimate.

TABLE 41—*Continued*

Food and description	Sodium (Mg.)	Potassium (Mg.)
Tangerines, raw (Dancy variety)	2	126
Tapioca, dry	3	18
Tapioca desserts, tapioca cream pudding	156	135
Tartar sauce, regular	707	78
Tea, instant (water-soluble solids) carbohydrate added:		
Dry powder	....	4,530
Beverage	....	25
Tomatoes, ripe:		
Raw	3	244
Canned, solids and liquid, regular pack	130	217
Tomato catsup, bottled	1,042[17]	363
Tomato juice:		
Canned or bottled:		
Regular pack	200	227
Special dietary pack (low-sodium)	3	227
Tomato juice cocktail, canned or bottled	200	221
Tomato puree, canned:		
Regular pack	399	426
Special dietary pack (low-sodium)	6	426
Tongue, beef, medium-fat, cooked, braised	61	164
Tuna, canned:		
In oil, solids and liquid	800	301
In water, solids and liquid	41[18]	279[18]
Turkey, all classes:		
Light meat, cooked, roasted	82	411
Dark meat, cooked, roasted	99	398
Turkey potpie, commercial, frozen, unheated	369	114
Turnips, cooked, boiled, drained	34	188
Turnip greens, leaves, including stems:		
Canned, solids and liquid	236[2]	243
Frozen, cooked, boiled, drained	17	149
Veal, retail cuts, untrimmed	80	500
Vinegar, cider	1	100
Waffles, frozen, made with enriched flour	644	158
Walnuts:		
Black	3	460
Persian or English	2	450
Watercress leaves including stems, raw	52	282
Watermelon, raw	1	100
Wheat flours:		
Whole (from hard wheats)	3	370
Patent:		
All-purpose or family flour, enriched	2	95
Self-rising flour, enriched (anhydrous monocalcium phosphate used as a baking acid)[19]	1,079	.........[20]
Wild rice, raw	7	220
Yeast:		
Baker's, compressed	16	610
Brewer's, debittered	121	1,894
Yogurt, made from whole milk	47	132
Zweiback	250	150

17. Applies to regular pack. For special dietary pack (low sodium), values range from 5 to 35 mg. per 100 grams.

18. One sample with salt added contained 875 mg. of sodium per 100 grams and 275 mg. of potassium.

19. The acid ingredient most commonly used in self-rising flour. When sodium acid pyrophosphate in combination with either anhydrous monocalcium phosphate or calcium carbonate is used, the value for calcium is approximately 120 mg. per 100 grams; for phosphorus, 540 mg.; for sodium, 1,360 mg.

20. 90 mg. of potassium per 100 grams contributed by flour. Small quantities of additional potassium may be provided by other ingredients.

APPENDIX 7

Mineral Elements and Excess of Acidity or Alkalinity

TABLE 42

Mineral Elements* and Excess of Acidity or Alkalinity† per 100 Gm. of Foods, Edible Portion

Food	Minerals					Excess‡	
	Magnesium (Gm.)	Potassium (Gm.)	Sodium (Gm.)	Chlorine (Gm.)	Sulphur (Gm.)	Acidity (Cc. of N Acid HCl)	Alkalinity (Cc. of N Alkali NaOH)
Almonds	0.275	0.756	0.024	0.037	0.164	2.2	12.0–18.3
Apples:							
fresh	0.006	0.116	0.015	0.004	0.004	....	0.8–3.7
dried	0.029	0.557	0.072	0.019	0.019	....	....
Apricots:							
fresh	0.012	0.370	0.021	0.004	0.006	....	4.8–8.4
dried	0.062	1.924	0.109	0.021	0.031	....	31.3–41.9
Asparagus	0.015	0.200	0.008	0.047	0.051	1.0	0.8
Bananas	0.024	0.412	0.023	0.163	0.013	....	4.4–7.9
Barley, entire	0.126	0.495	0.070	0.139	0.153	6.0–17.5	....
Beans:							
dried	0.165	1.281	0.189	0.007	0.004	....	18.9–43.0
Lima, fresh	0.067	0.606	0.089	0.009	0.068	....	14.0
dried	0.181	1.899	0.282	0.025	0.156	....	41.6
string or green	0.032	0.288	0.012	0.045	0.024	....	4.1–5.4
Beef	0.032	0.382	0.066	0.056	0.221	8.1–38.5	....
Beets	0.027	0.235	0.053	0.040	0.017	....	8.9–11.4
Beet greens	0.097	0.390	....	....	0.035	....	....
Brains	0.016	0.269	0.160	0.155	0.130	17.7–20.7	....
Bread, white	0.034	0.110	0.517	0.602	0.083	1.5–7.1	....
Broccoli	0.024	0.352	0.030	0.076	0.126	....	3.6–4.9
Brussels sprouts	0.015	0.375	....	....	0.098	....	0.8–4.3
Butter	0.002	0.019	§	§	0.009	0.4–4.3	....
Cabbage:	0.016	0.217	0.038	0.034	0.074	....	1.4–8.2
celery	0.011	0.400	0.028	0.023	0.013	....	....
Cantaloupe	0.016	0.243	0.048	0.048	0.016	....	7.5
Carrots	0.020	0.219	0.050	0.035	0.019	....	4.4–10.8
Cauliflower	0.023	0.292	0.048	0.038	0.074	....	1.4–5.3
Celery	0.025	0.320	0.101	0.225	0.021	....	2.5–11.1
Cheese, hard	0.031	0.116	0.900	0.972	0.214	0.3–11.8	3.6–5.1
Cherries	0.012	0.125	0.015	0.004	0.018	....	1.7–7.2
Chestnuts	0.048	0.415	0.037	0.010	0.049	....	7.4–11.3
Chicken	0.047	0.402	0.054	0.034	0.303	9.6–25.4	....
Chocolate	0.082	0.400	0.019	0.009	0.114	8.1	7.9
Cocoa	0.192	0.534	0.060	0.050	0.197	....	0.7
Coconut, fresh	0.040	0.360	0.040	0.120	0.044	....	4.1–7.0
Collards	0.017	....	....	....	....	....	....
Corn:							
field, mature	0.142	0.300	0.110	0.041	0.124	....	....
sweet							
fresh	0.047	0.278	....	....	0.037	1.8	....
mature	0.121	0.415	0.148	0.050	0.146	6.0	....
Cowpeas, dried	0.265	1.305	0.036	0.019	0.250	....	....
Crabs	0.117	0.271	0.366	0.570	0.255	39.5	....
Cranberries	0.005	0.056	0.002	0.004	0.008	....	3.2‖
Cream	0.006	0.112	0.031	0.067	0.033	....	0.4–3.2
Cucumbers	0.020	0.170	0.026	0.028	0.011	....	3.2–31.5

* W. H. Peterson, J. T. Skinner, and F. M. Strong, Elements of food biochemistry (New York: Prentice-Hall, Inc., 1944), pp. 262–65.

† M. A. Bridges and M. R. Mattice, Food and beverage analyses (Philadelphia: Lea & Febiger, 1942), pp. 200–214.

‡ The ranges indicated come from reports of several authors, in which variety and method of preparation influence the results in part. For individual studies and sources of data see Bridges and Mattice, *op. cit.*

§ Variable. ‖ Partly acid *in vivo*.

TABLE 42—*Continued*

Food	Minerals					Excess‡	
	Magnesium (Gm.)	Potassium (Gm.)	Sodium (Gm.)	Chlorine (Gm.)	Sulphur (Gm.)	Acidity (Cc. of N Acid HCl)	Alkalinity (Cc. of N Alkali NaOH)
Currants:							
fresh	0.031	0.208	0.015	0.010	0.021	...	0.7–8.8
dried	0.155	1.040	0.075	0.050	0.105	...	5.8–21.8
Dates	0.065	0.580	0.040	0.253	0.048	...	5.5–12.4
Eel	0.018	0.241	0.032	0.035	0.133	7.0–9.9	...
Eggplant	0.015	0.260	0.026	0.063	0.020	...	4.5
Eggs	0.009	0.149	0.111	0.100	0.233	11.1–24.5	...
Egg white	0.011	0.149	0.175	0.131	0.211	4.8–8.3	...
Egg yolk	0.013	0.110	0.078	0.067	0.214	25.3–51.8	...
Figs:							
fresh	0.020	0.205	0.043	0.037	0.017	...	...
dried	0.068	0.709	0.151	0.126	0.060	...	10.0–100.9
Fish (all kinds)	0.024	0.375	0.064	0.137	0.199	8.5–20.1	...
Flour, wheat, white	0.021	0.137	0.053	0.079	0.155	7.4–9.6	...
Frog	0.024	0.308	0.055	0.040	0.163	10.6–15.8	...
Garlic	0.008	0.130	0.009	0.004	0.318	...	...
Goose	0.031	0.406	...	...	0.326	7.7–24.5	...
Gooseberries	0.009	0.150	0.010	0.009	0.015	...	2.1–7.6
Grapefruit	0.007	0.164	0.006	0.007	0.005	...	6.4
Grapes	0.004	0.267	0.011	0.002	0.009	...	2.7–7.2
Haddock	0.017	0.334	0.099	0.241	0.225	8.5–19.7	...
Heart	0.035	0.329	0.102	0.204	0.151	27.6	...
Honey	0.004	0.051	0.006	0.015	0.003	1.1	0.4–4.6
Horse-radish	0.028	0.550	0.094	0.013	0.234	...	2.7–5.8
Kale	0.055	0.486	0.050	0.120	0.160	...	4.0–17.0
Kidney	0.019	0.240	0.238	0.376	0.148	8.4–31.0	...
Kohlrabi	0.052	0.370	0.050	0.050	0.039	...	6.0
Lamb (*see* Mutton)							
Leeks	0.037	0.380	0.036	0.110	0.056	...	5.5–11.3
Lemons	0.006	0.152	0.009	0.006	0.012	...	5.5–9.9
Lentils, dried	0.082	0.662	0.754	0.062	0.123	5.2–17.8	0.4–2.0
Lettuce	0.015	0.256	0.028	0.085	0.014	...	3.8–14.1
Liver	0.021	0.255	0.021	0.091	0.258	9.4–49.5	...
Lobster	0.022	0.258	...	...	...	38.4	...
Macaroni, dry	0.038	0.054	0.010	0.077	0.119	3.8–9.6	...
Milk:							
cow							
fresh	0.019	0.129	0.047	0.114	0.031	...	1.8–4.2
evaporated	0.038	0.258	0.094	0.228	0.067	...	4.6
powder	0.118	0.955	0.348	1.029	0.229	...	21.6
goat	...	...	0.026	0.163	...	...	...
human	0.005	0.055	...	0.058	0.142	...	...
Mushrooms	0.012	0.280	0.013	0.026	0.025	...	1.8–4.0
Mustard greens	0.016	0.330	0.020	0.090	0.142	...	...
Mutton	0.033	0.260	0.070	0.069	0.187	4.5–22.5	...
Oatmeal (rolled oats)	0.143	0.365	0.072	0.027	0.207	1.5–13.2	...
Oats, entire	0.150	0.450	0.168	0.089	0.187	...	...
Onions	0.016	0.200	0.020	0.053	0.065	...	0.2–8.4
Orange juice	0.014	0.200	0.006	0.008	0.005	...	4.5
Oranges	0.011	0.177	0.014	0.006	0.011	...	5.6–9.6
Parsnips	0.038	0.396	0.010	0.038	0.025	...	6.6–11.9

TABLE 42—*Continued*

Food	Minerals					Excess‡	
	Magnesium (Gm.)	Potassium (Gm.)	Sodium (Gm.)	Chlorine (Gm.)	Sulphur (Gm.)	Acidity (Cc. of N Acid HCl)	Alkalinity (Cc. of N Alkali NaOH)
Peaches:							
fresh	0.015	0.174	0.012	0.006	0.005	...	3.8–6.1
dried	0.087	1.009	0.070	0.035	0.029	...	4.1–12.1
Peanuts	0.169	0.706	0.052	0.040	0.276	3.9–16.4	...
Pears	0.005	0.110	0.010	0.004	0.010	...	1.5–3.6
Peas:							
green	0.035	0.259	0.024	0.049	0.035	1.4–2.9	1.2–5.2
mature	0.121	0.943	0.072	0.034	0.178	0.5–3.4	1.2–10.3
Peppers:							
green	0.025	0.270	0.015	0.031	0.030	...	...
red	0.013	0.120	0.006	0.014	0.030	...	...
Persimmons	0.005	0.170	0.013	0.009	0.011	...	...
Pike	0.031	0.416	0.029	0.032	0.218	2.8–19.5	...
Pineapple	0.014	0.230	0.008	0.038	0.003	...	2.2–7.00
Plums	0.010	0.212	0.003	0.002	0.004	...	4.8‖
Pork	0.027	0.415	0.081	0.040	0.216	7.7–28.6	...
Potatoes	0.027	0.498	0.030	0.048	0.033	...	7.0–12.8
Prunes, dried	0.032	0.845	0.101	0.004	0.024	...	7.8–20.3‖
Pumpkins	0.021	0.198	0.011	0.025	0.016	...	0.3–7.8
Rabbit	0.029	0.415	0.047	0.051	0.184	14.8–22.4	...
Radishes	0.014	0.166	0.083	0.056	0.038	...	2.9–7.2
Raisins	0.017	0.796	0.120	0.068	0.043	...	23.7–27.0
Raspberries	0.018	0.141	0.007	0.010	0.012	...	4.1–6.1
Rhubarb	0.015	0.392	0.010	0.070	0.008	...	8.6–13.0
Rice:							
entire	0.141	0.334	0.068	0.066	0.121	...	...
polished	0.033	0.046	0.012	0.056	0.114	2.5–9.0	...
Rutabagas	0.015	0.210	0.052	0.031	0.069	...	8.5
Rye, entire	0.136	0.477	0.060	0.043	0.152	11.3	...
Sardines, fresh	0.035	...	...	...	...	11.4–26.5	...
Shrimps:							
dried	...	...	...	...	...	...	...
salted	0.327	0.760	§	§	0.183	1.6	...
Soybeans, mature	0.287	1.693	0.280	0.007	0.269	...	...
Spaghetti (*see* Macaroni)							
Spinach	0.048	0.416	0.093	0.118	0.027	...	5.1–39.6
Squash	0.006	0.161	0.011	0.018	0.029	...	2.8
Strawberries	0.019	0.205	...	...	0.013	...	1.8–3.5
Sugar beets	0.041	0.440	0.130	0.180	0.021	...	3.3–9.4
Sweet potatoes	0.035	0.381	0.031	0.022	0.014	...	5.0–7.9
Tomatoes	0.016	0.277	0.013	0.048	0.017	...	5.6–13.7
Turkey	0.028	0.367	0.130	0.123	0.234	10.4–19.5	...
Turnip greens	0.079	0.300	0.260	0.390	0.051	...	2.3
Turnips	0.019	0.193	0.104	0.054	0.048	...	2.7–10.2
Veal	0.030	0.380	0.086	0.073	0.199	9.8–28.5	...
Venison	0.029	0.336	0.070	0.041	0.211	23.8	...
Walnuts	0.132	0.606	0.013	0.030	0.120	7.9–9.2	...
Watercress	0.010	0.100	0.031	0.059	0.071	...	...
Watermelon	0.006	0.071	0.012	0.006	0.005	...	1.8–2.7
Wheat:							
entire	0.163	0.409	0.106	0.088	0.175	9.7–12.0	...
bran	0.420	1.252	0.007	0.042	0.245	...	...
Yams	0.015	0.290	0.015	0.037	0.013	...	...

APPENDIX 8

Weight and Height Tables

TABLE 43

Desirable Weights for Men and Women, According to Height and Frame, Ages 25 and Over*

Height (in Shoes)		Weight in Indoor Clothing		
		Small Frame	Medium Frame	Large Frame
		MEN		
Feet	Inches	Pounds	Pounds	Pounds
5	2	112–120	118–129	126–141
5	3	115–123	121–133	129–144
5	4	118–126	124–136	132–148
5	5	121–129	127–139	135–152
5	6	124–133	130–143	138–156
5	7	128–137	134–147	142–161
5	8	132–141	138–152	147–166
5	9	136–145	142–156	151–170
5	10	140–150	146–160	155–174
5	11	144–154	150–165	159–179
6	0	148–158	154–170	164–184
6	1	152–162	158–175	168–189
6	2	156–167	162–180	173–194
6	3	160–171	167–185	178–199
6	4	164–175	172–190	182–204
		WOMEN		
4	10	92–98	96–107	104–119
4	11	94–101	98–110	106–122
5	0	96–104	101–113	109–125
5	1	99–107	104–116	112–128
5	2	102–110	107–119	115–131
5	3	105–113	110–122	118–134
5	4	108–116	113–126	121–138
5	5	111–119	116–130	125–142
5	6	114–123	120–135	129–146
5	7	118–127	124–139	133–150
5	8	122–131	128–143	137–154
5	9	126–135	132–147	141–158
5	10	130–140	136–151	145–163
5	11	134–144	140–155	149–168
6	0	138–148	144–159	153–173

* Derived from data of the 1959 Build and Blood Pressure Study, Society of Actuaries. Developed by the Metropolitan Life Insurance Company, Statistical Bureau.

APPENDIX 9

Energy Expenditure

Passmore and Durnin (1) have compiled more than five hundred values representing energy expenditures while carrying out personal necessities: sitting and walking at different speeds; during children's recreation; light indoor recreation of adults; domestic work; mental work; office work; during such "moderate" exercise as canoeing, horseback riding, cycling; during "heavy" exercise, such as football, swimming, skiing, cross-country running, fishing; in various types of light and heavy industry, agriculture, lumber work, and the various activities of soldiers.

TABLE 44

Daily Energy Expenditure of the Reference Man and Woman (2)
(Mean Annual Temperature 10° C.)

		Calories
Man, 65 Kg.		
A. 8 hr. *working activities:* mostly standing, over-all rate: 2.5 cal/min		1,200
B. 8 hr. *non-occupational activities*		
1 hr. washing, dressing, etc., at 3.0 cal/min	180	
1½ hr. walking at about 6 k.p.h. at 5.3 cal/min	480	
4 hr. sitting activities at 1.54 cal/min	370	
1½ hr. active recreation and/or domestic work at 5.2 cal/min	470	1,500
C. 8 hr. *rest in bed* at basal metabolic rate		500
Total		3,200
Woman, 55 Kg.		
A. 8 hr. *working activities* in the home or in industry, mostly standing, over-all rate: 1.83 cal/min		880
B. 8 hr. *non-occupational activities*		
1 hr. washing, dressing, etc., at 2.5 cal/min	150	
1 hr. walking about 5 k.p.h. at 3.6 cal/min	220	
5 hr. sitting activities at 1.41 cal/min	420	
1 hr. active recreation and/or domestic work at 3.5 cal/min	210	1,000
C. 8 hr. *rest in bed* at basal metabolic rate		420
Total		2,300

The unit used in expressing energy expenditure is in terms of the *total* energy expenditure in calories per minute rather than in *net* energy expenditure above basal calories. This unit has been recommended by the Committee on Calorie Requirements of the Food and Agriculture Organization in 1957 (2). Table 51 presents an example of how the energy expenditure may be distributed during the day.

REFERENCES

1. PASSMORE, R., and DURNIN, J. V. G. A. Human energy expenditure, Physiol. Rev., **34**:801–40, 1955.
2. FOOD AND AGRICULTURE ORGANIZATION OF THE UNITED NATIONS. Calorie requirements. ("FAO Nutritional Studies," No. 15.) Rome, 1957.

GLOSSARY OF DIETETIC TERMS REVISED, 1965

In 1931, members of The American Dietetic Association were actively working on the complexities of diets named after doctors, diseases, and many miscellaneous symptoms. The lack of consistent principles, nutritional inadequacies, and overlapping produced much confusion, controversy, and strain in the dietetic services. At that time, Grace Bulman, as chairman of a committee of the Diet Therapy Section, began collecting routine hospital diets used in sixty-five Class A hospitals in various parts of the country. With characteristic understatement, she reported: "These show a wide variation as to nomenclature and type of foods included" (1). Margery Ardrey, as chairman in the following year, carried on with some description of diets (2).

By 1939 the situation had reached the place where members felt the need for further revisions in nomenclature and descriptions of therapeutic diets that, among other things, would reflect the principle propounded earlier by Dr. Ruth Wheeler—that such diets should be regarded as modifications of the normal diet. At this time, Sister Jeanne d'Arc was appointed chairman of a committee to develop a glossary of dietetic terms. After two years of serious effort, a mimeographed list of terms was compiled and submitted to over two hundred members of the Association for review (3, 4). In the end, much order had been brought about by naming and describing diets in terms of dietetic principles rather than after doctors and diseases. Official use was made of this "Glossary of Dietetic Terms" in the first edition of the *Handbook of Diet Therapy* compiled for The American Dietetic Association in 1946 (5). Diets were named, defined, and described as set forth in this Glossary.

By 1948 rapid strides in diet therapy made members realize that corrections of inaccuracies, deletions, and additions were in order. Dr. Hazel Hauck as chairman and Dr. Helen Pilcher and Beatrice Finkelstein took the matter in hand, making extensive changes to bring the Glossary more closely in line with the newer findings in nutrition and with the wishes of the members. At this time the committee stated:

> In general the terms selected for inclusion in the Glossary of Dietetic Terms fall into the following categories: terms relating to the field of dietetics or the work of the dietitian; therapeutic diets; nutrients, or classes of nutrients required by man or thought to be useful in the human dietary; terms used in describing diets or foods, or relating to food composition; diseases associated with dietary deficiency or conditioned malnutrition; and some terms relating to digestion. The reader should consult a medical dictionary and appropriate texts for terms which are outside the scope of this glossary.

This revision was completed in 1950 and was used in naming and describing diets in the revised edition of the *Handbook of Diet Therapy* in 1952 (6). The complete Glossary appeared in this edition.

In 1956, members were again ready to reconsider the content of the Glossary. Under the chairmanship of Lorraine Weng, a committee of the Diet Therapy Section solicited recommendations from the state diet therapy sections regarding revisions in the *Handbook* which were incorporated in the third edition (7). In response to a question, "Do you use the Glossary of Dietetic Terms in naming and defining diets in your hospital manual?" approximately 70 per cent replied that they used it in some degree; 30 per cent that they did not.

The most recent revision of the Glossary was completed in 1965. Important contributors to this revision were: Elisabeth Yearick, Ph.D.; Annie Galbraith, Chairman, Diet Therapy Section, The American Dietetic Association; and Marion Seymour Noland, past-Chairman, Diet Therapy Section, The American Dietetic Association.

Since the purpose of the Glossary is to provide aid in the naming and the description of diets as well as in the use of other related terminology in diet manuals, recommendations from this committee have been included in the Glossary. In addition, recent findings relating to the chemical structure and function of certain nutrients have been incorporated from the National Academy of Science–National Research Council Publication No. 1164 (sixth revised edition). However, the guide lines established in 1950 have been retained.

REFERENCES

1. Waller, D. S. Report of Diet Therapy Section chairman, J. Am. Dietet. A., 7:292, 1931.
2. Digest of committee reports, Diet Therapy Section. *In* American Dietetic Association Reports for 1931–32, J. Am. Dietet. A., Suppl. 8, p. 21, 1933.
3. Committee reports, Diet Therapy Section. *In* Annual Reports, 1939–40, and Proceedings New York meeting, J. Am. Dietet. A., **16**:1015, 1940.
4. Committee report, Diet Therapy Section. *In* Annual Reports, 1940–41, and Proceedings St. Louis meeting, J. Am. Dietet. A., **17**:999, 1941.
5. Glossary of dietetic terms. *In* Turner, D. Handbook of diet therapy. Chicago: University of Chicago Press, 1946.
6. Revised glossary of dietetic terms. *In* Turner, D. Handbook of diet therapy. 2d ed. Chicago: University of Chicago Press, 1952.
7. Revised glossary of dietetic terms. *In* Turner, D. Handbook of diet therapy. 3d ed. Chicago: University of Chicago Press, 1959.

GLOSSARY OF DIETETIC TERMS, REVISED 1965

ACID, ARACHIDONIC—*See* Acids, Fatty, Essential.

ACID, ASCORBIC ($C_6H_8O_6$)—Vitamin C. A water-soluble vitamin destroyed by irreversible oxidation which is hastened by heat, light, and alkalinity. Occurs in metabolically active plant and animal tissues in two biologically active forms: ascorbic acid (reduced), and dehydroascorbic acid (oxidized). Essential for the formation of collagen of fibrous tissue, vascular endothelium, and matrices of bone and dentine; participates in biological oxidations and reductions. Certain clinical and biochemical manifestations occur well in advance of the deficiency disease, scurvy (1, 2).

ACID, DEHYDROASCORBIC ($C_6H_6O_6$)—The reversibly oxidized form of ascorbic acid; biologically active.

ACID, FOLIC—*See* Folacin.

ACID, FOLINIC ($C_{20}H_{24}N_7O_7$)—Citrovorum factor, formyl tetrahydrofolic acid; one of the functionally active forms of the folic acid group of vitamins. *See* Folacin.

ACID, LINOLEIC—*See* Acids, Fatty, Essential.

ACID, LINOLENIC—*See* Acids, Fatty, Essential.

ACID, NICOTINIC—*See* Niacin.

ACID, OXALIC ($C_2H_2O_4$)—A dicarboxylic acid which occurs as a result of metabolic processes in the body, and which is found in certain foods (especially cocoa, rhubarb, spinach, and certain other greens). Oxalic acid forms insoluble salts with calcium, magnesium, and iron.

ACID, PANTOTHENIC ($C_8H_{16}O_3NCOOH$)—A member of the B complex, thought to be essential for man; water-soluble, thermolabile. A constituent of coenzyme A which is essential for transacylations occurring in the energy cycle, in lipid synthesis and degradation, and in porphyrin synthesis. A deficiency has not been recognized in man on a natural diet; fatigue, gastrointestinal and neuromuscular disturbances have been observed after administration of an antagonist. It is distributed widely in plant and animal foods, synthesized by intestinal bacteria. Daily requirements appear to be provided by the average diet supplying 10–15 mg. (1, 4).

ACID, PARA-AMINOBENZOIC ($NH_2C_6H_4COOH$)—A component of the folacin molecule; a member of the B complex; originally considered to be a vitamin essential to humans.

ACID, PHYTIC ($C_6H_66H_2PO_4$)—Inositol hexaphosphoric acid; a phosphoric acid ester of inositol; occurs in nuts, legumes, and outer layers of cereal grains; the insoluble calcium-magnesium salt is called phytin. Because phytic acid forms insoluble salts with calcium, iron, and magnesium, it interferes with the intestinal absorption of these minerals.

ACID, PTEROYLGLUTAMIC—*See* Folacin.

ACID ASH RESIDUE—The preponderance in a food of inorganic (fixed) acid radicals, chiefly chloride, sulfate, and phosphate, which form acid ions (anions) in the body. The value is computed and expressed as the amount of 0.1N alkali which would be required for neutralization (5). See Table 42.

ACID-FORMING FOODS—Foods in which acid ash residue exceeds alkaline ash residue are meat, fish, poultry, eggs, cereals, and some nuts. Certain fruits, such as cranberries and some varieties of prunes and plums, although they have a predominantly alkaline residue, are acid-forming because the organic acids in them are not metabolized by the body. Pure starches, sugars, and fats, which produce carbonic acid during metabolism, are not included as "acid-forming" since carbonic acid is readily excreted by the lungs, without affecting alkaline reserve. *See* Acid Ash Residue.

ACIDOSIS—A condition caused by the abnormal accumulation of acids in the body or an excessive loss of base from the body; usually accompanied by a lowered alkali reserve. Acidosis may result from the accumulation of ketone bodies (diabetes), insufficient removal of acids (renal failure), inadequate removal of carbon dioxide (pulmonary), or excessive loss of alkaline intestinal secretions (diarrhea).

ACIDS, AMINO—Any one of a class of organic compounds containing the amino (NH_2) group and the carboxyl (COOH) group; the chief components of protein material.

ACIDS, AMINO, ESSENTIAL—Some twenty-two amino acids are known to be physiologically important. Of these, eight have been demonstrated to be dietary essentials for the adult human, since they are synthesized in inadequate quantity by the body. This group of "essential" amino acids includes isoleucine, leucine, lysine, methionine, phenylalanine, threonine, tryptophan, and valine. Dietary sources of a ninth amino acid, histidine, are probably necessary to maintain growth during childhood. The diet must include adequate sources of the essential amino acids and sufficient amounts of the other amino acids for maintenance in the adult and growth in children. Estimates of human requirements (6) appear in Table 45. Amino acids in foods (7) appear in Table 40.

ACIDS, FATTY—Any of a homologous series of open-chain monocarboxylic acids, containing only carbon, hydrogen, and oxygen. The saturated fatty acids ($C_nH_{2n}O_2$) of food fats are chiefly lauric (C_{12}), palmitic (C_{16}), and stearic (C_{18}). Mono-unsaturated fatty acids, such as oleic, have a single double bond ($C_nH_{2n-2}O_2$); polyunsaturated fatty acids, such as linoleic, have more than one double bond per molecule.

ACIDS, FATTY, ESSENTIAL—A group of unsaturated fatty acids, of which linoleic ($C_{17}H_{31}COOH$), and arachidonic ($C_{19}H_{31}COOH$) have been shown to be essential for growth and dermal integrity in human infants. Linolenic acid ($C_{17}H_{29}COOH$), formerly considered to be essential, does not prevent the dermatitis of fatty acid deficiency, nor is it as effective as linoleic in promoting growth. An intake of 1–3 per cent of total calories in the form of linoleic acid appears to meet the infant and probably adult needs. Excellent sources are corn, cottonseed, safflower, and soybean oils. The fatty acid content of additional foods appears in Table 36.

ADEQUATE—An amount sufficient to meet a specific requirement. The term "adequate diet" is often incorrectly used in reference to an individual diet which provides the dietary allowances of nutrients as recommended by the Food and Nutrition Board of the National Research Council. *See* Dietary Allowances, Recommended; Balanced Diet.

ALCOHOL—Ethanol. A term usually applied to ethyl alcohol (C_2H_5OH) which is distilled from the products of anaerobic fermentation of carbohydrate; yields about 7 calories per gram, of which more than 75 per cent is available to the body.

ALKALINE ASH RESIDUE—The preponderance in a food of the elements sodium, potassium, calcium, and magnesium, which form basic ions (cations) in the body. The value is computed and expressed as the amount of 0.1N acid which would be required for neutralization. *See* Table 42.

ALKALOSIS—A condition resulting from the abnormal accumulation of base or the excessive loss of acid from the body. Alkalosis may result from excessive administration of absorbable alkali, from prolonged vomiting of acid gastric juice, and from hyperventilation.

ALLERGEN—Any substance capable of inducing a condition of allergy or specific hypersensitiveness.

ALLERGY, FOOD—Hypersensitiveness to a substance (probably protein) in food which is ordinarily harmless in similar amounts for the majority of persons.

ANEMIA—A deficiency of hemoglobin in the blood, associated with either a decreased number of red blood cells, reduced corpuscular hemoglobin, or an abnormal type of hemoglobin. In the macrocytic anemias of folacin and B_{12} deficiency, the red cells are large, immature, and few in number; in the microcytic hypochromic anemia of iron deficiency, the red cells are small and contain insufficient hemoglobin.

ANOREXIA—Lack or loss of appetite for food.

ANTIVITAMIN—Any substance that interferes with the synthesis or metabolism of a vitamin—for example, avidin, which combines with biotin and prevents its absorption; thiaminase in certain raw fish, which destroys thiamine; and sulfanilamide, which interferes with the synthesis of folic acid in the intestinal tract by competing with para-aminobenzoic acid for a place in the molecule.

APPETITE—A natural desire for food.

ARIBOFLAVINOSIS—A disease resulting from the deficiency of riboflavin; characterized by lesions of the tongue and at angles of the mouth, dermatitis, and ocular changes.

ARTERIOSCLEROSIS—A generic term which includes a variety of conditions which cause the artery walls to become thick and hard and lose elasticity. *See* Atherosclerosis.

ARTIFICIAL SWEETENERS—*See* Saccharin, Sulfamate, Sorbitol.

AS PURCHASED (A.P.)—Refers to food as offered for sale on the retail market. In tables which give nutritive value for food "as purchased," the nutrient content is stated in terms of the weight of the food before inedible portions usually discarded are removed; i.e., the nutritive value of refuse is not included. *See* Edible portion.

ASH—The total mineral matter residue after ignition of a food; always either neutral or alkaline, since acid in excess of that which can be neutralized is volatilized.

ATHEROSCLEROSIS—A kind of arteriosclerosis in which the inner layer of the artery wall is made thick and irregular by deposits of a fatty substance. These deposits (called atheromata) project above the surface of the inner layer of the artery, and thus decrease the diameter of the internal channel of the vessel. *See* Arteriosclerosis.

AVAILABLE—A nutrient is available to the body when it is in the form that can be absorbed from the digestive tract and then used for its intended function in the body.

AVIDIN—A glycoprotein in raw egg white which binds biotin and prevents its absorption from the intestinal tract. Avidin is rendered inactive by heating.

AVITAMINOSIS—A disease due to the dietary deficiency of a vitamin or vitamins or to failure of absorption or utilization of the vitamin.

BALANCE—In nutrition, the term balance refers to that condition in which the nutrients taken into the body are balanced by corresponding excretions. When the intake and output are the same, the condition is described as balance or equilibrium. When the intake exceeds the output, the balance is positive, and retention of the nutrient has occurred. A negative balance describes the state in which the intake is less than the output, and the body stores have been used. The balance study has been a useful tool for measuring protein and mineral metabolism, although the balance is greatly affected by other dietary components and by body stores.

BALANCED DIET—The term "balanced diet" has been loosely or incorrectly used to imply ideal proportions of all proteins, minerals, fats, and carbohydrates for "optimum" nutrition or that two or more food essentials are ideally proportioned to meet "optimum" nutritional needs. Since no one "diet" can be quantitatively "balanced" for "optimum" needs of all individuals, the term "balanced diet" should be used only in properly informative statements where its meaning is plainly evident and free of misleading implications.

BERIBERI—A deficiency disease due to lack of thiamine, and endemic in areas in which polished rice is the chief item of the diet; characterized by multiple peripheral neuritis, with paralysis, edema, or cardiac failure.

β-Carotene—*See* Carotene.

BIOLOGICAL VALUE—*See* Protein, Biological Value of.

BIOTIN ($C_{10}H_{16}O_3N_2S$)—Vitamin H, a vitamin of the water-soluble B complex. Occurs bound in nature in at least two active forms; participates in carbon dioxide fixation reactions associated with fatty acid synthesis and energy utilization. Deficiency states have been recognized in man only when the absorption of dietary biotin has been prevented by the ingestion of large amounts of avidin. Widely distributed in plant and animal foods, and synthesized by intestinal bacteria; daily requirements seem to be provided by an average diet supplying 150–300 μg.

BULK—*See* Carbohydrate, indigestible, which is the preferred term.

CALCIFEROL ($C_{28}H_{44}O$)—Vitamin D_2; a fat-soluble antirachitic factor, formed by the irradiation of ergosterol.

CALORIE (LARGE OR KILO-CALORIE)—The unit used to express food energy; the amount of heat required to raise the temperature of 1 kg. water 1° C.

CARBOHYDRATE, AVAILABLE—This term represents the portion of the carbohydrate of foods which is available to the human body for glycogen formation. It includes starch, dextrins, glycogen, maltose, sucrose, lactose, as well as the monosaccharides glucose, fructose, galactose, mannose, and pentoses.

CARBOHYDRATE, INDIGESTIBLE—Substances which make up the cell-wall structure of plants, consisting of varying amounts of cellulose, hemicellulose, lignin, pectin substances, gums, mucin, etc.; not hydrolyzed by enzymes of the human gastrointestinal tract.

CARBOHYDRATE, TOTAL, BY DIFFERENCE—Solids in foods other than protein, fat, and ash; includes both available and indigestible carbohydrates and some organic acids.

CAROTENE—Provitamin A. A group of yellow-red plant pigments which yield vitamin A upon oxidative scission. β-carotene ($C_{40}H_{56}$) is the most abundant form in green leafy and yellow vegetables. Because of inefficient conversion of carotene to vitamin A in the body, 2 I.U. of β-carotene are considered equivalent to 1 I.U. vitamin A in man; approximately two-thirds of the vitamin A activity of the average diet is provided by carotene.

Cellulose ($(C_6H_{10}O_5)_n$)—A polysaccharide made up of beta-glucose units; constituent of the cell walls of plants. *See* Carbohydrate, indigestible; Fiber, crude.

Cellulose, Methyl—A methyl ester of cellulose which swells in water to produce a colloidal solution; used as a thickening agent, an emulsifier, and as a non-caloric source of bulk.

Cholesterol ($C_{27}H_{45}OH$)—A fat-like steroid alcohol found in animal tissues; may be synthesized in the body; excreted in the bile, but largely reabsorbed from the digestive tract in the presence of fat. Transported in serum attached to specialized proteins (lipoproteins). See Table 39 for food sources.

Choline ($C_5H_{15}NO_2$)—A component of lecithin and acetylcholine; often considered a member of the B complex; necessary for fat transport in the body; acts as donor of labile methyl groups.

Cook Manager—One who by training and/or experience is qualified to assume the responsibility for food and beverage preparation of the food service in a hospital, nursing home, school food service, and other institutions.

Also supervises and instructs all personnel in food service, maintains and establishes standards of sanitation, safety, and housekeeping. May also be responsible for scheduling of work and hours for personnel; maintaining records including food costs, meal census, and personnel records; planning of menus and routine modified diets; and purchasing of food and supplies. The services of a qualified dietary consultant or a shared dietitian should be available.

Cyanocobalamin—One form of vitamin B_{12}. *See* Vitamin B_{12}.

Cyclamates—The sodium or calcium salts of cyclohexylsulfamic acid; water-soluble, with a sweet taste (30 times that of sucrose). Used as non-caloric sweeteners.

Diet—Daily allowance of food and drink.

Diet, Balanced—*See* Balanced Diet.

Diet, Bland—A diet composed of mild-flavored foods. (See pp. 43-44 in text.)

Diet, Caloric, High—A diet* which has a prescribed caloric value above the total energy requirement.

Diet, Caloric, Low—A diet* which has a prescribed caloric value below the total energy requirement.

Diet, Cholesterol, Low—A diet* in which the intake of total cholesterol is restricted. The dietary prescription should include the permissible amounts of fat, and cholesterol. *See* Diet, Fat Modified, page 62 in text.

Diet, Elimination—An allowance of foods which do not commonly produce sensitivity in human patients. Used for the diagnosis of food allergy.

Diet, Fat Modified—A diet* prescribed to meet a specified level of fat in the diet, a percentage of fat calories, or specified amounts or ratios of fatty

* This diet is one planned to approximate the Recommended Dietary Allowances of the Food and Nutrition Board, National Research Council (1968), for healthy persons.

acids. When used for regulation of abnormal serum lipids or in treatment of patients with vascular disease, fat modification may be combined with cholesterol restriction. *See* Diet, Cholesterol, Low; Polyunsaturated: Saturated (P/S) Fatty Acid Ratio.

DIET, FIBER, HIGH—A normal diet,* including an additional 2–3 servings of foods high in indigestible carbohydrate and an unrestricted amount of connective tissue.

DIET, FIBER, LOW—A diet* which contains a minimum of indigestible carbohydrates and no tough connective tissue.

DIET, FULL HOSPITAL—A normal diet* for patients who do not require dietary modifications for therapeutic purposes; also known as House, Regular, or General diet.

DIET, GALACTOSE FREE—A diet which has been made almost free of galactose by the elimination of milk and milk products; or those containing complexed forms. Peas, Lima beans, and beets contain raffinose and stachyose which may release galactose. *See* text page 000.

DIET, GENERAL—*See* Diet, full hospital.

DIET, GLIADIN-RESTRICTED—A diet without wheat, rye, oats, and barley. (See pp. 78–79 in text.)

DIET, "GLUTEN-FREE"—*See* Gliadin-restricted diet.

DIET, HOUSE—*See* Diet, full hospital.

DIET, KETOGENIC—A diet in which the ratio of fatty acid (ketogenic) value to glucose (antiketogenic) value equals 2 or more, i.e., is sufficiently high to produce ketosis. It provides small amounts of carbohydrate, approximately 1 gm. protein per kilogram of body weight, and sufficient fat to meet full caloric requirements.

DIET, LIQUID, CLEAR—This diet is most often used pre- and postoperatively. It supplies fluids but is of little importance nutritionally. Only fat-free broth, tea, and coffee with sugar but without milk or cream are allowed. Occasionally small amounts of ginger ale, clear fruit or vegetable juice, and gelatin may be added.

DIET, LIQUID, FULL—A diet* consisting of a variety of foods that are liquid or liquefy at body temperature.

DIET, MODIFIED—A diet based on the normal diet and designed to meet the requirements of a given situation. It may be modified in individual nutrients, caloric value, consistency, flavor, techniques of service or preparation, content of specific foods, or a combination of these factors. A diet is described as "high" in a specific nutrient when it provides substantially more of the nutrient than is ordinarily required; the converse is true of a diet which is "low" in a specific nutrient. A diet can be called "free" of a nutrient only if that nutrient has been completely eliminated from the diet. The adjectives "restricted" and "controlled" are applied to a diet in which the specific nutrient is provided in amounts less than usually consumed. See text for specific modifications.

DIET, PHENYLALANINE-RESTRICTED—A diet in which phenylalanine is limited to a prescribed amount (p. 71 in text) by the use of selected natural foods and a specially prepared commercial product (p. 73 in text).

DIET, PROTEIN MODIFICATIONS—A diet* prescribed to provide a specified level of protein, or protein fraction, or a specified ratio or amount of amino acids.

DIET, PURINE, LOW—A diet* in which the chief sources of purines, such as glandular organs, dried legumes, and meat extractives are eliminated. Other meat and fish may be restricted to 4 oz. weekly, thus reducing the daily intake of uric acid equivalent to approximately 35 mg. *See* Purines, pages 116–19.

DIET, REGULAR—*See* Diet, full hospital.

DIET, SALT, LOW—*See* Diet, sodium-restricted.

DIET, SODIUM-RESTRICTED—A diet in which the sodium content is limited to a prescribed level. (See pp. 104–15 in text.)

DIET, SOFT—A diet* modified in consistency, i.e., including liquid foods and those solid foods which contain a restricted amount of indigestible carbohydrate and connective tissue. (See pp. 39–46 in text.)

DIET, TEST—A meal or meals used as part of a diagnostic procedure (9). See *Annual Reports and Proceedings, American Dietetic Association,* (1945–46), p. 35.

DIET, THERAPEUTIC—*See* Diet, modified.

DIETARY ALLOWANCES, RECOMMENDED (R.D.A.)—The amounts of various nutrients recommended by the Food and Nutrition Board of the National Research Council as normally desirable objectives toward which to aim in planning practical dietaries in the United States; enough higher than the minimal requirements of average individuals to cover substantially all individual variations in the requirements of persons in normal health. Allowances are related to body size and are stated for the reference men and women at moderate physical activity; for pregnancy and lactation; and for children and adolescent boys and girls of various age groups. "Comparative Dietary Standards for Adults in Other Countries," appears in tabular form in Publication 1146, NAS-NRC. *Recommended Dietary Allowances*, 1964 (1).

DIETARY CONSULTANT (ALSO CONSULTANT DIETITIAN)—One who has followed a prescribed academic program resulting in a baccalaureate degree from an accredited College or University and has satisfactorily completed an approved dietetic internship or qualifying experience. Advises and assists public and private establishments, such as child care centers, hospitals, nursing homes, and schools in food service management and nutritional problems in group feeding. Plans, organizes, and conducts such activities as in-service training courses, conferences, and institutes for food service managers, food handlers, and other workers.

Develops and evaluates informational materials. Studies food service practices and facilities, and makes recommendations for improvement. Confers with architects and equipment personnel in planning for building or remodeling food service units.

DIETARY HISTORY—An informative description of an individual's food intake over a period of time. Should include socioeconomic factors affecting food habits. Usually serves as a basis for planning individualized dietary therapy and education. For use in research, specialized information may be included in detail.

DIETARY STATUS—Summation of information received in dietary history. *See* Dietary History.

DIETETIC INTERN—One who has followed a prescribed academic program resulting in a baccalaureate degree from an accredited College or University and is completing an approved dietetic internship. Learns to function as a professionally qualified dietitian while following the planned internship program. Gains professional and practical experience as requirement for positions in dietetics.

Dietetics—The combined science and art of feeding individuals or groups under different economic or health conditions according to the principles of nutrition and management.

Dietitian—One who has followed a prescribed academic program resulting in a baccalaureate degree from an accredited College or University and has satisfactorily completed an approved dietetic internship or qualifying experience. Plans and directs food service programs in hospitals, schools, restaurants, and other public or private institutions. Plans menus and modified diets providing required food and nutrients to feed individuals and groups. Supervises workers engaged in preparation and serving of meals. Purchases or requisitions food, equipment, and supplies, and develops and analyzes food-cost control records. Inspects work areas and storage facilities to insure observance of sanitary standards. Counsels individuals and groups in application of principles of nutrition to selection of food. May prepare educational materials on nutritional value of foods and methods of preparation.

Dietitian, Administrative—One who has followed a prescribed academic program resulting in a baccalaureate degree from an accredited College or University and has satisfactorily completed an approved dietetic internship or qualifying experience. Organizes, plans, and directs food-service programs, applying principles of nutrition and management to menu planning, food preparation, and service. Develops standards for selecting, purchasing, and inspecting food, equipment, and supplies. Develops standards of sanitation. Supervises selection and training of nonprofessional food-service personnel. Prepares reports of financial management, safety practices, and program efficiency. Evaluates physical layout and equipment, employee utilization, and work procedures, and coordinates dietary services with those of other departments to increase effectiveness of program.

Dietitian, Director—One who has followed a prescribed academic program resulting in a baccalaureate degree from an accredited College or University and has satisfactorily completed an approved dietetic internship or qualifying experience. Administers, plans, and directs activities of department providing quantity food service. Establishes policies and procedures, and provides administrative direction for menu formulation, food preparation and service, purchasing, sanitation standards, safety practices, and personnel utilization. Selects professional dietetic staff, and directs departmental educational programs. Coordinates interdepartmental professional activities, and serves as consultant to management on matters pertaining to dietetics.

Dietitian, Teaching—One who has followed a prescribed academic program resulting in a baccalaureate degree from an accredited College or University and has satisfactorily completed an approved dietetic internship or qualifying experience. Plans, organizes, and conducts educational programs in dietetics and nutrition, nursing, medical and dental students, and other personnel. Prepares manuals, visual aids, course outlines, and other material used in teaching. May provide dietary counseling for patients in hospital or public health center. May engage in research.

DIETITIAN, THERAPEUTIC—One who has followed a prescribed academic program resulting in a baccalaureate degree from an accredited College or University and has satisfactorily completed an approved dietetic internship or qualifying experience. Plans and directs preparation and service of modified diets prescribed by the physician. Consults medical, nursing, and social service staffs concerning problems affecting patients' food habits and needs. Formulates menus for therapeutic diets based upon indicated physiologic and ethnic needs of patients and integrates them with basic institutional menus. Establishes and maintains standards of palatability and appearance of patient meals. Counsels patients and their families on the requirements and importance of their modified diets, and on how to plan and prepare the food. May engage in research. May teach nutrition and diet therapy to dietetic, medical, dental, and nursing students.

DIGESTIBILITY, COEFFICIENT OF APPARENT—The percentage of an ingested nutrient which cannot be recovered in the feces; hence, the percentage of an ingested nutrient which is assumed to have been absorbed. The coefficients of digestibility of protein, fat, and carbohydrate in a mixed American diet have been estimated to be 92 per cent, 95 per cent, and 97 per cent, respectively.

DIGESTION—The process of converting food into substances which can be absorbed by the body.

EDIBLE PORTION (E.P.)—As used in food tables, this term refers to that part of a food which is most commonly eaten. Some parts, such as parings of potatoes, which are edible but not usually eaten, are excluded.

ENERGY, FOOD—Expressed in terms of calories per unit weight; represents the energy available after deductions have been made for losses in digestion and metabolism. Energy values stated in food composition tables have been computed on the basis of the specific fuel factors for the individual foods. The commonly used physiological fuel factors, when applied to the total daily intake of protein, fat, and carbohydrate from a typical American diet, provide a good estimate of the energy value of the diet. *See* Fuel factors, physiological and specific.

ENRICHED BREAD—May be made from enriched flour or by the addition of the required substances to the baker's formula or by the use of special high-vitamin yeast and iron. *See* Enriched flour.

ENRICHED FLOUR—White flour enhanced in thiamine, riboflavin, niacin, and iron value by changing the milling process to retain these constituents or by the addition of chemicals to white flour. The minimum levels specified in the standards of identity promulgated under the Food, Drug, and Cosmetic Act are: thiamine, 2.0 mg.; riboflavin, 1.2 mg.; niacin, 16 mg.; and iron, 13 mg. per pound. Certain levels of vitamin D and calcium are permitted as optional ingredients. States which require enrichment of white flour have generally been guided by federal legislation.

ENRICHMENT—A food may be labeled "enriched" if it contains added nutrients in kinds and amounts meeting standards established by the Food and Drug Administration; usually applied to addition to nutrients of cereal products.

EXCHANGES—*See* Food Exchanges.

ERGOSTEROL ($C_{28}H_{44}O$)—Provitamin D_2; a plant sterol found chiefly in yeast, which, upon irradiation, forms calciferol (vitamin D_2).

EXTRINSIC FACTOR—A term applied by Castle to the hemopoietic factor in foods. *See* Vitamin B_{12}.

FAT—A glyceryl ester of fatty acids, which on hydrolysis yields three molecules of fatty acids to one of glycerol. In food tables, figures for fat include, in addition to true fats, other ether-extractable substances (3).

FIBER—As used in reference to therapeutic diets, this term includes indigestible organic tissue, either plant or animal.

FIBER, CRUDE—Made up largely of cellulose, those hemicelluloses which are not readily soluble, and lignin; as usually determined, that portion of a food sample which resists solution when boiled in dilute acid and dilute alkali.

FOLACIN ($C_{19}H_{19}N_7O_6$)—Folic acid, pteroylglutamic acid; a vitamin of the B complex sparingly soluble in water; functionally active forms are formyl derivatives of reduced folic acid, among them, folinic acid. Essential to the transfer of single carbon units in amino acid metabolism and nucleoprotein syntheses. Deficiency occurs in sprue and other malabsorption syndromes, frequently in combination with deficiencies of vitamin B_{12} or ascorbic acid; manifested by macrocytic megaloblastic anemia, glossitis, and gastrointestinal disturbances. Daily needs seem to be met by the average diet supplying 0.15–0.3 mg. of folic and folinic acid conjugates (0.05–0.1 mg. folacin); major sources (11) are liver, yeast, kidney, and green leafy vegetables; additional vitamin is synthesized by intestinal micro-organisms. Because folacin therapy promotes blood regeneration in pernicious anemia without correcting the neurological complications, sale without prescription of vitamin preparations recommending more than 0.1 mg. folic acid a day is prohibited.

FOOD EXCHANGES—Lists of foods grouped in terms of approximate equivalents in carbohydrate, protein, and fat content; as well as minerals and vitamins. Used for the purpose of planning diabetic, low-calorie, and other quantitative diets.

FOOD SERVICE SUPERVISOR—One who by education and/or successful completion of a planned in-service training program trains and supervises employees engaged in serving food in a hospital, nursing home, school or university food service department, and similar institutions. Supervises maintenance of established standards of cleanliness for food service areas, equipment, and dining areas. May assist in the direction of food and beverage production and in preparation of employee schedules. Instructs workers in methods of performing duties, assigns and coordinates work of employees to promote efficiency of operations. Maintains records such as food costs, meal census, and personnel records. Other duties may be performed as delegated by dietitian or food service director. In smaller institutions may be responsible for daily routine food service.

FORTIFICATION—The addition of a nutrient or nutrients to a food in amounts sufficient to make the total content larger than that contained in any natural (unprocessed) food of its class—for example, vitamin D milk, fortified margarine, fortified fruit juices. In general, no standards of identity have to be met when a food is labeled "fortified."

FORTIFIED MARGARINE—Most of the margarine on the market in the United States is fortified with 15,000 I.U. of vitamin A per pound.

FUEL FACTORS, PHYSIOLOGICAL (ATWATER)—The general energy values of protein, fat, and carbohydrate (4, 9, and 4 calories per gram, respectively) which are applicable to the total nutrient intake of the mixed American diet. These factors allow for incomplete oxidation of protein in the body, and for average losses in digestion. They are not applicable to specific foods which differ in their coefficients of digestibility.

FUEL FACTORS, SPECIFIC (ATWATER)—The energy values of protein, fat, and carbohydrate, expressed as calories per gram, determined for individual foods on the basis of the coefficients of digestibility which are specific for each food.

GALACTOSEMIA—The accumulation of the monosaccharide galactose in the blood, owing to a hereditary lack of an enzyme involved in the conversion of galactose to glucose; mental and growth retardation; liver enlargement and cataracts occur. *See* Diet, Galactose Free.

GLYCOGEN—A polysaccharide, also known as "animal starch," which yields glucose on hydrolysis; found in liver, muscle, and other tissues.

GOITER, SIMPLE—Enlargement of the thyroid gland, caused by an absolute or relative deficiency of iodine.

HEMICELLULOSE—A group of polysaccharides forming part of the cell wall of plants; indigestible, but may be broken down to a considerable extent by intestinal micro-organisms. It also absorbs water. *See* Fiber, crude.

HYDROGENATED FAT—Food fats commercially processed to harden fat by eliminating part of double bonds. Some of the natural cis double bonds change to the trans form.

INORGANIC ELEMENTS—*See* Ash; Minerals.

INOSITOL—$C_6H_6(OH)_6$ is an alcohol allied to the hexoses. It occurs in many foods, particularly bran of cereal grains. Inositol in combination with six phosphate molecules forms the compound phytic acid which hinders absorption of calcium and iron. *See* Acid, Phytic.

INSULIN—The hormone derived from the beta cells of the islands of Langerhans of the pancreas; essential for normal carbohydrate metabolism. Seven forms of insulin are now commercially available, each havings its own time effect ranging from rapid to very slow and prolonged. Products include Crystalline Insulin (regular), Semi-Lente, Globin Insulin with Zinc, Insulin Isophane (NPH), Lente Insulin, Protamine Zinc Insulin, and Ultra-Lente Insulin.

INTRINSIC FACTOR—A mucoprotein enzyme present in normal gastric juice; essential to the efficient intestinal absorption of dietary vitamin B_{12}; deficient in the gastric juice of the patient who has pernicious anemia.

IODINE VALUE (IODINE NUMBERS)—The number of grams of iodine absorbed by 100 grams of fat. One of several ways of expressing amounts of fatty acids in foods. A measure of total double bonds in a fat, but does not indicate particular fatty acids present. Ranges from about 10 for coconut oil to about 200 for safflower oil. *See* Polyunsaturated, Saturated Fatty Acid Ratio; Diet, Fat Modified.

KETOSIS—A condition in which there is an accumulation in the body of ketone compounds (beta-hydroxybutyric acid, acetoacetic acid, and acetone) as a result of incomplete oxidation of fatty acids; occurs when the amount of fat being oxidized is excessive, as with the use of ketogenic diets, in semistarvation, and uncontrolled diabetes.

KWASHIORKOR—A nutritional deficiency syndrome observed in children subsisting on low-protein, cereal diets; owing chiefly to protein malnutrition, but complicated by deficiencies of other nutrients; characterized by edema, dermatitis, dyspigmentation of hair and skin, growth failure, and liver damage.

LIGNIN—A constituent of crude fiber, occurring in the cell wall of plants; resistant to hydrolysis by digestive enzymes, strong acids, and alkalis; not attacked to any extent by intestinal micro-organisms. *See* Carbohydrate, indigestible; Fiber, crude.

LIPIDS—Fat or fat-like substances, including fatty acids, soaps, triglycerides, sterols, waxes, and phosphatides.

MALNUTRITION—A condition of the body resulting from an inadequate or excessive supply, or impaired utilization of one or more of the essential food constituents.

MALNUTRITION, CONDITIONED—Deficiency or excess of one or more nutrients in the tissues, caused by factors other than diet alone; for example, deficiencies caused by factors which interfere with ingestion, digestion, absorption, or utilization of essential nutrients or by factors that increase their requirement, destruction, or excretion.

MALABSORPTION SYNDROME—A term used to grossly describe such conditions as the sprues; celiac disease, idiopathic steatorrhea which have in common the failure to absorb various nutrients as fats, calcium, and other minerals, as well as certain vitamins, notably the fat-soluble ones.

MARASMUS—Severe malnutrition characterized by extreme emaciation. Incidence is highest in young children who are not eating or utilizing sufficient amounts of food.

MENADIONE ($C_{11}H_8O_2$)—A synthetic compound, having greater vitamin K activity than the naturally occurring vitamin; used as a reference standard for biological assays of vitamin K. In large doses, synthetic vitamin K has produced toxic effects; consequently, a dose in excess of 5 mg. should be avoided.

METABOLISM—A general term to designate all chemical changes which occur to substances within the body after absorption. These changes include constructive (anabolic) and destructive (catabolic) processes.

MICRONUTRIENTS—Nutrients present in very small amounts in food; as applied to mineral elements, the term usually refers to those present in the body in amounts less than that of iron, as manganese, copper, iodine, cobalt, molybdenum, and zinc.

MINERALS—"Inorganic" elements. The following are known to be present in body tissue: calcium, cobalt, chlorine, fluorine, iodine, iron, magnesium, manganese, molybdenum, phosphorus, potassium, selenium, silicon, sodium, sulfur, zinc. It is generally accepted that a requirement exists for most of these. Mineral constituents, obtained from food, aid in the regulation of the acid-base balance of body fluids and of osmotic pressure, in addition to the specific functions of individual elements in the body. Some minerals are present in the body largely in organic combination, as iron in hemoglobin and iodine in thyroxin; others occur in the body in inorganic form, as calcium salts in bone, sodium and chlorine in sodium chloride. The terms "minerals" and "inorganic elements" do not imply that the element occurs in inorganic form in food or body tissue. *See* Ash.

NIACIN (C_5H_4NCOOH)—Anti-pellagra factor, nicotinic acid. A water-soluble, heat-stable vitamin of the B complex. Functionally active as the niacinamide coenzymes; essential to cell respiration, carbohydrate and protein metabolism, and lipid syntheses. Deficiency results in the skin lesions, gastrointestinal and cerebral manifestations which characterize pellagra. Dietary sources include preformed niacin and the precursor tryptophan; human requirements are expressed in terms of niacin equivalents and are related to caloric consumption (1, 2, 3).

NIACINAMIDE ($C_5H_4NCONH_2$)—Nicotinamide, the amide of niacin; principal form of the vitamin occurring in tissues; a component of the coenzymes nicotinamide-adenine-dinucleotide (NAD) and nicotinamide-adenine-dinucleotide phosphate (NADP), which are essential to cell respiration.

NIACIN EQUIVALENT—The Recommended Dietary Allowances for niacin are expressed by the Food and Nutrition Board of the National Research Council as niacin equivalents, on the assumption that 60 mg. tryptophan may be converted to 1 mg. niacin (1).

NICOTINAMIDE—*See* Niacinamide.

NUTRIENT—Any substance useful in nutrition; for example, proteins, fats, carbohydrates, minerals, vitamins, water. *See* Nutrition.

NUTRITION—The combination of processes by which the living organism receives and utilizes the materials necessary for the maintenance of its functions and for the growth and renewal of its components.

NUTRITION HISTORY—An informative and comprehensive description of laboratory, and clinical findings as well as dietary history of an individual. *See* Dietary History; Nutritional Status.

NUTRITION, NORMAL—A condition of the body resulting from the efficient utilization of sufficient amounts of the essential nutrients provided in the food intake.

NUTRITIONAL STATUS—The condition of the body resulting from the utilization of the essential nutrients available to the body. Nutritional status may be good, fair, or poor, depending not only on the intake of dietary essentials but also on the relative need and the body's ability to utilize them. *See* Nutriture.

NUTRITIONIST—One who has followed a prescribed academic program and received a Master's degree in public health nutrition from an accredited College or University. Organizes, plans, and conducts programs concerning nutrition to assist in promotion of health and control of disease. Instructs auxiliary medical personnel and allied professional workers on food values and utilization of foods by human body. Advises health and other agencies on nutritional phases of their food programs. Conducts in-service courses pertaining to nutrition in clinics and similar institutions. Interprets and evaluates food and nutrient information designed for public acceptance and use. Studies and analyzes scientific discoveries in nutrition for adaptation and application to various dietary problems. May be employed by voluntary or public health agency.

NUTRITIONIST-PUBLIC HEALTH—One who has followed a prescribed academic program and received a Master's degree in public health nutrition from an accredited College or University. In a public health agency, interprets and applies scientific knowledge of nutrition to planning, organizing, and carrying out or directing programs for the promotion of positive health, the prevention of chronic and debilitating diseases, and the treatment and rehabilitation of individuals. Consults with administrators, medical, and para-medical personnel on current scientific findings in food and nutrition and their application to agency programs. Conducts or participates in pre-service and in-service education of professional staff of own and related agencies. May design, conduct, or participate in dietary and nutrition studies, and other studies with a nutrition component. Prepares and evaluates technical and popular educational material. Cooperates with other agencies in the formulation and coordination of nutrition programs involving professional or lay groups. Should have post-graduate education in nutrition as it relates to public health and qualifying experience for the responsibilities entailed.

NUTRITIONIST-TEACHING—One who has followed a prescribed academic program and received a Master's degree in public health nutrition from an accredited College or University. Plans, organizes, and conducts education programs in nutrition for the preparation of professional workers as well as for the public. Develops curricula, course outlines, visual aids, pamphlets, and other materials used in teaching. The nutritionist in the college teaches the basic science and application of science of food and nutrition. Often engages in research. The nutritionist in the Extension Service advises agency administrators and county home economists and participates with the agent in training lay leaders. In business, the nutritionist gives technical advice and guidance in preparing and conducting consumer education programs. Should have post-graduate education in nutrition as it relates to public health, research, and teaching and qualifying experience.

NUTRITURE—Condition as to nourishment, either with respect to all nutrients (general nutriture) or to one nutrient at a time.

OXALIC ACID—*See* Acid, Oxalic.

PELLAGRA—A multiple deficiency disease caused by the lack of niacin or its equivalent, and associated with deficiencies of other B vitamins. Signs and symptoms involve the skin, gastrointestinal tract, and nervous system.

PHENYLKETONURIA—The excretion of phenylpyruvic acid and other phenyl compounds in the urine, resulting from the hereditary lack of an enzyme necessary for the conversion of the amino acid phenylalanine to tyrosine; phenylalanine accumulates in blood and tissues, and mental retardation occurs.

POLYUNSATURATED: SATURATED (P/S) FATTY ACID RATIO—One of several ways to express relative amounts of fatty acids in foods or diets. Usually refers to linoleic acid (polyunsaturated) and total saturated fatty acids. Mono-unsaturated fatty acids (chiefly oleic) are not considered in this ratio. *See*: Diet, Fat modified.

PROTEIN—Any one of a group of complex nitrogenous compounds (approximately 16 per cent nitrogen) which yields amino acids upon hydrolysis; widely distributed in plant and animal tissues; essential constituents of the cell protoplasm. Protein values as stated in food composition tables are generally computed from total nitrogen content and include, in addition to true protein, other compounds such as amino acids and purine bases.

PROTEIN, BIOLOGICAL VALUE OF—The percentage of absorbed nitrogen that is retained by the body. The numerical value obtained varies with the conditions of the experiment.

PROTEIN HYDROLYSATE—A mixture of amino acids and polypeptides prepared by the digestion of proteins by acids, alkalies, or proteolytic enzymes. Properly prepared hydrolysates may be used for either oral or parenteral administration. Some methods of hydrolysis lead to the destruction of certain essential amino acids.

PROVITAMIN—The precursor of a vitamin; for example, carotene, ergosterol.

PROXIMATE COMPOSITION—As applied to food, the term usually includes the percentages of protein, fat, total carbohydrate, ash, and water; calorie values may also be included.

PURINES—Purine bases; compounds which contain heterocyclic nitrogenous purine structure ($C_5H_4N_4$); catabolized to uric acid; dietary purines are supplemented by endogenous synthesis. *See* Diet, Purine, Low (text, pp. 116–19).

PYRIDOXINE—*See* Vitamin B_6.

REFUSE—That portion of foods which is inedible (as bones, pits, shells) or usually discarded in preparation of food for the table (as potato parings and tough outer leaves of vegetables). In food values expressed on the "as purchased" basis, the nutrients in refuse have been disregarded.

REQUIREMENTS—Although the average minimal requirements for various nutrients cannot be stated with accuracy, certain "minimum daily requirements" for food-labeling purposes have been designated in regulations for enforcement of the Federal Food, Drug, and Cosmetic Act (Table 46). These should not be confused with the Recommended Dietary Allowances.

RESEARCH NUTRITIONIST (MAY BE DESIGNATED AS RESEARCH DIETITIAN)—One who has followed a prescribed academic program and received a Master's degree in public health nutrition from an accredited College or University. Originates or assists in planning, organizing, and conducting programs in nutritional research. Performs research in improvement of food as related to appearance, palatability, and nutritional value. Studies and analyzes recent scientific discoveries in nutrition for application in current research, for development of tools for future research, and for interpretation to the public (10).

RESIDUE, FECAL—The total solid of feces made up of undigested and unabsorbed food and metabolic and bacterial products. Some foods, such as milk, or fats which contain no fiber, may significantly increase fecal residue under abnormal conditions.

RIBOFLAVIN ($C_{17}H_{20}N_4O_6$)—A vitamin of the B complex; sparingly soluble in water, decomposed by exposure to light, heat-labile in alkaline solutions. Functions biologically as the coenzymes flavin mononucleotide (FMN), and flavin adenine dinucleotide (FAD), which are components of the flavoproteins, essential to protein and energy metabolism; participates in biological oxidations and reductions. The deficiency disease, ariboflavinosis, is frequently associated with deficiencies of other B vitamins. Human requirements are now considered to be more closely related to energy expenditure than to protein intake; recommended allowances have been computed on the basis of caloric intake (1, 2).

RICKETS—A condition, caused chiefly by deficiency of vitamin D in infancy and childhood, in which calcification of the growing bone does not occur normally; marked by softening and bending of the long bones, delayed closure of the fontanelles, and other deformities. The effects of hypovitaminosis D may be influenced by other factors affecting calcium absorption.

SACCHARIN—Ortho-benzosulfimide; usually marketed as the sodium or calcium salt of saccharin; 300 times as sweet as sucrose.

SALT, IODIZED—Table salt (sodium chloride) to which has been added 1 part per 10,000 of iodine as potassium iodide.

SATIETY VALUE—That quality of food contributing to satisfaction and resulting in a sustained sense of comfort or well-being.

SCURVY—A disease resulting from the relative or absolute deficiency of ascorbic acid; characterized by hemorrhage, anemia, delayed wound healing, and defective skeletal growth in children.

SORBITOL ($C_6H_{14}O_6$)—A hexahydric alcohol. Imparts a sweet taste; used in maintaining moisture and in inhibiting crystallization of certain commercial products. Contains 4 calories per gram.

STANDARD OF IDENTITY OF FOODS—The U.S. Food, Drug, and Cosmetic Act as Amended authorizes the U.S. Food and Drug Administration to establish food standards. Under this authority, the FDA has promulgated definitions and standards of identity, also standards of quality and fill of container, for approximately 200 foods. These standards apply to foods shipped in interstate commerce. Food standards have also been established by the Department of the Interior, Bureau of Commercial Fisheries, the Department of Agriculture, the Department of Defense, the Department of Commerce, the Federal Trade Commission, the Veterans Administration, and the General Services Administration.

SUPPLEMENT, NUTRITIONAL—A general term which usually refers to a concentrated source of nutrients, prescribed in addition to the daily diet to increase the nutrient intake. A supplement may be a food such as yeast or wheat germ, a concentrate such as cod liver oil, or a pharmaceutical preparation of vitamins or minerals.

SWEETENERS, NON-NUTRITIVE, ARTIFICIAL—Artificial sweetening ingredients are saccharin, sodium saccharin, sodium cyclamate, potassium cyclamate, calcium cyclamate, or any combination of these. *See* Saccharin; Cyclamates.

THIAMINE ($C_{12}H_{17}N_4OS$)—Antiberiberi factor, vitamin B_1; water-soluble, heat-labile in neutral or alkaline solution. Active form is thiamine pyrophosphate (TPP) or cocarboxylase, a constituent of the carboxylase and transketolase enzymes which function in carbohydrate metabolism. Thiamine deficiency results in polyneuritis (beriberi). Human requirements are related to carbohydrate utilization, recommended allowances are based upon caloric intake.

TOCOPHEROL—Vitamin E; a group of four phenolic compounds (designated α, β, γ, and δ) with vitamin E activity; fat-soluble, sensitive to oxidation and to ultraviolet light. As antioxidants, the tocopherols may retard oxidation of other fat-soluble vitamins and lipoperoxidation in adipose tissue associated with a high intake of polyunsaturated fatty acids; they may also be involved in cell respiration and in nucleoprotein synthesis. Evidence is accumulating that the tocopherols, long recognized as having vitamin activity for animals, may play an essential role in human nutrition. Richest sources are the vegetable oils, whole grains, and eggs; the average daily intake has been estimated at 24 mg. tocopherol (14 mg. α tocopherol). Human needs are related to the intake of polyunsaturated fatty acids and may vary between 10 and 30 mg. per day for adults (1, 12).

TRACE ELEMENTS—Minerals occurring in small amounts in food or body tissues; those which are known to be dietary essentials are also called "micronutrients."

TRIGLYCERIDES—Glyceryl esters of fatty acids. *See* Fat.

TRYPTOPHAN ($C_8H_6NCH_2CHNH_2COOH$)—An essential amino acid; a constituent of body proteins, a source of the vitamin niacin and of the vasoconstrictor serotonin. Animal protein contains approximately 1.4 per cent and vegetable protein 1 per cent tryptophan; an average daily diet may provide 500–1,000 mg. tryptophan. The dietary tryptophan available over and above the body's requirement (approximately 500 mg. for young men) may be converted to niacin in a proportion of 60 mg. tryptophan to 1 mg. niacin.

UNIT, INTERNATIONAL VITAMIN (I.U.)—A definite quantity of each International Standard of Reference, used for expressing the content of the respective vitamins in foods and other materials. Such units have been established for vitamins A, C, D, and thiamine but are used principally for vitamins A and D, since values for thiamine and vitamin C can now be conveniently expressed in weights. Originally established by a committee appointed by the Health Organization of the League of Nations, standardization of vitamin units is now under the supervision of subcommittees of the World Health Organization.

UNIT, INTERNATIONAL VITAMIN A—The activity of 0.300 μg. vitamin A alcohol (equivalent to 0.344 μg. vitamin A acetate, or to 0.550 μg. vitamin A palmitate), equal to 0.600 μg. of the provitamin β-carotene.

UNIT, INTERNATIONAL VITAMIN B_1—The vitamin B_1 activity of 3.0 μg. of the International Standard crystalline thiamine hydrochloride (vitamin B_1), therefore 1 mg. thiamine equals 333 I.U.

UNIT, INTERNATIONAL VITAMIN C—The vitamin C activity of 0.05 mg. of the International Standard crystalline ascorbic acid (vitamin C).

UNIT, INTERNATIONAL VITAMIN D—The vitamin D activity of the International Standard solution of irradiated ergosterol in oil, containing 0.025 μg. of calciferol.

UNIT, U.S.P. (UNITED STATES PHARMACOPEIA)—Equal to the corresponding International Units.

VIOSTEROL—A general name for preparations of irradiated ergosterol in oil, in which the active agent is calciferol (vitamin D_2).

VITAMIN—An organic substance occurring in minute quantities in plant and animal tissues; must be either supplied in the diet of animals or synthesized from essential dietary or metabolic precursors; essential for specific metabolic functions or reactions to proceed normally.

VITAMIN A ($C_{20}H_{29}OH$)—A fat-soluble vitamin occurring in several biologically active forms; sensitive to oxidation and exposure to light; an unsaturated alcohol which may be found as an aldehyde or an ester; synthesized in animal tissue from plant precursors (carotenes). Functions in the development of normal skin and bone and in the maintenance of scotopic vision; essential for regeneration of visual purple, participates in synthesis of mucopolysaccharides. Deficiency may be manifested by night-blindness, keratinization of epithelial tissue, and xerophthalmia. Excessive doses of the vitamin produce toxic effects (1, 2).

VITAMIN A VALUE—The combined potency of a food or diet, represented by its content of vitamin A, carotene, and other plant precursors (1, 3).

VITAMIN B_1—*See* Thiamine.

VITAMIN B_2—An obsolete term for riboflavin.

VITAMIN B_6—A collective term which includes three water-soluble, heat-stable pyridine derivatives: pyridoxine ($C_8H_{11}O_3N$) in plant products, pyridoxal ($C_8H_9O_3N$) and pyridoxamine ($C_8H_{12}O_2N_2$) in animal products; all exhibit activity in humans, functioning as the phosphorylated derivatives. Principally concerned with the metabolism of amino acids, as a coenzyme in transaminations, deaminations, and decarboxylations, and in the metabolism of tryptophan; also involved in carbohydrate and fat metabolism. Symptoms attributed to a vitamin B_6 deficiency in humans include convulsions in infants receiving a synthetic diet, lesions of the skin and mucous membranes of adults receiving an antagonist. Widely distributed in plant and animal foods, excellent sources include yeast, wheat germ, liver, kidney, and muscle meats. Although there is evidence that vitamin B_6 requirements increase with protein intake, the needs seem to parallel those of thiamine; a tentative adult allowance of 1.5–2.0 mg. per day is readily provided by ordinary mixed diets.

VITAMIN B_{12}—Animal protein factor, anti-anemic principle, extrinsic factor; a group of cobalt-containing compounds (cobalamins) with hemopoietic activity, of which cyanocobalamin ($C_{69}H_{90}N_{14}O_{14}PCo$) is the prototype; soluble in water, relatively stable to heat; occurs bound to protein in animal tissues. Functions in nucleic acid and protein syntheses; facilitates reduction reactions; necessary for activity of folic acid coenzymes. Deficiency occurs in the absence of the gastric intrinsic factor (pernicious anemia, post-gastrectomy syndrome), in the malabsorption syndromes, and as a consequence of a strict vegetarian diet; manifested by a macrocytic megaloblastic anemia, spinal cord degeneration, and gastro-intestinal changes. Daily needs are met by the average diet supplying 3–5 μg. vitamin B_{12}; major sources are liver, kidney, and muscle meats (13).

VITAMIN B COMPLEX—As originally used, this term referred to the water-soluble vitamins occurring in yeast, liver, meats, and whole-grain cereals, but some of the newer B complex vitamins, for example, folic acid and Vitamin B_{12}, do not correspond to this distribution; includes a number of compounds which have been identified, isolated, and synthesized, viz., thiamine, riboflavin, nicotinic acid, vitamin B_6, pantothenic acid, biotin, folic acid, inositol, and choline; vitamin B_{12}, the structure of which has been determined; and others which have been only partially demonstrated or identified.

VITAMIN C—*See* Ascorbic Acid.

VITAMIN D—A group of fat-soluble factors which have antirachitic activity; structurally related to the sterols. Vitamins D_2 and D_3 are derived from their respective provitamins ergosterol and 7-dehydrocholesterol by ultraviolet irradiation. Vitamin D increases the availability, retention, and utilization of calcium and phosphorus for proper mineralization of the skeleton. Deficiency of vitamin D is a major cause of rickets in the infant, and one of the causes of osteomalacia in the adult. The requirements of infants are generally met through the use of vitamin D milk; the needs of adults are probably supplied by the average diet and casual exposure to sunshine. Excessive doses of the vitamin produce toxic effects (1, 2).

VITAMIN D_2—*See* Calciferol.

VITAMIN D_3 ($C_{27}H_{44}O$)—A fat-soluble antirachitic factor, obtained by ultraviolet-ray activation of 7-dehydrocholesterol; occurs in fish-liver oils and in irradiated foods of animal origin; termed "natural" vitamin D.

VITAMIN D MILK—May be produced by three different methods: (1) "fortified" milk, which is now more generally distributed than the other types, is that to which a vitamin D concentrate has been added; (2) "metabolized" milk is produced by feeding the cows irradiated yeast; and (3) "irradiated" milk has been exposed directly to ultraviolet rays. The standard amount used for fortification is 400 I.U. vitamin D per quart of fresh or reconstituted milk.

VITAMIN E—*See* Tocopherol.

VITAMIN INHIBITORS—*See* Antivitamins.

VITAMIN K—"Koagulationsvitamin." A group of fat-soluble, light-sensitive vitamins possessing a common naphthoquinone structure; natural forms include vitamin K_1 ($C_{31}H_{46}O_2$) occurring in green leaves, and vitamin K_2 ($C_{41}H_{56}O_2$) produced by intestinal bacteria; synthetic forms, such as menadione, are available as water-soluble esters. Vitamin K is required for the maintenance of normal prothrombin time; it may be involved in cell respiration and associated phosphorylations. Deficiency, which is characterized by hemorrhagic tendencies, may result from reduced synthesis by intestinal bacteria or poor intestinal absorption; prophylaxis is achieved with 1–2 mg. vitamin K, administered orally.

VITAMINS, FAT-SOLUBLE—Vitamins A, D, E, and K, which are extractable from foods with fat solvents.

VITAMINS, WATER-SOLUBLE—Members of the B complex and vitamin C which can be extracted from foods with water as the solvent.

WATER, ENDOGENOUS—Water which is provided by metabolic processes.

WATER, EXOGENOUS—Water ingested as such or as a component of food. In food composition tables, "water" includes volatile substances in addition to free water.

WATER, REQUIREMENT—Determined by body heat production, amounts of dissolved materials to be excreted by the kidney and its concentrating capacity, and losses due to sweating. Water and salt requirements are intimately related. Under ordinary environmental conditions, the daily requirement of a 70-kg. man on a 3,200-calorie diet is about 2,300–3,100 ml., much of which is contained in foods as eaten.

TABLE 45

Tentative Minimum Requirements of Amino Acids by Young Adults

Amino Acid	Minimum Requirements* (gm. per day)	
	Women	Men
Isoleucine	0.45	0.70
Leucine	0.62	1.10
Lysine	0.50	0.80
Methionine } Cystine }	0.55	1.10
Phenylalanine	0.22 }	1.10
Tyrosine	0.90 }	
Threonine	0.31	0.50
Tryptophan	0.16	0.25
Valine	0.65	0.80

* Values for women are from R. M. Leverton in *Protein and Amino Acid Nutrition*, ed. A. A. Albanese. New York: Academic Press, 1959, p. 504. Values for men are from W. C. Rose, Fed. Proc., **8**: 546, 1949.

TABLE 46

Minimum Daily Requirements of Certain Vitamins and Minerals*

Established by the Food and Drug Administration for Labeling of Special Purpose Foods. If a food or food supplement is represented to be for special dietary use by man by reason of its vitamin or mineral properties, the label must bear a statement of the proportion of the minimum daily requirement for such vitamins or minerals supplied by the food or food supplement when consumed in specified quantity during the period of 1 day. For the purpose of regulation, the minimum daily requirements are stated as follows:

	Infants under 1 Year	Children 1–5	Children 6–11	Children 12 yrs. and Over	Adults	Pregnancy or Lactation
Calcium, gm.	....	0.75	0.75	0.75	0.75	1.5
Phosphorus, gm.	....	0.75	0.75	0.75	0.75	1.5
Iron, mg.	....	7.5	10.0	10.0	10.0	15.0
Iodine, mg.	....	0.1	0.1	0.1	0.1	0.1
Vitamin A, U.S.P. units	1,500	3,000	3,000	4,000	4,000	....
Thiamine, mg.	0.25	0.5	0.75	1.0	1.0	....
Riboflavin, mg.	0.5	....	....	2.0	2.0	....
Niacin, mg.	5.0	5.0	7.5	7.5	10.0	....
Ascorbic acid, mg.	10.0	20.0	20.0	30.0	30.0	....
Vitamin D, U.S.P. units	400	400	400	400	400	....

* Food and Drug Administration, U.S. Department of Health, Education, and Welfare: Title 21, Code of Federal Regulations and 21 CFR, 1959 Supplement, and amended as in Federal Register, June 1, 1957.

REFERENCE LIST FOR GLOSSARY

1. National Academy of Sciences, National Research Council. Recommended Dietary Allowances. 6th revised ed. Washington, D.C.: National Academy of Sciences, National Research Council Publication 1146, 1964.
2. U.S. Food and Drug Administration. Minimum Daily Requirements of Certain Vitamins and Minerals. U.S. Department of Health, Education, and Welfare, Food and Drug Administration, Federal Register, **22**:3841, 1957. Also in Code of Federal Regulations, Title 21, and 21 CFR Supplement 1959. (See Table 46.)
3. Watt, B. D., and Merrill, A. L. Composition of Foods—Raw, Processed, Prepared. U.S. Department of Agriculture Handbook No. 8, revised 1963.
4. Zook, E. G., MacArthur, M. J., and Toepfer, E. W. Pantothenic Acid in Foods. U.S. Department of Agriculture Handbook No. 97, 1956.
5. Mattice, M. R. Bridges' Food and Beverage Analyses. Philadelphia: Lea and Febiger, 1950, pp. 201–15.
6. Leverton, R. M. Amino Acid Requirements of Young Adults. In Protein and Amino Acid Nutrition, ed. A. A. Albanese. New York: Academic Press, 1959, p. 504.
7. Orr, M. L., and Watt, B. K. Amino Acid Content of Foods. U.S. Department of Agriculture, Home Economics Research Report No. 4, 1957. (See Table 40.)
8. Nutritive Value of Foods, U.S. Department of Agriculture, Home and Garden Bulletin No. 72, Washington, D.C., revised September, 1964.
9. Annual Reports and Proceedings, American Dietetic Association, 1945–46, p. 35.
10. Occupational Analysis Branch, U.S. Employment Service, Dictionary of Occupational Titles, Second Ed., Suppl. I. (Washington: U.S. Department of Labor, Bureau of Employment Security, Division of Placement Methods, March, 1955.)
11. Toepfer, E. W., Zook, E. G., Orr, M. L., and Richardson, L. R. Folic Acid Content of Foods. U.S. Department of Agriculture Handbook No. 29, 1951.
12. Harris, P. L., Quaife, M. L., and Swanson, W. J. Vitamin E content of foods. J. Nutr., **40**:367, 1950.
13. Lichtenstein, H., Beloian, A., and Murphy, E. W. Vitamin B_{12}—Microbiological assay methods and distribution in selected foods. U.S. Department of Agriculture, Home Economics Research Report No. 13, 1961.

INDEX